A DRUG-FREE APPROACH TO HEALTHCARE
Disease Prevention – Not Symptom Suppression
* 2009 Revised Edition *

The Soaring Heights Series

In order to avoid disease, prevention absolutely must take priority, and can't possibly be accomplished with medications.

By Dr. David W. Tanton, Ph.D.

DISCLAIMER:

Every effort has been made by the author to ensure that the information in this book is as complete and accurate as possible, although the author cannot, and does not render judgment or advice regarding a particular individual. As our bodies are each unique, we will not always experience the same results that another might from the very same therapy.

The author believes in both prevention and the superiority of a natural non-invasive approach over drugs and surgery.

The information herein is presented by an independent research scientist, whose sources of information include nearly a half-century of his own personal experiences, and decades of researching the world's medical and scientific literature, patient records, and other clinical and anecdotal reports.

The leading cause of death and disability today appears to be the lack of awareness of natural therapies, by both doctors and their patients, known to prevent and treat many common degenerative diseases. This book is dedicated to making as many as possible aware that they no longer need to suffer and die needlessly from diseases that may already have cures. Unfortunately, the general public is seldom aware of many valuable resources available for preventing or effectively eliminating serious health conditions, as they are often suppressed due to their lack of profitability.

Those who read this book and make decisions regarding their health or medical care based on ideas contained in this book, do so as their constitutional right. Please do not use this book if you are unwilling to assume responsibility for results that arise from the use of any of the suggestions, preparations or procedures in the book. The author and publisher are not responsible for any adverse effects or consequences resulting from the use of any of the suggestions or information contained in the book, but offer this material as information that the public has a right to hear and utilize at their own discretion.

This Revised Edition, Published by *Soaring Heights Publishing* 2009

Library of Congress Control Number: 2005907716
ISBN: 978-0-9772703-3-0
SAN: 257-1641

Printed in the United States by Morris Publishing
3212 East Highway 30
Kearney, NE 68847
1-800-650-7888

Additional copies of this book can be ordered at http://www.drtanton.com.

For single book purchases, send check or money order for $27.95 to:
Soaring Heights Publishing
PO Box 2138
Jasper, OR 97438

For wholesale prices or quantity purchases:
Email: books@drtanton.com
Or Call: (541) 726-5959

TABLE OF CONTENTS

INTRODUCTION

What You Can Expect To Learn From Reading This Book

This could very well be one of the most valuable books you will ever invest in regarding your future health (especially if you are taking medications). You will soon discover that this book is actually quite unique. It's not just a book that you will read only once, but instead be a valuable resource you will be constantly referring to, as many serious health issues are addressed. By following the many recommendations within, you should begin experiencing a profound improvement in your overall health and energy level, as well as a much greater potential for longevity, and overall quality of life. You will encounter many comprehensive in-depth explanations (in simple terms) regarding the causes of various diseases and poor health in general. Although poor dietary habits are an obvious contributor to less than optimum health, you will soon discover that in many instances, your medications are quite often the greatest concern of all. Your body immediately recognizes them as the toxic chemicals they are. Drugs are typically designed to override important bodily functions in order to suppress symptoms. Only when we begin employing natural organic substances that our body instantly recognizes as beneficial, can true healing possibly take place.

It's important you understand that the symptoms we may experience are an important part of our body's communication system, (or its cries for help), and thus **symptoms should never be suppressed with any drug!** If it wasn't for pain or discomfort, how could we possibly know when a problem exists, or when it is finally resolved? If we were not somehow alerted when a concern exists, the condition would gradually continue to worsen, although we would obviously be totally unaware of the fact. That is exactly what we are doing when we resort to symptom suppressing drugs, which basically makes a bad condition even worse. Unfortunately, we soon forget that a problem ever existed, thus allowing the problem to continually worsen undetected. Medications are notorious for creating other uncomfortable symptoms (side effects), which normally results in one or more prescriptions for additional medications (basically the domino affect). Drugs not only create many side effects, but they also deplete many important nutrients critical to our health in the process. The more medications you are relying on, the greater the risk will be.

You will soon discover that no two people will actually assimilate, and thus receive the same amount of any medication as another person might, even on the very same dosage. This is an issue the companies producing your medications are actually fully aware of, although something they have absolutely no way of controlling. Even your own effective dosage can easily vary considerably, based on several factors. How many drugs you might be taking, as well as how many other toxins (such as alcohol) your body is dealing with on a particular day, will have an influence. This is why you see so many potential side effects associated with many medications. How many you might experience depends upon how much of each drug is able to effectively get around your best friend – your liver (the detoxifier). Many other variables, such as your size, your gender, your age, and especially your metabolism, will play a part as well, although most doctors seldom consider these issues when drugs are prescribed. In my opinion, drugs are inherently unpredictable, basically unhealthy, and most importantly, seldom necessary.

You will learn how Mary Lou successfully went from nine medications (including a 16-year dependency on Prozac™), to none, in only 60 days! The most amazing part is, it was surprisingly easy to accomplish, and she is now feeling terrific, losing weight, and no longer dependent on all those medications (including two for depression). An added bonus was, all those uncomfortable side effects soon begin disappearing. She was totally amazed at how terrific she felt, and says it's such a relief to finally be free from a lifetime dependency on all those medications. **From nine to none in only 60 days (quite amazing)!**

You will also meet the retired professor and body-builder named Al, who mysteriously lost a tremendous amount of muscle in only a couple years. After a little detective work, I discovered it was due to his oxygen-suppressing and CoQ_{10}-depleting medications. They destroyed years of hard-earned muscle when he continued working out as he had his entire adult life. He also lost his strength, his endurance, as well as his energy, (and even his memory). Within two weeks after stopping his medications, he was already making dramatic improvements, and as you will soon learn, continued doing so. When Al attempted to share this newfound discovery with his doctor, he was surprised to learn that he really wasn't the least interested. His doctor likely didn't want to admit that those drugs he prescribed were not only unnecessary, but also very destructive. That is especially a concern regarding the heart, which is also a muscle that depends even more on an adequate level of both oxygen and CoQ$_{10}$ than any other muscle in the entire body.

You will find that this book is actually two-books-in-one, as the last half of the book basically focuses on some of the conditions or diseases most prevalent in the nation today. You will learn what the various contributors to many **"supposedly incurable" diseases** are, and how they can be easily avoided, and often resolved. You will also discover that although most doctors' typical resources (drugs and surgery) seldom provide an effective solution, that doesn't necessarily hold true when the proper natural approach is taken. Just because a "disease" is considered as incurable by traditional medicine, doesn't necessarily hold true if true when proper healing principles are applied. Natural solutions are often so surprisingly simple that it's difficult to believe they could possibly be effective (but they are). Although Our Creator provided us with a very complex yet extremely efficient body, He in turn provided us with many simple solutions for maintaining its health. Even though the various nutrients are relatively easy to use, they are actually very complex, (just like our body). Fortunately, we don't have to fully understand their complexity in order to benefit from their use. Many herbs and plant extracts have hundreds of constituents, many that scientists are still unable to identify, although they have proven benefits.

Just learning how you can stop either a stroke or heart attack in a matter of minutes (sometimes seconds), and do so very easily would in itself be well worth your investment. I learned this amazing discovery from a brilliant doctor who claimed that it worked hundreds of times with his patients, and never once failed. I also discovered some additional supplements that would provide the additional benefit of rapidly increasing the delivery of oxygen to both the heart and brain. I call this my **"Stroke / Heart Attack Emergency Kit."**

My objective is to unravel the many seemingly unexplainable mysteries of both the body and brain, in order to provide you with an in-depth explanation of each one, as we progress. In "*The Soaring Heights Series,*" you will discover many things that even most medical doctors are totally unaware of. While designing a computer operating system over forty years ago, I accomplished something the IBM engineers assigned to the project considered as impossible. Their conclusion was based on the complexity of the task, and the fact that it involved employing an unproven theory, (something no one had ever attempted). To me, no task is too daunting or impossible, but just another challenge to solve. As I continue uncovering new mysteries, by following my series you will be the very first to know. Together we will go on an amazing journey, making new life-changing discoveries along the way, and optimum (drug-free) health and longevity will be our final destination, although we will make many interesting and informative stops along the way.

Important Questions That You Will Find Answers For:

Following are some questions we must ask ourselves. My objective is to provide the answers:

- Should I take more responsibility for my own health?
- Does my doctor not necessarily have all the answers?
- If others never take medications, why must I continue doing so?
- If others eliminated their medications, why can't I do the same?
- If it doesn't seem logical, is it possibly not, in spite of what I was told?
- Why is it that the longest living people have never used drugs?
- Did My Creator make mistakes that I somehow need drugs to fix?
- Were the scriptures wrong in recommending the use of herbs for healing?
- Should I continue taking medications if they just make me feel worse?
- Is my body trying to tell me something I'm ignoring?
- Isn't prevention the most logical approach to avoiding disease?
- Is there some reason the average doctor lives only 58 years?
- Could it be that doctors are taking advantage of all those free samples?
- If my doctor insists that drugs are the only solution, is it time for a change?
- Will I suddenly die if I stop taking my medications?
- If my body is organic, why should I continue ingesting chemicals?
- Whose example should I follow? The most healthy or least healthy?
- Have I considered praying for guidance regarding my health?
- If drugs are so cheap to produce, how come they cost so much?
- If drugs fix problems, why must I continue taking them?
- Could my drugs be the problem behind my unexplainable symptoms?
- Why are those taking the most medications, experiencing the worst health?
- Why have I continually exposed my body to toxic chemicals?
- Shouldn't we take Hypocrites' advice and let food be our medicine?
- Doesn't Hypocrites' advice "First do no harm" seem logical?

CHAPTER ONE
A DRUG-FREE APPROACH HAS PROVEN EFFECTIVE FOR ME

At 75 years of age, I use absolutely no prescription or over-the-counter drugs, and find no reason what so ever for doing so. In 1962, at the age of 28, I weighed 205 pounds, had allergies, and often caught colds. Today I weigh 175 pounds, and have approximately the same muscle-to-fat ratio as I did at 18. I have very fast reflexes, and my memory appears to be better than at any time in the past. I also have excellent vision without glasses, and the last time I checked my blood pressure, it was 110/70. I have never checked my cholesterol, and see absolutely no reason to do so. If we just learn the rules of health and show our body the respect it deserves, it is perfectly capable of efficiently managing the details, and there will be absolutely no reason to stress about all those levels.

Although many people tend to believe that disease is just the result of getting older, that doesn't necessarily have to be the case. Disease is normally the result of an unhealthy condition in the body, (not the result of our age), and something we all can control. We just need to learn what our body really needs and then provide it, and stop abusing it with all those potentially dangerous and unnecessary drugs.

If perchance you might possibly question any of the statements made by either myself or the many other doctors I have quoted in this book, I would suggest you resort to prayer, that you might have the power of discernment and recognize the real truth. I do not take my responsibility to mankind lightly, and thus depend upon daily prayer and a great deal of research, for the answers to questions that so many are desperately looking for.

Hypocrites, known as the father of medicine, once said, *"Let your food be your medicine."* That was over 2,000 years ago, and his theory has not only proven true, but should be obvious. You can't just suppress symptoms with drugs (which are foreign to the body), and eat processed foods devoid of nutrients, and somehow expect to maintain health. How we look, feel, and perform, is influenced much more by our lifestyle and dietary habits than our genetic inheritance, which people sometimes attribute their poor health to. Children born of the same parents often experience overall health that varies considerably, which is much more of a reflection of their diet and lifestyle than their DNA.

You can't always blame your doctor for lack of effective solutions either, as he only knows what he was taught in medical school. Most medical doctors were trained to treat symptoms with drugs, rather than using natural nutrients for prevention. Your doctor likely devoted many years of his or her life, and a great deal of money, getting a medical degree. If an M.D. chose to use a natural therapy (unapproved by the American Medical Association), he or she could help save a life yet jeopardize their license to practice medicine in doing so. Conversely, if a patient dies as the result of a therapy or drug approved by the U.S. Food and Drug Administration (FDA), it would be considered perfectly acceptable.

Avoiding disease by prevention obviously makes much more sense, and thus should be our first line of defense, as well as the primary objective of medicine. A friend of mine said her doctor indicated that he was taking a statin (cholesterol lowering) drug just for prevention, even though his cholesterol was not elevated. He suggested that she also take the drug just for prevention. **That is definitely not preventative medicine**, which will soon become quite obvious. She decided that a change of doctors was in order (a wise decision, I might add).

Another concern regarding modern medicine today is the approximate 10 minutes many clinics allot doctors to spend with their patients, and they normally schedule appointments accordingly. It would obviously be very profitable, and certainly makes good business sense, but what about the patients' welfare? Although it doesn't take long to write a prescription, it would normally take a medical doctor considerably longer to adequately diagnose and properly resolve a particular health issue, as well as evaluating the potential interactions of the drugs the patient might already be taking. Most natural practitioners normally spend approximately one hour on the patient's first visit, and allow approximately thirty minutes on follow up visits. This approach may not be nearly as profitable, but is obviously much more effective. The same also applies to natural supplements versus drugs. The ingredients in natural supplements normally cost more than prescription drugs, although they sell for **far less**.

I believe that many doctors are totally unaware of the serious implications associated with many of the drugs they prescribe daily. The drug commercials imply that your doctor will know if you should be using their particular drug, and that he is basically an authority with all the answers. They then focus on convincing your doctor that many patients could benefit from their drug (even for unapproved uses). There are more drugs being continually added, and many are just variations of the same basic class of drug. Although similar, they often vary in potency and potential for interactions with other drugs. And as you will soon find out, your doctor is normally so busy with his practice, and dealing with many different patients on a daily basis that he unfortunately has very little time left for research or evaluation.

Natural medicine is in my opinion a true science, as the basic ingredients normally used were created by Our Creator, (who is much more brilliant than man), and whose major concern is our welfare, rather than the most profitable solution. Natural foods are far more complex than any drug produced in a laboratory, and organic (as is our body). We must basically decide where we will place our trust, in man or in Our Creator who also created our body. He is obviously in a far better position to understand our body's needs, and has provided many natural resources for our benefit.

Our body always knows exactly what it is doing and why. The only thing we need to concern ourselves with is providing adequate resources to allow it to do the job it was very efficiently designed by Our Creator to do. We must stop trying to second-guess our body's intentions by using drugs to override our body's very efficient functions. Modern medicine seems to hypothesize that our body somehow has some major design flaws that must be suppressed and controlled at all costs through the use of high-tech drugs. Our bodies were obviously designed to withstand a tremendous amount of abuse, but there is a limit. Unfortunately, we sometimes exceed that threshold, and many diseases continue to evolve as a result. This basic problem will not go away unless we drastically change our course of action. One thing that should be obvious to all of us is: **We cannot continue doing the same things, and somehow expect to get different results!**

The study of health can be very fascinating, as well as rewarding. I will do my very best to share my knowledge from years of research with you. Although modern medicine tends to categorize and label specific diseases, and assign a title to each, such as diabetes, cardiovascular disease, or cancer, they are often interconnected and normally have one basic common denominator – unhealthy cells. There are two primary contributors to unhealthy cells. The first contributor is an excessive accumulation of toxins (the cells are basically surrounded by toxins). The other is an inadequate supply of nutrients. As stated by Dr. Joel Wallach, B.S., D.V.M., N.D., well-known for his *Dead Doctors Don't Lie* audiotape series, quite simply the problem stems from doing too many of the bad things, and not enough of the good things. My objective is to teach you what they both are (good and bad). Many of the toxins are actually a bi-product of drugs, while others are the result of normal respiration (the production of energy). There are also toxins produced by viruses, or the candida yeast infection (often the result of antibiotic drugs). The most difficult toxins of all to eliminate are the multitude of environmental toxins we are exposed to on a daily basis, and there is absolutely no way to avoid them all. Many are inorganic (man-made chemicals) that the liver has no enzymes to effectively detoxify. By using prescription or over-the-counter drugs, we are also unnecessarily adding to the body's toxic burden, and that is something we can avoid if we so choose.

The continual accumulation of toxins over the years is one reason people are more prone to experience disease as they age. But don't panic! There is an effective solution to this problem. In my forthcoming book on healthy weight loss, I will be explaining what I consider to be the most effective overall detoxification program, with multiple solutions available. I believe that anyone who seriously evaluates the major health concerns associated with their medications would be sufficiently motivated to begin phasing them out of their life forever. Unfortunately, most people have no idea there is a viable alternative, and that a dependency upon these potentially dangerous drugs actually contributes to disease, and is totally unnecessary. My objective is to show you exactly how that can be accomplished.

A major deterrent is the unfair advantage created by the drug manufacturers' influence on your insurance coverage. Most people who prefer healthier solutions to prescription medications find they have no choice in the matter for financial reasons. Many people in the nation are currently taking medications costing hundreds, and at times thousands of dollars a month. Even though many of their drugs, upon close evaluation, are over-prescribed and definitely not justifiable, they are nonetheless covered by their insurance. Yet any nutritional supplement, no matter how important to your health or survival, will not be covered. Even a woman who becomes pregnant, and thus should be taking prenatal vitamins to prevent the possibility of a birth defect, will find they will not be covered by her insurance!

I am quite amazed that the drug industry has continually been effective in totally controlling our healthcare choices, for decades. This obvious injustice absolutely must be addressed and resolved. This problem, if allowed to continue, will have a tremendous negative impact on the health of the entire nation (but especially the poor). Currently, having good insurance coverage can actually be very detrimental to your health (except for dental coverage). The lower your co-pay, the more drugs you will likely to be taking. People are less inclined to question the importance, or benefit of a particular drug that their doctor might possibly recommend, if someone else is paying the bill.

My two primary objectives are to show why medications are seldom necessary, and to cover in detail the major healthcare concerns in the nation today. With a couple exceptions, you can easily evaluate your progress yourself. Absolutely no one can evaluate better than you, the level of depression you might be experiencing. You would also know if there might be a valid reason for your depression, and if it might possibly be a temporary event that you should soon recover from. A medical doctor, on the other hand, might give the grieving person a prescription for one or more antidepressants. In some cases, antidepressants are contra-indicated (not recommended), yet something far too many doctors are either unaware of, or just choose to ignore. Many are also placed on antidepressants following a divorce, or the death of a loved one, and left on them for years. Although psychiatrists are taught that it's not appropriate to prescribe antidepressants under those circumstances, the majority of prescriptions are written by General Practitioners who are totally unaware, and thus continue doing so.

Only you know exactly how much pain you might be experiencing at any one time, as well as where it might be located, and when it is subsiding. You will also learn why a thyroid disorder is not only a major contributor to depression, but also intimately connected with both diabetes and cardiovascular disease.

With today's modern conveniences available at most any drug store, you can easily take your own blood pressure, and check your blood sugar level, and all in the privacy of your own home. Monitors for testing blood pressure are inexpensive and relatively easy to use. Every diabetic must normally monitor their blood sugar level regularly, and can also easily recognize the typical symptoms associated with hypoglycemia (low blood sugar). If not, we will show you how to identify them.

So as you can easily see, these common conditions that plague millions of people in the nation, conditions that many are currently taking medications for, can be quite easily and safely self-evaluated. And as you will soon discover, these same conditions can very effectively be resolved without the use of drugs. The savings could be tremendous, as well as reducing the concern of the shortage of nurses and doctors that we are currently experiencing. As the baby boomers continue to age, (if unnecessarily placed on more drugs), the problem would just worsen, as would the cost of Medicare and Medicaid. Something obviously must be done to stop the current trend in our healthcare system, or in the near future we could easily be facing a major dilemma. The longer we procrastinate, the greater the cost in lives, as well as threatening the solvency of both Medicare and Medicaid, which are already at risk.

Eliminating your unnecessary dependency upon a lifetime of prescription medications could quite possibly be one of the most important decisions you will make regarding your future health. What are we waiting for?

CHAPTER TWO
WHAT IS WRONG WITH OUR CURRENT HEALTHCARE SYSTEM?

For far too long, we the public have somehow allowed the very powerful and extremely profitable pharmaceutical giants, with their crafty commercials, to basically insult our intelligence, and attempt to treat us as a bunch of adolescents rather than rational adults. They somehow manage to turn symptoms into a disease with a label (i.e. *"acid reflux disease"* – often the result of poor dietary habits). Many people are then led to believe that their health, and possibly even their life, is somehow dependent upon these potentially dangerous and outrageously inflated drugs, or that they shouldn't have to live with the pain. The proponents deviously evaluate exactly what it might be worth to a person to somehow make a particular symptom such as pain go away. The established retail price that the consumer is normally charged has little to do with the actual cost of producing the drug. Also, according to a *USA Today* study, more than half of the experts hired to advise the FDA on the safety and effectiveness of medicine have financial ties to the pharmaceutical companies that will be helped or hurt by their decisions.

The following was posted on the Internet at http://medicaltruth.com/FDA-AMA/home.htm:

> *The sincerest motives of the medical **PROFESSION** are derailed by the greed and power of the medical **INDUSTRY**.*
>
> *For Example: if you are ever diagnosed with cancer, you need to know that your MD or Oncologist is **legally forbidden from curing your cancer**. Their hands are tied by the FDA and AMA, who have used their power to pass legislation forbidding any licensed MD from treating cancer with anything other than treatments that have never proven to work – surgery, radiation, and chemotherapy.*
>
> *"The thing that bugs me is that **people think the Food and Drug Administration is protecting them – it isn't**. What the FDA is doing and what the public thinks it's doing are as different as night and day."*—Dr. Herbert L. Ley, **former Commissioner of the FDA**.
>
> *Did you know? **The average lifespan of the average American is 75 years, while the average lifespan of your MD is 58 years! Following your doctor's advice can cost you 17 years of your life (if you're lucky)!!** Is there something our Doctor's are not being taught?*
>
> *In spite of our supposedly superior medical technology**, the USA is #1 in the world in degenerative disease** and the 20th in life expectancy. – World Health Organization.*
>
> *"Heart disease, cancer, stroke are the top 3 killers in our country [Despite the fact that **all 3 of these diseases have been curable for decades]. The 4th major killer in the US is prescription drugs." – USA Today***
>
> ***Any treatment that you can obtain and self-administer threatens to remove your doctor from the treatment program.** Although your doctor may not object to this, **the American Medical Association (AMA) is strongly opposed to such a trend.** For this reason **the American Medical Association has pushed for legislation to prevent the public from ever being exposed to alternatives.***

And, the following was taken from http://medicaltruth.com/FDA-AMA/story2.html:

> *It has come to light that **the FDA and the Pharmaceutical Advertising Counsel ("PAC"), which represents some 35 major drug companies, have formed and co-funded a corporation under a joint letterhead, calling itself the National Council Against Health Fraud ("NCAHF").** Under this questionable aegis, William Jarvis, MD,*

and Stephen Barrett, MD, and others, **are paid to publicly discredit as unscientific or unknown any or all viable herbs, vitamins, homeopathic remedies or non-allopathic therapies, particularly those that are proven to have the most promise and present the greatest threat to the PAC members.**

The FDA regularly approves dangerous, often lethal pharmaceuticals. Most of the time, the side effects of these drugs can only be fully discovered by widespread use.

Typically, after one of these highly publicized "wonder" drugs fails, causes death or serious side effects, no FDA official nor PAC member company president, research assistant, corporate official, company doctor nor testing lab will be subjected to raid, investigation, indictment or jail term as often happens to "alternative" practitioners.

In his March 2003 newsletter, Dr. James F. Balch, M.D. stresses his concern regarding the increasingly aggressive marketing techniques employed by the pharmaceutical sales reps to encourage a broader use for their products as follows:

WARNING! Drug Companies Illegally Push "Innovative Treatments" That Kill!

Drug company sales reps are secretly selling your doctor a bill of goods and the result could seriously harm your health or even kill you. I'm talking about the deliberate misuse of prescription drugs by doctors who are prescribing those drugs for off-label uses.

Unapproved prescriptions are soaring. Between the summer of 2002 and the summer of 2003, over 115 million such prescriptions were written. That's double the number from just five years earlier. This increase is driven by the aggressive marketing of pharmaceutical sales reps who are carefully trained to sidestep FDA regulations against promoting off-label uses!

The drug companies are breaking the law and it's happening in doctors' offices and at medical conferences every day!

Prozac is just one of the drugs being touted for everything from weight loss to pain management. **In one year, 500,000 Prozac prescriptions were written for off-label reasons.**

After 13 days on Prozac, one man in Tennessee hung himself. He was a happy person looking forward to both retirement and moving into a new home.

The antidepressant Prozac was not given to him by a psychiatrist, it had been given to him by his heart specialist to help ease his chest pain. This is a use for which Prozac was never approved! (*Prescriptions for Healthy Living*, p. 4)

I might just interject my observation regarding the above incident. Although Prozac™ will eventually dull the senses, as well as the emotions, it can in no way stop the chest (angina) pain this individual had been experiencing. But first, regarding the suicide: In her book *Prozac – Panacea or Pandora?* (1991/1994), antidepressant authority Dr. Ann Blake Tracy cited many cases where, shortly after being placed on Prozac™, and with no apparent provocation, people suddenly committed suicide. Many times the Prozac™ was actually prescribed for symptoms other than depression (often unapproved uses), as was this particular individual. Even worse, some even killed others, such as a spouse, or even their own children (Andrea Yates is a prime example). Everyone doesn't respond in the same way to antidepressants, or in the same time frame. From years of use, they have proven time and again, to be potentially dangerous, and as you will soon discover, totally unnecessary.

Now, back to the angina pain that the heart specialist placed this man on Prozac™ for. Angina pain is a warning signal that the heart muscle is starving for oxygen. Any effort to ignore the pain, rather than resolving the critical issue at hand, is in my opinion inexcusable. Prozac™ could actually contribute to an already serious concern (ignoring the unfortunate suicide). The potential problem stems from the fact that, according to Dr. Tracy, just one 30 mg dose of Prozac™ increases the stress hormone cortisol by 200%! Stressors, be they physical or hormonal, stimulate an increase in the heart rate, and thus an even greater demand for oxygen to the already deficient heart muscle.

Unfortunately, far too many doctors have only a superficial knowledge of the many medications they prescribe daily, and not only in this instance, but also in far too many cases. We will soon evaluate some typical examples of drugs that were all too often prescribed in potentially dangerous combinations, where apparent oversight seems to be obvious.

Now, with the assistance of the late news anchor Peter Jennings, we will evaluate the opinions of some medical experts that appear to have a conscience. These are medical doctors who are totally aware of the corruption in the very powerful and profitable (legal) drug industry, and are not afraid to express their opinion. The following excerpts were taken from the *ABC News Special Report - Bitter Medicine: Pills, Profit and the Public Health*. The report by Peter Jennings aired on Wednesday, May 29, 2004 on ABC.

> **Peter Jennings** – *...Dr. Drummond Rennie is an editor at The Journal of the American Medical Association. He says* **researchers who are critical get attacked all the time.** *Do you actually believe, Dr. Rennie, that drug companies are intent on keeping the consumer on drugs, which are not as good as older drugs, for the simple requirement of profit?*

> **Dr. Drummond Rennie** – *Yes. Yes, very much so. Absolutely. ....***They've got to be prevented.**

> **Peter Jennings** – *... The top 10 drug companies combined made profits of more than $37 billion in the year 2001. And* **you, the taxpayer, are subsidizing research that benefits the drug industry.**

> **Peter Jennings** – *The majority of the drugs approved by the FDA are simply modifications of old drugs...***Consumers spend $90 billion more on prescription drugs last year than was spent just six years ago.** *And are we $90 billion healthier? ...But what critics call this 'gaming of the system' may have a much more damaging result.*

> **Dr. Sharon Levine, Kaiser Permanente Medical Group** - *If I'm a manufacturer, and I can change one molecule and get another 20 years of patent life and convince physicians to prescribe and consumers to demand ... then why would I be spending money on a lot less certain endeavor, which is looking for brand new drugs?*

> **Peter Jennings – The pharmaceutical industry has more registered lobbyists than the number of senators and congressmen combined.**

> **Dr. Jerry Avorn, Brigham and Women's Hospital** – *I think there's a sense that, for example, when the FDA approves a drug, everything that needs to be known about it is known. I think patients believe that. I think doctors sometimes believe that. And that is not true.*

> **Dr. Matt Handley, Group Health Cooperative** – *I would personally wait years for long-term safety from the FDA's monitoring program before I'd consider taking them. If they were free, I would do that same thing.*

Peter Jennings – *What does this say about the social responsibility of the pharmaceutical industry? Or is the pharmaceutical industry supposed to have a social responsibility?*

Dr. Sharon Levine – *That's a very good question that the American people need to answer, do we want to entrust critical elements of the public health to an industry whose purpose, whose mission is to earn return for shareholders?*

Peter Jennings – *Congress has never required the FDA to routinely compare new drugs with older drugs. This is costing consumers billions of dollars that we do not need to spend. And in some cases, it could be costing lives. …There is no law that says new drugs have to be proven 100 percent safe. … The government says they must be relatively safe, which means that **every drug comes with risks.** And the result of that is that sometimes new drugs turn out to be more dangerous than old drugs.*

Dr. Jerry Avorn, Harvard Medical School – *If patients were aware of the limitations that all of us physicians have in terms of what we know and what we wish we knew and what we don't know, they would be more scared than they are at present. …The saying that a lot of doctors use sometimes in jest is, **'Always wait a year before prescribing a new drug. And if it's for a family member, wait five years.'** And that's an awful thing to say, but it reveals a perception that we really don't know as much as we would like to know about a drug until it's been around. **INSERT: In other words, tested on the public.***

Peter Jennings – *The fact is, drugs can be used for years before we really know how safe they are. …Dr. Drummond Rennie is an editor at The Journal of the American Medical Association. **He says researchers who are critical get attacked all the time. Why do you think the industry is able to get away with what you have in the past called 'bullying tactics'?***

Dr. Drummond Rennie, Journal of the American Medical Association – *Money. Because if the shareholders are happy, whom else do they have to answer for? **These are multinationals. They have no masters.***

Peter Jennings – ***Can we trust studies funded by companies that have a vested interest in the results?** …Will the pharmaceutical industry do whatever it takes to get the results it wants from research?*

Dr. Drummond Rennie – *The temptation to spin those results is always there, and it's frequently used. Frequently.*

Peter Jennings – ***For nearly every drug on the market, doctors must wrestle with conflicting and sometimes inaccurate information.***

Dr. Drummond Rennie – *If only the good news about a drug is published, and never the bad news, then a false impression is given of the quality, effectiveness of that drug. It may be entirely false.*

Peter Jennings – ***Does the drug industry, on occasion or regularly, suppress data?***

Dr. Drummond Rennie – ***Oh, we suspect, and rather know, that this happens all the time.***

Peter Jennings – *Does a drug company ever not publish the results of a trial because it doesn't like the results?*

Dr. Drummond Rennie – *Yes.*

Peter Jennings – *Do you actually believe, Dr. Rennie, that drug companies are intent on keeping the consumer on drugs, which are not as good as older drugs, for the simple requirement of profit?*

Dr. Drummond Rennie – *Yes. Yes, very much so. Absolutely. …* **They've got to be prevented.**

Peter Jennings – *There is one last thing this evening which we believe is important for all of us. The questions about what we are getting for our money cannot and must not be answered only by the drug companies. Virtually everyone we talked to for this broadcast agrees on that.* **The rules by which this hugely profitable industry operates do not always serve consumers adequately. And nothing is going to happen, no matter how angry consumers get, unless the Congress and the president decide that the time is come. The country can do better.** *I'm Peter Jennings. Thank you for joining us. Good night.*

I can't help but respect Peter Jennings for conducting the interview to help us better understand the corruption in medicine that I am fully aware of, although many in the nation are not. All too often we see announcements in the national news promoting the use of drugs in deceptive ways, and at times for unapproved uses. A prime example is the woman who was interviewed on the national news, claiming that after stopping Hormone Replacement Therapy (HRT), she discovered that Paxil™ seemed to help reduce her hot flashes. That announcement was aired shortly after it was announced that HRT had many potential associated problems, so many women stopped their HRT drugs. Although there are natural supplements proven to resolve the hot flashes, taking Paxil™ is much more of a serious threat than HRT.

Paxil™ is a very serious antidepressant never approved for hot flashes, or anything other than depression. Paxil™ is the same basic class of antidepressants as Prozac™, but an even more potent version. One woman was actually prescribed Paxil™ to **help her stop biting her fingernails!** She soon discovered that biting her nails was minor compared to the major problem she experienced from the use of Paxil™. For over a year she could no longer control her movements, and as a result was unable to work.

I would guess that after the interview on the national news indicating that Paxil™ might possibly help prevent hot flashes, many women likely asked their doctor if they could try Paxil™. Unfortunately, many doctors would likely accommodate them, and write a prescription for Paxil™, just like the doctor did for the lady who was biting her fingernails. Hot flashes are basically a walk in the park compared to the many potential side effects associated with this serious class of antidepressants (diabetes being just one).

There is often a cascade effect from drug use, resulting from both drug interactions, and the nutrient depletion they cause. A prime example: The high blood pressure and congestive heart failure that results from the use of drugs used to lower cholesterol. Your doctor would likely then place you on anti-hypertensive (blood pressure) medication for that problem. There are several blood pressure medications, each with their own set of problems (discussed later in this book). They are often prescribed in tandem (combination) today. Incidentally, there are over 20 brands of beta-blockers, a popular blood pressure medication, and they all just happen to deplete the very same critical nutrient CoQ_{10} that is also depleted by the statin (cholesterol lowering) drugs, which would just make a bad problem even worse.

CoQ$_{10}$ is a natural and extremely critical enzyme used in every cell of the body for energy production. We will soon be discussing the importance of CoQ$_{10}$ in considerable detail.

Although the combination of many prescription medications may be very profitable for some, it just increases the potential for side effects for the recipients. The congestive heart failure that can also be caused by statin drugs and results in edema (fluid retention) is then treated with diuretics. The problem with the diuretics is that they remove critical vitamins and minerals along with the excess body fluids. The most critical mineral depleted is magnesium, which often results in an irregular heartbeat, for which your doctor might then recommend installing a pacemaker. That might sound like a stretch, but that is often standard protocol for modern medicine that considers drugs and surgeries as the only available options.

Regarding the pacemaker implant to resolve a temporary mineral deficiency, my aunt Daisie is a prime example. Over 50 years ago her doctor indicated that she needed a pacemaker. When she refused, he insisted that he would no longer be her doctor unless she agreed to the implantation. Fortunately, she didn't give in, and lived without one until age 93, and without a pacemaker!

The question remains: Just how long can we allow this obvious deception to continue? Millions of lives were already at stake, and even millions more are now with the more aggressive measures regarding cholesterol-lowering drugs in place. We will soon experience a dramatic increase in not only strokes and heart attacks, but also kidney failures requiring dialysis or transplants (if any available kidneys can be found).

Sadly, we are not the only country having this particular problem. The following article, regarding the frustrations of doctors in Britain, was taken from an emailed issue of *the McAlvany Health Alert* (October 23, 2004):

The Royal College of General Practitioners has accused drug companies of "disease-mongering" in order to boost sales.

*The college, whose members include many of Britain's 37,000 GPs, says **the pharmaceutical industry is taking the National Health Service to the brink of collapse by encouraging unnecessary prescribing of costly drugs.***

In evidence to a parliamentary inquiry, the college accuses the companies of over-playing the dangers of conditions such as mild depression or slightly raised blood pressure.

Dr. Maureen Baker, the college's honorary secretary, wants the Commons health inquiry to investigate the companies' practices.

"It would be fruitful to look into the increase in disease-mongering by them," she told The Sunday Telegraph.

"It is very much in the interest of the pharmaceutical industry to draw a line that includes as large a population as possible within the 'ill' category. The bigger this group is, the more drugs they can sell. If current trends continue, publicly funded health-care systems will be at risk of financial collapse with huge cost to society as a whole."

The college lists hypertension, high cholesterol, osteoporosis, anxiety and depression as examples of common conditions that, in mild forms, are often inappropriately treated with drugs.

Sound familiar? I can only add "Amen!" That is my sentiments also. Britain is apparently experiencing the very same problems associated with the pharmaceutical industry that we in the U.S. have been dealing with. Apparently, they are now attempting to deal with the issue head on, and the problem in this nation will not go away unless we address this critical issue also.

CHAPTER THREE
THE COST: WHO BENEFITS AND WHO PAYS THE PRICE?

There is absolutely no condition I am aware of that can't be more easily avoided, and often resolved, by effectively using God's natural pharmacy, rather than man's chemicals. Herbs, for instance, normally contain hundreds of organic ingredients that our body can instantly recognize and effectively utilize, and are far more complex than any drug that man could possibly produce in a laboratory. The myriad of constituents in herbs, for instance, works synergistically throughout the body. Herbs, as well as vitamins, minerals, and amino acids, are all involved in many important functions throughout our body and brain. However, many preferring an alternative approach to healthcare, of practicing prevention and truly resolving the basic underlying problem, have absolutely no choice in the matter. Their insurance provider, along with the financially biased experts, are responsible for determining just what is or is not considered acceptable coverage. The pharmaceutical industry is also very adept at placing individuals in key positions to assure that **only those highly inflated drugs, (and not natural supplements), are covered by the insurance providers.**

Dr. Sherry A. Rogers, M.D., in her book *Detoxify or Die* (2002), helps identify the basic underlying problem when she quotes an article from the *Journal of the American Medical Association* (*JAMA*) that *"documented how **over 87% of physicians who make up the panels of 'experts' who determine the practice guidelines for medicine receive compensation from the drug industry. These are the guidelines that your doctors and insurance companies follow"** (JAMA 287: 6,12-6 17, 2002).* Unfortunately, **we are not even allowed to enjoy the basic freedom we should all enjoy,** which is **the freedom of choosing our own healthcare.** That is especially true regarding the poor, or the many senior citizens with limited incomes who are on Medicare or Medicaid. They are often not even sure what the drugs they are taking are actually for, or their potential side effects and interactions. Some will even attempt to reduce their food budget just so they can somehow afford to pay for their medications.

An article in the September 2004 issue of the *AARP Bulletin* sheds light on the serious over-medication of our seniors in both our nursing homes and long-term care facilities. The article focuses on a 66-year old gentleman named Armon Neel who tells patients how they can both save money and possibly their lives. Neel however isn't a doctor, but rather a pharmacist whose specialty is determining whether people are taking the right medications – and in the right doses – for their ailments. Apparently Neel hasn't worked behind a prescription counter since the early 1970s, when he gave up dispensing drugs for a career that would often put him on a collision course with the doctors who prescribe them.

He told one of his patients that the blood pressure medication she had been taking isn't the drug of choice, but in her case may in fact be responsible for some of her other health problems. He looked through her records and discovered that her doctor, in an attempt to control her hypertension, had tried four different ACE inhibitors, two beta-blockers and two alpha-blockers. Nothing worked, and she had allergic reactions to every one of them. Neel seemed stupefied. *"There wasn't a need to go to the second one after the first one did you harm,"* he notes. *"They're in the same family. You need a calcium channel blocker instead."*

In my opinion, that is not a good option either. Even most pharmacists can't possibly keep up with all the drugs' many interactions and side effects. According to Dr. Sherry A. Rogers, M.D., in her book *Detoxify or Die* (2002), **"Calcium channel blockers, the number one prescribed drug by cardiologists, have been proven with MRI (special x-rays) to cause shrinking and deterioration of the brain."** Dr. Rogers indicates that **this eventually leads to a loss of function, which in a few short years is then** *"dismissed as 'normal aging' or later, Alzheimer's"* (pp. 172, 188).

Although Neel appears to be very knowledgeable in regard to prescription medications, most pharmacists have no training in nutrition, or in the use of natural therapies. For example, the mineral magnesium works very well as a natural calcium channel blocker and without the potentially dangerous side effects. Magnesium basically causes the muscles in the arteries to relax and dilate, thus reducing the blood pressure. Incidentally, adequate magnesium levels along with calcium is also important for maintaining a regular heart rhythm, as well as strong bones. As usual, natural supplements normally have many additional benefits, versus drugs' many side effects.

Neel indicated that almost 100 percent of the people he saw as out patients were overmedicated, as they were the ones having problems. He also noted that even in a long-term care environment, it is still about 80 percent. In his opinion, **Neel feels that medication levels in nursing homes could be cut in half or even better.** Neel stresses that: *"If I can get the drug therapy management correct, there are fewer hospital stays, fewer hospital admissions, lower labor costs involved in care and a better quality of life for residents."* Certainly a tremendous benefit, if he could just get the doctors' cooperation, which according to Neel seldom happens.

For each patient that Neel evaluates, he types up his recommendations for what he considers are properly prescribed medications, **according to Neel, the medical director rejects his recommendations almost without exception.** The doctors basically tend to resent being second-guessed by a pharmacist. Although many doctors hate to admit the fact, pharmacists are normally much more knowledgeable regarding prescription medications, their interactions, and potential side effects, than doctors are. That is basically their specialty. None of us are perfect, and anyone can make a mistake, but when someone's life is at stake, pride should never get in the way of making a rational decision.

Pharmacists are sometimes the patient's last line of defense in a nation of doctors who, more often than not, don't know a great deal about the drugs they are prescribing, or the geriatric patients they are treating who normally have different concerns and requirements than the general population. This is contrary to the results we should all be able to expect from the very doctors that we are placing our complete trust in. Although the pharmacist Armon Neel is obviously heading in the right direction by identifying inappropriately prescribed drugs, my objective is to go a step further, by providing natural solutions to replace drugs. Many doctors are unknowingly depriving their patients of the potential for good health that we all desire.

Are We Also Needlessly Drugging Our Children?

The answer is yes, beyond a doubt, and it absolutely must be stopped! We are not only overmedicating adults, but also very young children, our nation's future. Far too many children are needlessly being placed on some of the most potentially dangerous drugs currently on the market.

Following is an extract from an article found in the June/July 2004 issue of the *Let's Talk Health* newsletter, by Dr. Kurt W. Donsbach, D.C., N.D., Ph.D.:

AN OUTRAGE, AN INSULT TO OUR INTELLIGENCE, A DANGER TO OUR CHILDREN!

Quote: 'Blood pressure screening for children should start at age 3, according to the latest government diagnosis and treatment guidelines that were presented at the American Society of Hypertension's Nineteenth Annual Scientific Meeting.'

Dr. Kurt W. Donsbach's observation: "I am fearful the next move will be to suggest doctors check children for possible cholesterol problems and start prescribing statin drugs. I ask you in all sincerity – How long are you going to take this before you rebel?????"

As you can see, the improper and excessive prescribing of drugs is actually quite common, and not just limited to those in nursing homes and long-term care facilities. If we also consider the addition of the over-the-counter medications that many people are also taking, the potential for serious interactions is even greater. That is something many doctors quite often fail to consider (usually the result of the average 10-minute office call).

A prime example is my assistant's 9-year-old son named Jeffrey, who was diagnosed with ADHD at the age of 3. Almost daily he would completely terrorize his preschool classroom, often biting and hitting other children and the teachers, to the point that his teachers strongly suggested medication. Just after turning 4, Jeffrey was put on Ritalin™, three times a day, under the direction of his pediatrician. When that didn't succeed in calming his outbursts, his dosage was increased, to the point that his pediatrician indicated it was standard protocol to try a stronger drug, as Jeffrey was already taking the highest dosage of Ritalin™ allowed. Thus, time-release Dexedrine™ was prescribed, which resulted in many serious side effects. He had difficulty staying awake, appeared more like a zombie when he was awake, and complained of terrible headaches. Not only was the Dexedrine™ also unsuccessful in calming Jeffrey, but within one week of changing his medication, Jeffrey was kicked out of preschool due to his uncontrollable behavioral problems. After observing the many severe and varied side effects Jeffrey was experiencing, his mom decided to stop giving him the Dexedrine™.

By May of his first grade year (age 6), the County Mental Health counselor announced, after just **one** visit, that Jeffrey's problems were actually "emotional" and that a new drug Zoloft™ was especially beneficial for that sort of problem. Jeffrey took Zoloft™ through the summer until November of that year, a total of 6 months. During this time, he continued to complain of terrible headaches on a daily basis, began to experience difficulty in remembering things, and also wet the bed nightly.

After my assistant went to work for me, we were discussing Jeffrey's behavior and problems with bed-wetting, as well as his difficulty remembering. A milk allergy is often the underlying cause of bed-wetting, as well as headaches, and after discovering he was also on Zoloft™, that would likely explain his difficulty remembering. Together we decided to wean Jeffrey off Zoloft™, eliminate both milk and excess sugar from his diet, and give him a calming herb called Valerian Root. Although calming, Valerian will not (and did not) cause drowsiness, but instead helps in staying focused, which is important to a child with ADHD. Jeffrey is now in the 3rd grade, doing 4th grade math and 5th grade reading, and his memory is just fine. He now goes months with only an occasional short-lived *"fit"*, and is no longer troubled with any headaches or bed-wetting, which is much more relief than any prescription drug ever provided.

Although Jeffrey is just one prime example, there are many more children in the nation needlessly placed, and often left on these potentially dangerous drugs for years. A food allergy is quite often the underlying problem, and sugar, milk, and sometimes wheat are the most common allergens. Although the natural solution is often very simple, it is seldom considered, but as usual with our broken healthcare system, it is instead just treated with drugs.

The long-term potential for children taking these serious drugs cannot be overstated. Zoloft™ and Prozac™ are the same basic class of SSRI antidepressants, known for creating havoc with people's lives in general. And we are even giving them to our very young children. What a terrible way to destroy a life at such an early age!

From their long-term use, these antidepressants soon create an imbalance of neurotransmitters in the brain, leading to worse depression and mood swings. According to Dr. Ann Blake Tracy, the elevated stress hormone (cortisol) produced by these drugs can result in brain damage, adrenal fatigue, and even diabetes. More and more children are being placed on these drugs, and at a very young age, which would help explain the dramatic increase in the rate of diabetes experienced by children today.

We must seriously ask ourselves why years ago, no one ever heard of giving children drugs to control their behavior, or for depression. Back then, we somehow did just fine without them. Just a slight diet modification is normally all that is necessary to resolve the same problems that children are being placed on potentially dangerous drugs every day. As most doctors were never trained in nutrition, that is something they seldom consider, although that should always be the very first consideration.

In my opinion, the greatest potential problem regarding our future financial burden, involves the largest single group of people in the nation, (the baby boomers), who are just beginning to fit into that category. These expensive drugs nearly bankrupt many people (especially the elderly), not only financially, but also physically (basically stealing their health).

Following is a list of just a few of the more common prescription drugs on the market today, comparing the consumer price with the actual cost of the generic ingredients. The list was compiled by the non-profit organization *The Life Extension Foundation* (April 2002, p. 15), which has extensive laboratory facilities and an advisory panel of some of the more respected and knowledgeable doctors in the world. I would assume for that reason that they are a credible source of information. I can only add that the following figures obviously speak for themselves, both loud and clear.

What Drugs Really Cost

BRAND NAME	CONSUMER PRICE (For 100 tabs/caps)	COST OF GENERIC (For 100 tabs/caps)	PERCENT MARKUP
Celebrex 100 mg	$130.27	$0.60	21,712%
Lipitor 20 mg	$272.37	$5.80	4,696%
Paxil 20 mg	$220.27	$7.60	2,898%
Prevacid 30 mg	$344.77	$1.01	34,136%
Prilosec 20 mg	$360.97	$0.52	69,417%
Prozac 20 mg	$247.47	$0.11	224,973%
Xanax 1 mg	$139.79	$0.024	569,958%
Zocor 40 mg	$350.27	$8.63	4,059%
Zoloft 50 mg	$206.87	$1.75	11,821%

If you have you ever wondered how the companies that produce these drugs can possibly afford to continually advertise these drugs on TV every day, often several times a day, considering the high cost of TV advertising, you now have the answer. And it is obviously working!

Promoting Medications To The Public Results in Inappropriate Prescribing of Drugs

Following is an article from the front page of the *Eugene Register Guard*, (April 27, 2005), as printed in the *Los Angeles Times*, by Alan Zarembo:

Primary care doctors are easily persuaded to prescribe antidepressants – even unnecessarily – when a patient mentions having seen television advertisements for them, researchers reported Tuesday.

In an unusual experiment in which actresses posed as mildly depressed patients who did not need medication, doctors were five times more likely to write them prescriptions when an ad for a specific drug was mentioned.

Drug companies spend about $3 billion a year on direct-to-consumer advertising, fomenting sharp debate over how much sway the advertisements have over doctors. The study showed the effect is significant.

"When patients ask for a drug, they tend to get a drug regardless of whether it is appropriate for them," said Joel Weissman, a health policy expert at Harvard Medical School who was not involved in the research. "That is a fascinating finding."

Surveys have shown that in up to 7 percent of doctor visits, a patient requests a prescription based on an ad – a rate that experts say can significantly boost sales.

In the study, published in the current issue of the Journal of the American Medical Association, **the patients were actresses all playing the same part: a 45-year-old divorcee who had recently lost her job and was suffering from stress, fatigue and back pain. Those are symptoms of adjustment disorder, a mild, event-induced depression in which medications are thought to be of little value.**

Each actress used these lines to request Paxil, a popular antidepressant: "I saw this ad on TV the other night. It was about Paxil. Some things about the ad really struck me. I was wondering if you thought Paxil might help me."

Out of 49 such visits, 27 – or 55 percent – resulted in a prescription for an antidepressant, *most often Paxil.*

By comparison, patients who did not mention an ad were prescribed antidepressants just 10 percent of the time.

Critics of direct-to-consumer advertising say **it leads to needless prescribing.**

Considering how many people in the nation are actually on several drugs, we can easily identify the basic problem behind the tremendously inflated cost of our healthcare. Any company should normally expect to make a significant profit, even at a reasonable profit margin, providing the volume of customers is fairly broad based. The pharmaceutical industry not only attempts to create a lifetime dependency on their drugs with a very extensive base of customers, but they are also determined to make an outlandish profit on each and every customer. Absolutely no other industry in the world comes close to that kind of profitability. In my opinion, this is basically extortion, and a crime against humanity just for the sake of exorbitant profits.

Although the Canadian pharmaceuticals make a substantial profit on their drugs, the companies in the U.S. are intent upon nearly doubling the price that Americans pay for the very same drugs. Now that the decision that cholesterol levels should be reduced even further (as was the case with the blood pressure recommendations), that will open the door for doctors to prescribe increasingly dangerous dosages of statin drugs, and to prescribe the drugs to patients whose cholesterol was considered normal in the past. As these drugs are one of the most expensive and most profitable, we can easily see how our already tremendously inflated healthcare costs could easily spiral out of sight. This kind of irresponsibility and manipulation for the sake of profit, if allowed to continue, could quite easily bankrupt the nation. The longer we continue to overlook the problem and allow it to continue, the worse both the health and financial structure of our nation will become.

To make matters even worse, as of July 2004 "obesity" (which has become an epidemic) became classified as a *"disease"* by the surgeon general. Considering that more than half of the population is currently overweight, that could easily result in yet another exponential rise in the cost of healthcare. Furthermore, it opens the market for a whole new class of weight loss drugs, which is something some drug companies were likely already working on. A clue was when the herb ephedra, used by the Chinese for thousands of years and an ingredient in many weight loss formulas to stimulate the metabolism, was pulled by the FDA. A major issue was made over the fact that an athlete, who suffered from a heat stroke, had taken ephedra. Many had used the herb for years, and without incident. In excessive doses it could possibly over stimulate, but Tylenol™, sold over-the-counter, and in some children's remedies, could easily result in liver failure in high doses. If all the drugs currently on the market were no more dangerous than ephedra, there would be much less concern than there is regarding their safety. The basic difference is that ephedra is a natural herb, and not approved by the FDA **(for our protection, of course).**

The FDA has had far better reasons for stopping the use of many potentially serious drugs still on the market today, such as some of the antidepressants. Incidentally, **shortly before the antidepressant Prozac™, with its hundreds of associated side effects, was about to be announced, the FDA somehow deemed it necessary to pull the natural amino acid L-tryptophan from the market.** The only excuse was that a tainted batch was imported from overseas. It is just a safe and natural substance that our body needs, but was becoming too popular as a natural treatment by many doctors for depression! The timing is amazing, and the motive quite obvious. I believe we can all recall when there was a problem with Tylenol™ that was also tainted, although that somehow that didn't prove to be a threat, and has thus continued to be available to the public ever since.

We are all very fortunate to live in a country that has been blessed beyond measure. The question we must seriously ask ourselves is: Can we continue to stand idly by and allow our nation's very financial structure to be destroyed. I believe the majority of people in the nation are both honest and caring, and that is what makes the United States such a great nation. Any time we see such an obvious injustice, or basic lack of freedom in a particular area, I believe we must do our utmost to fight injustice and defend our right to freedom. Can we, in good conscience, continue to allow our basic freedom of healthcare to be withheld, due to the influence of a few very powerful, and extremely profitable multi-national corporations? The best solution is to just say *"no"* to a lifetime of drug dependence. We all have much better options available, and they do not require a prescription by your doctor.

CHAPTER FOUR
ARE ALL THESE DRUGS REALLY NECESSARY?

I truly believe that the excessive and unnecessary use of prescription and over-the-counter drugs in the nation is far more pervasive, and an even more serious problem than all the illegal drugs combined, due to their extensive use. Quite often, drugs are prescribed just to deal with side effects associated with the other drugs a person might already be taking. For example, you will learn about Al (the professor/body-builder) who was totally shocked to learn that his memory loss, terrible fatigue, and extensive muscle loss was actually caused by his medications. He couldn't believe how much improvement he had already made in just two weeks, after stopping his medications. I gave Al some information on what these drugs were actually doing and exactly how. He took the information to his doctor, and left it with his secretary. He also told his doctor how much improvement he had made since stopping the medications. At the next visit he asked his doctor what he thought about the information. His doctor's response was *"I don't have time to read all that stuff,"* which means **you** must take the time to read this stuff, just for your own protection.

Many are taking drugs that are contra-indicated (a potential risk when combined), and are totally unaware of the potential risk they are being subjected to. You will also hear Mary Lou's story. She had no idea that the lithium, the ACE inhibitors, and her diuretic, all cause dehydration. She was not aware that the Prozac™ she had been on for 16 years, was just attempting to resolve the typical symptom of depression (caused by her hypothyroid condition). She also had no idea that one problem associated with Prozac™ is thyroid suppression, which made the problem even worse. And another problem associated with the long-term use of Prozac™ is diabetes, which Mary Lou also developed, as well as the bipolar disorder, which she was then given lithium for. Also, one more potential side effect of Prozac™ is **depression!** This results from the overstimulation of serotonin in the brain, which begins shutting down the serotonin receptors (similar to the insulin resistance in the body). For this she was given a second antidepressant. One thing the lithium carbonate is also known for is thyroid suppression (compounding the original problem), as well as permanent kidney scarring. The kidney scarring then leads to hypertension, for which she was given medications for also. Then **six of her medications** caused chest congestion, chest tightness, or asthma as side effects. She was then given **three more medications for asthma!**

Somewhere along the line, some doctor recognized that she obviously had a thyroid problem, and thus prescribed the typical artificial form of T_4 thyroid (called Synthroid™). As usual, because Synthroid™ seldom works, (as was the case with Mary Lou), this typical scenario could have been avoided if Mary Lou had found a good doctor initially, who would have recognized the low thyroid condition early on, which is often brought on by a stressful event (which was true in Mary Lou's case). If he had just prescribed Armour™ Thyroid (a natural thyroid that also contains T_3), and that **does work**, the whole nightmare of years of unnecessarily taking medications (nine total) could have been avoided. Although Mary Lou is now totally drug-free, she was still needlessly forced to deal with many drug-related side effects for years, not counting the money she was required to spend on her medications for so many years. Mary Lou even began losing excess weight with no dietary changes, following her successful withdrawal from nine medications! You will learn more about Mary Lou later, under "Mary Lou's Story".

By far the most important issue of all, aside from all the drugs' seriously potential dangers, and their unreasonably inflated cost, is that they are in my opinion seldom even necessary. This viewpoint is not just mine alone, but also shared by many other doctors who were not trained in natural medicine, but actually received traditional medical training.

Some Expert Opinions On The Subject

To help substantiate this claim, let's take a look at what some medical experts have to say about pharmaceutical drugs. The following comments were extracted from an undated newsletter provided by Paul Oberdorf of NMS Publishing. Keep in mind that the following doctors are all M.D.s, who are normally taught the use of prescription medications in medical school.

- *"The cause of most disease is in the poisonous drugs physicians superstitiously give in order to affect a cure."* **Charles E. Page, M.D.**

- *"The person who takes medicine must recover twice, once from the disease and once from the medicine."* **William Osler, M.D.**

- *"If all the medicine in the world were thrown into the sea, it would be bad for the fish and good for humanity."* **O. W. Holmes, Professor of Medicine. Harvard University**

- *"The greatest part of all chronic disease is created by the suppression of acute disease by drug poisoning."* **Henry Lindlahr, M.D.**

- *"Drug medications consist in employing as remedies for disease, those things which produce disease in well persons... all are poisons."* **R. T. Trall, M.D. lecture to Congress and medical profession**

- *"Every drug increases and complicates the patient's condition."* **Robert Henderson, M.D.**

- *"Drugs never cure disease. They merely hush the voice of nature's protest, and pull down the danger signals she erects along the pathway of transgression. Any poison taken into the system has to be reckoned with later on even though it palliates* present symptoms. Pain may disappear, but the patient is left in a worse condition, though unconscious of it at the time."* **Daniel H. Kress, M.D.**

- *"Every educated physician knows that most diseases are not appreciably helped by medicine."* **Richard C. Cabot, M.D., Mass. General Hospital**

- *"Why would a patient swallow a poison because he is ill, or take that which would make a well man sick."* **L. F. Kebler, M.D.**

- *"What hope is there for medical science to ever become a true science when the entire structure of medical knowledge is built around the idea there is an entity called disease which can be expelled when the right drug is found?"* **John H. Tilden, M.D.**

- *"We are prone to thinking of drug abuse in terms of the male population and illicit drugs such as heroin, cocaine and marijuana. It may surprise you to learn that a greater problem exists with millions of women dependent on legal prescription drugs."* **Robert Mendelsohn, M.D.**

- *"The necessity of teaching mankind not to take drugs and medicines is a duty incumbent upon all who know their uncertainty and injurious effects; the time is not far distant when the drug system will be abandoned."* **Charles Armbruster, M.D.**

In the December 2000 issue of the *Prescriptions for Healthy Living* newsletter, Dr. James F. Balch, M.D. stated that **the side effects of prescription drugs result in 106,000 deaths each year!** He went on to point out that **if adverse reactions to medications were classified as disease, it would rank as the fifth leading cause of death in the United States.** And, he goes on to note that you may wonder how a drug can be approved for use when it is so potentially dangerous and its list of ominous side effects is longer than its list of benefits. He warns:

> *If the side effects of these "approved" medications don't kill you, they can cause severe intestinal trouble, liver or brain damage, stroke, insomnia, vertigo, psychosis, rapid heartbeat, shortness of breath, tremors, dizziness, impotence, migraines, deafness, blindness... the list goes on and on* (p. 1).

Regarding prescription drugs, the authors of the book *Breaking Your Prescribed Addiction* (Sahley & Birkner, 1998) put it this way:

> *Everyone has problems.* **Drugs make these problems unmanageable, unresolvable, and unbearable. Drug therapy is very hazardous to one's mental and physical health.** *Drug users are thirty times more likely to commit suicide than the norm.* **No one ever fully recovers from anxiety, insomnia, or depression while on drugs, whether they take drugs in the form of alcohol, or recreational or pharmaceutical drugs** (p. 7).

> **There are no drugs in pharmacology which cure** *anxiety, panic, phobias, insomnia, depression, allergies, arthritis, asthma, cardiac disorders, diabetes, hypertension, hyperactivity, or inflammatory conditions, chronic pain, or disease* (p. 12).

> *There are many drugs which* **treat the symptoms** *of these disorders. However,* **many prescription drugs have significant potential for long-term adverse or permanent drug side effects** (p. 12).

> **Using prescription drugs ranks as one of the most hazardous activities in the world today. There is no such thing as a safe prescription medication.** *In his best seller, Prescription for Disaster, Thomas J. Moore states, "more than a million prescriptions are written every hour of the working day; in a year's time 8 prescriptions have been written for every man, woman, and child in the United States." All research statistics on medication abuse demonstrate a major problem in this country with prescription medication abuse* (p. 19).

In an article in his December 2001 issue of *Health Alert* newsletter, Dr. Bruce West, D.C. tells us:

> *The real truth is that* **the hundreds of thousands of people killed and maimed by doctors and drugs are only the medical "accidents" that are recorded and occur in hospitals. All others are not counted,** *which makes the full tally monumental to say the least. This is particularly true with mind-altering prescriptions. Just as in the case of Andrea Yates, the mother who drowned her five children, these drugs can be fraught with very serious delusional side effects. She was reported to have begun psychiatric drugs*

*after her fourth pregnancy, ending up with many – including Haldol, Effexor, Wellbutrin, Remeron, and **several used in combination*** (p. 6).

The side effects associated with some drugs actually produce symptoms or conditions that are much worse than the problem they were prescribed for in the first place. One such example is, during one of my lectures at a local senior center, a lady in the class indicated that her husband had Parkinson's disease, and that his doctor had placed him on the SSRI antidepressant Zoloft™. She basically wondered if that was a good idea. I showed her the book *Prozac Backlash* (2000) by Joseph Glenmullen, M.D., indicating that both Prozac™ and Zoloft™ are known to produce an approximate 50% decrease in dopamine levels, which has long been associated with the loss of motor control. Zoloft™ would obviously worsen Parkinson's disease symptoms, as a dopamine deficiency is normally the underlying problem behind the disease. I asked her if her husband might also be on blood pressure medication, and she indicated that he was. I suggested that she check with her husband's doctor to determine if his Parkinson's-like symptoms might possibly be a side effect of his blood pressure medication.

Dr. West further confirmed this, as he indicated that blood pressure medication could sometimes be the underlying cause of what appears to be Parkinson's disease. He cited a particular case regarding a new patient who was diagnosed with Parkinson's disease 10 years prior, and was taking medication for Parkinson's. He discovered it was just the symptoms from her blood pressure medication. By phasing out her blood pressure medication, the symptoms resolved, and she was able to discontinue her Parkinson's medication also.

In my opinion, many people's poor health is to a large degree due to their medications, and the more medications a person is taking, the worse their health is likely to be. Although poor dietary habits are also a concern, unnecessarily overloading the body with chemicals is an even greater concern. If we then combine the two (a poor diet and unnecessary medications), we now have a prescription for poor health, and a greatly increased risk of eventually contracting one or more major diseases.

Considering that drug toxicity damages the immune system and central nervous system, it should come as no surprise that **many powerful drugs are also the main contributor to CFS and FM. Complete immune system damage or dysfunction is a common cause of CFS and FM, and with today's drugs and steroids, immune system damage occurs more and more often.** According to an article in *CURES Vol. 1 - A Special Report from Health Alert*, titled *"Chronic Fatigue Syndrome and Fibromyalgia"* (2003, p. 53): *"It is no longer unusual for kids to have ten or more series of antibiotics before they are two years old. This takes its toll not only in childhood but in later years too. They are typically in a weakened and achy state."*

By unnecessarily overloading the body with drugs, we are basically reducing the liver's ability to effectively remove other toxins from normal metabolism, food additives, and the many environmental toxins we are all exposed to. This resultant buildup of toxins is a major contributor to all disease, but especially cancer. This extremely critical issue absolutely must be addressed and effectively resolved, and the longer we procrastinate, the more lives will be needlessly lost.

A Closer Look At Some Critical Issues

It was stated in the book *Constant Craving* (Doreen Virtue, 1995) that ***"We are not meant to live our lives dependent upon prescription medication"*** (pp. 108-109), and I whole-heartedly agree with that observation. I believe that very few people would continue taking drugs if they were fully aware of the potential damage that could result from their use. Most importantly, there is normally a much better natural solution for any underlying problem, and the use of prescription and over-the-counter medications is seldom (if ever) necessary. Drugs basically place an added burden on the liver, and just how extensive the damage they can potentially create (especially in combination) might be very difficult to accurately predict. Drugs are actually chemicals (or toxins) that the liver does everything within its power to eliminate, which has been proven. I personally consider them as poisons that I would never expose my body to. I have too much respect for my body to subject it to that kind of abuse.

You will find that natural supplements normally have multiple benefits throughout the body, which is especially true of all vitamins, minerals, and herbs. I personally am not aware of any condition that can't be more effectively resolved without the use of potentially dangerous drugs. Our body is organic, and anything that can truly help us resolve a particular health issue will be also. Drugs are patentable and thus very profitable, but basically foreign to our body, which is the very reason behind their associated side effects, and why the liver attempts to eliminate them.

While evaluating the many benefits of natural supplements is quite uplifting and very encouraging, just the opposite is true regarding the prescription drugs that far too many people today unknowingly depend upon. There is a very large textbook called the *Physicians' Desk Reference* (PDR), which lists prescription drugs, their potential side effects, and their many interactions with other drugs (and occasionally even some foods or natural supplements). I happen to own the 35th edition, published in 2001. It contains over 3,500 large pages of very fine print which few doctors have the time to read. It is rather scary reading, when you consider that for any particular symptom a drug might be attempting to suppress, many of these drugs can potentially create an extensive list of side effects (some extremely serious). As we will discuss later, they also deplete many vitamins and minerals critical to our health. The question we must seriously ask ourselves is: Are they really worth the potential danger they pose?

Just one prime example is the SSRI antidepressant, Prozac™ (which we will be discussing further). Dr. Ann Blake Tracy states in her book *Prozac – Panacea or Pandora?* (1991/1994), ***"Although Prozac was reported to have fewer side effects than most anti-depressants, and this was the basis for the aggressive marketing that has pushed Prozac to the top of the charts, <u>the FDA lists approximately 575 side effects</u>"*** (p. 54). If anything would be depressing, wondering which ones you might be forced to deal with in the future would unquestionably be.

The MAO Inhibitors, another class of antidepressants (also discussed later in this book), is another prime example. There is a very extensive list of contra-indications (things you must avoid) when using the drug. You would basically be forced to eliminate most of the foods your body needs to produce healthy cells and important enzymes, as well as the critical neurotransmitters. By using these potentially dangerous drugs, you are basically borrowing from the future, and some day the debt must be paid, and with interest.

If you are still not convinced that you should consider phasing the drugs out of your life forever, I recommend you make a list of all the drugs you are currently taking, along with the manufacturer's name, to make them easier to locate in the PDR. Then go to your local library and look each one up. You might take along a magnifying glass, a pen, and a notepad, because you will likely discover a lot of fine print that can be a real eye opener. **You then need to find a good doctor, knowledgeable in nutrition,** to help you identify and resolve any basic underlying problems so each drug (one by one) can be safely eliminated, although the causes of and solutions to the majority of conditions most people experience are covered in considerable detail in this book. You will find that most of them you can resolve yourself, if you so choose. Your liver will be eternally grateful for lightening its load, as it is fully aware that these drugs are considered toxins, and consequently it does its very best to eliminate them.

One major concern regarding medications is that some can be lethal if you receive an overdose. Even an overdose of the pain medication Tylenol™, which is sold over-the-counter and even included in many cold remedies, can lead to liver failure. Seldom, if ever, will two different people, prescribed the very same drug at the exact same dosage, actually receive the same effective dosage.

The Many Contributors To Drug Overdose – Can They Be Prevented?

A few years ago, I attended a lecture in Seattle by the doctor who was conducting genetic research for a pharmaceutical company. He indicated that they were looking at the reason behind fast and slow metabolizers. Scientists sometimes tend to complicate relatively simple issues. Normally, scientists spend years of research, along with a tremendous amount of money, in an attempt to resolve something, when the solution should be obvious. A prime example is the microchip, produced by the pharmaceutical giant Roche Molecular Systems, called Ampli chip 450. Its primary objective is to evaluate a person's rate of metabolism. Your metabolism actually has a considerable bearing on just how much of your medications can actually get around your defense mechanism, the P450 enzyme in your liver. The simple truth is, it depends upon several factors that can easily be identified without researching your DNA and looking at the two genes, 2D6 and 2C9 they are focusing on.

As you will soon discover, there is considerably more to the concern regarding the potential for a drug overdose. A primary goal of the drug companies is likely to avoid being required to withdraw a profitable drug from the market, due to serious reactions, often the result of an unanticipated overdose. This would also increase the potential for litigation (law suits) filed for serious medical problems, (or sometimes even death), which actually happens more often than most people realize.

Unfortunately, There Are Many Unpredictable Variables

We will now attempt to identify several factors that can easily influence the level or active dose of your medications you will actually be getting. As with drugs in general, this particular issue is far from an exact science. Several factors determine exactly how much of your medications will be able to get around your best defense (your liver). Your body considers any inorganic substance as a chemical toxin, which absolutely must be eliminated. With that in mind, **it greatly depends on just how many toxins your liver might be exposed to on any particular day, and how efficient it might be in eliminating them.** The fast or slow metabolism they are dependant on, although an important issue, is actually determined by the efficiency of your thyroid function, which should be the primary focus. Unfortunately, there just happens to be a conflict of interest in that respect.

1. Where the conflict of interest comes into play, is in regard to the very common **hypothyroid condition** that results in reduced metabolism, increasing the risk for a drug overdose. The pharmaceutical industry makes sure, by its influence on your doctor's training, that the condition will seldom be identified, due to the standard protocol that most doctors are trained to follow. The standard blood test for TSH (and sometimes T_4 thyroid) will seldom detect the true problem. If the doctor still suspects a thyroid deficiency, the artificial T_4 (Synthroid™) that most doctors insist on prescribing, will seldom resolve the true problem (that of a T_3 thyroid deficiency).

In the majority of cases, only an inexpensive form of the natural thyroid, called Armour™ thyroid, will be effective. If unresolved, you can potentially suffer from thirty or more symptoms due to the reduced metabolism, and consequentially the suppression of all 3,000 enzymes in the body. Many of the very profitable antidepressants such as Prozac™ are prescribed for a one common condition associated with a hypothyroid condition (depression). Fatigue and fluid retention are also typical symptoms. For years, elevated cholesterol had been considered an indication that you were hypothyroid, and once resolved, the cholesterol level would usually normalize. Fibroid tumors are also the result of reduced metabolism (one common cause of the many unnecessary hysterectomy surgeries preformed). I could easily go on, but I believe you get the point. The objective is to promote the sale of as many profitable drugs as possible. Thus by choosing to ignore, or improperly treat a common thyroid condition, it creates a huge market for billions of dollars worth of drugs to treat the hypothyroid symptoms, (and billions of dollars is definitely not an exaggeration), and that amount could easily apply to just the cholesterol lowering medications alone. And of course in traditional medicine, any natural solution for resolving a condition is basically off limits, and not to be even considered.

And then, as the thyroid pioneer Dr. Broda Barnes discovered over forty years ago, **when he gave his diabetic patients Armour™ thyroid, <u>their diabetes symptoms resolved</u> (an amazing discovery)!** Even though we just scratched the surface on the typical hypothyroid symptoms that could, as you can see, be easily resolved, we can't help but recognize the tremendous financial potential for very profitable antidepressants and cholesterol medications, as well as medications for diabetes and fluid retention. Each medication then results in side effects and the depletion of valuable nutrients, which as we have seen, just leads to more medications. And we can't forget the unnecessary surgeries for tumors on the ovaries, or in the breast, which are very common for women with the undiagnosed thyroid condition.

The people behind this obvious profit-motivated conspiracy to get you on as many of their overly inflated drugs as possible, are actually not stupid. Although I'm sure they are very aware of the true solution for resolving the thyroid condition, unfortunately that's something you will likely never hear of from them. Neither will your doctor be alerted by the drug representatives, regarding any of the serious side effects associated with their drugs.

2. In addition to the metabolism, **a person's age and gender also come into play.** Women's livers for instance, are not as efficient as men's. And as we age, our liver function gradually becomes less effective. Also, as people age they tend to forget if they took their medication, and they could as a result take one or more drugs more often than recommended. The elderly are the most likely to have a lower-than-normal metabolism, and also be on more medications than others (a bad combination).

3. A person's size is also a factor that should obviously be considered. Just as a smaller person requires less food, the same would apply to drugs. Many older people tend to be smaller, unless they are overweight.

4. Then there is the issue regarding **the <u>number</u> of drugs you might be taking, as well as the prescribed dosage of each,** which would also come into play. For instance, you will learn in "Al's Story" that he was initially placed on 20 mg of Zocor™, but eventually ended up on 80 mg (four times the original dosage). Any time another drug is added, or a drug's dosage is increased, the risk for overdose would obviously increase, (more work for your liver). Our liver performs over 500 vital functions, thus unnecessarily adding to its burden is definitely not a good idea.

5. Grapefruit juice is a concern that few are aware of. Drugs, be they legal or illegal, prescription or over-the-counter, are basically chemicals foreign to the body, and thus treated as the toxins they are by the liver. The liver will not attempt to eliminate anything beneficial to the body, (that is not its function). We now have absolute proof that this is true, and in the Spring 2003 issue of the *Consumer's Guide to Health*, Dr. Stephen Sinatra, M.D. helps explain how a common citrus fruit helps prove it's not just a theory. According to Dr. Sinatra, it has now been confirmed that **grapefruit can actually multiply the effect of certain drugs up to ten times.** Grapefruit juice suppresses an enzyme in the liver that metabolizes these drugs, and without the P450 enzyme system, the drugs accumulate in our body at high, toxic levels, and the effects can last up to 24 hours.

Just a few of the dozens of drugs that grapefruit affects include:

* **Anti-anxiety drugs**
* **Viagra™**
* **Statin cholesterol-lowering drugs**

* **Calcium channel blockers**
* **Blood thinners, such as Warfarin**
* **SSRI antidepressants**

Women taking Hormone Replacement Therapy are also especially at risk, as **grapefruit juice increases the amount of estrogen available to your cells. This may result in acute estrogen imbalance**, causing all the side effects of elevated estrogen to be more potent, possibly even increasing your risk of breast cancer. Elevated estrogen also suppresses the thyroid function, thus reducing the metabolism.

Be cautious of grapefruit seed extract, too. Definitely don't risk ingesting grapefruit juice, the raw fruit, or even the extract if you are taking ANY prescription drug. This is very convincing evidence that our liver is totally aware that these prescription drugs are basically toxins that must be eliminated. The best solution is to not subject our liver to these potentially dangerous toxins in the first place. Incidentally, **that very same P450 enzyme suppressed by grapefruit, is also responsible for detoxifying alcohol!**

6. Some drugs also place a greater burden on the liver than others. That is especially true regarding the SSRI antidepressants such as Prozac™, Paxil™, Zoloft™, etc., as they are highly protein-binding, and thus extremely difficult for the liver to detoxify. A good example of the problem is reflected in their influence on the body's ability to detoxify alcohol (the same P450 enzyme is responsible for detoxifying both). That certainly should be telling us something. As Dr. Ann Blake Tracy tells us, drinking just one drink of alcohol while also taking Prozac™ is like drinking ten drinks, and with Paxil™ it is even worse. So we can easily see the major influence that combining these antidepressants with other medications would have on the effective dosage you might be getting. Over-the-counter medications such as cold or pain medications are also toxic chemicals, and thus compete to get around your liver as well.

7. If you also drank **alcohol**, that would just compound the problem even more. And, anyone who has the **Candida yeast infection**, (actually quite common), is producing alcohol, along with a very toxic metabolite in their intestine called acetaldehyde, from sugar in its various forms.

8. Even **the food you have just eaten** (especially processed foods with preservatives), or **the environmental toxins** we are all exposed to daily, will increase your liver's load.

The drug companies are currently facing a real dilemma, as more and more people are experiencing serious reactions to their medications. The problem stems from the aggressive promotion of drugs to both the doctors and the general public. As people are being placed on more medications, their risk of overdose dramatically increases.

In spite of the tremendous expense involved in the development of DNA technology, such as the Ampli chip 450, in an attempt to evaluate a person's metabolism, (which could vary daily), it still falls far short of truly resolving the real issue. Our metabolism depends upon many different factors, which can influence either the thyroid or the liver, as both are involved in regulating the metabolism. So as you can see, just one single factor is far from adequate to accurately predict anyone's overall potential for a drug overdose.

If you consider the many different variables that are impossible to predict or control, and thus accurately evaluate, there appears to be only one safe, yet effective solution. Just remember, **the healthiest, longest living people in the world never use drugs**, (legal, illegal, prescription, or over-the-counter). They are all considered as toxins by the body, and something we obviously can do without.

CHAPTER FIVE
THE AGGRESSIVE MARKETING OF CHOLESTEROL-LOWERING DRUGS

Statin drugs are a class of drugs widely prescribed for lowering high blood cholesterol, claiming they reduce the risk for heart disease. Unfortunately, they instead deplete a very important coenzyme known as CoQ_{10}, and as you will soon discover, their influence is not just localized, but actually very extensive. The most obvious concern is the major cardiovascular risk factors they are known to produce, rather than resolve.

Regardless of their tremendous risk, it seems as though approximately half the people I talk to these days are either taking these statin drugs, or their doctor has suggested they begin doing so, or recommended doubling their dosage. The aggressive promotional campaigns seem to be working, and it could quite easily result in a potential disaster for those who are being taken in. An article from *The New York Times*, published in the *Eugene Register Guard,* July 20, 2004, sheds light on the issue, as follows:

> *Among cardiologists, it has become a running joke: Maybe the powerful drugs known as statins should be added to the water supply.*
>
> *"I'm pro-statin, but I don't want to go beyond what the evidence says," said Dr. Beatrice Golomb, an associate professor at the University of California, San Diego, and the principal investigator of a large federally financed study of the effect of statin use in cognition, mental state and other noncardiac processes.*
>
> *"There's a multibillion-dollar industry ensuring that you hear all the good things, but no corresponding interest group ensuring that you hear the other side,"* Golomb said.
>
> *One statin, Bayer's Baycol,* was removed from the market in 2001 after reports that *31 people taking it had died from rhabdomyolysis, a disorder involving muscle-tissue breakdown that can lead to kidney failure.*
>
> *Another statin, Crestor, has come under attack by Public Citizen, a Washington consumer group.*
>
> *In a letter published in April in The Lancet, Dr. Sidney Wolfe, director of Public Citizen's health research group, asserted that Crestor had caused 18 cases of severe muscle deterioration and a dozen cases of kidney damage since it went on the market. The organization has petitioned the Food and Drug Administration to ban Crestor.*
>
> *"The renal toxicity, high rate of cases of rhabdomyolysis compared with other statins, and lack of unique benefit are compelling reasons to remove rosuvastatin (Crestor) from the market before additional patients are injured or killed,"* Wolfe wrote.

Interestingly, the study was federally financed (paid for by the tax payers), and the doctor selected to conduct the study just happened to be, by her own admission, *"pro statin".*

In spite of the preponderance of evidence just noted, if you just watch the evening news, you likely have seen several commercials promoting the statin drug, Crestor™. The main character in the plot of an older commercial was told by his doctor that he should start taking Crestor™, which of course he promptly does. He then goes joyfully and enthusiastically walking through *"the land of success,"* which appears to be an upscale neighborhood, spreading the word. You get the impression that your life will somehow begin to improve once you begin taking Crestor™. Even though it appears that they are obviously insulting our intelligence, apparently it actually worked. According to Gary Bruell, a spokesman for the drug manufacturer AstraZeneca, *"We've not seen anything to indicate that the safety profile is any different from the other marketed statins."* As you noticed, he didn't say it was proven safe. Crestor™ just happens to produce the same basic problems that other statin drugs do, although at an accelerated rate, so you won't have to wait so long to discover that taking the drug was a big mistake.

Continued from the article previously referred to, in the *New York Times*:

> *AstraZeneca, Crestor's maker, says that the drug is safe and dismisses the accusations made by Public Citizen as groundless.*
>
> *Golomb said she has been documenting cases of adverse events associated with statin use.*
>
> *Golomb said, the problems resolved after the patients stopped the statin and came back if they went back on the drug or took another statin.*
>
> *One participant in Golomb's study, Jane Brunzie, 66, of Vista, Calif., said she began having frequent "senior moments" while on a regimen of 30 milligrams of Lipitor.*
>
> *"I was constantly struggling to remember a person, a place, an event, a word," Brunzie said.* **"I'd get lost driving to familiar places. It got so bad I couldn't carry on a normal conversation. But my doctor wanted to raise my Lipitor because my cholesterol was still high."**
>
> *At her son's prompting, Brunzie said, she stopped the medication several months ago and the problem cleared up within a week.*

The following excerpt from an article titled "Therapeutic-Class Wars—Drug Promotion in a Competitive Marketplace", was published in the *New England Journal of Medicine* (1994 November 17, Vol. 331, pp. 1350-1353), written by former FDA commissioner Dr. David A. Kessler, Janet L. Rose, Robert J. Temple, Renie Schapiro, and Joseph P. Griffen:

> *Pharmaceutical companies are waging aggressive campaigns to change prescribers' habits and to distinguish their products from competing ones, even when products are virtually indistinguishable. Victory in these therapeutic-class wars can mean millions [billions today] of dollars for a drug company. But* **for patients and providers it can mean <u>misleading promotions, conflicts of interest, increased costs for health care,</u> and ultimately, <u>inappropriate prescribing.</u>**

In October 2003, Dr. Richard Horton, editor of the *Lancet*, published a scathing critique of Crestor's marketing, stating that the manufacturer's tactics *"raise disturbing questions about how drugs enter clinical practice and what measures exist to protect patients from inadequately investigated medicines."*

Even though the FDA has repeatedly cautioned doctors about using new drugs when older, better-known drugs are available, the onslaught of drug reps and intensive advertising pushing Crestor™ worked. *The Wall Street Journal* reported that **by early 2004, 27 percent of all new prescriptions for statin drugs were for Crestor™.**

AstraZeneca sales force (Crestor™) was making more calls to doctors than any of its competitors. Beginning in late February 2004, reflecting the sales calls, new prescriptions of Crestor™ began to rise and overtook Lipitor™ by the beginning of March. Once again, <u>intensive marketing trumps medical science – and patient safety. Is this how we want our health care system to run?</u> The bottom line is to recognize that you should seek natural therapies that address the cause of the disease before choosing a drug-based solution – no matter what the dose.

Baycol™, another statin, was withdrawn because of dozens of deaths, and Crestor™ has already been linked to <u>numerous cases of severe muscle breakdown, kidney toxicity, and deaths.</u> Liver injury, liver toxicity, and death are also concerns with statins. Like other statin side effects, these reactions are dose-related: **the greater the dose, the greater the risk.** Dr. W. C. Roberts, the editor-in-chief of the ***American Journal of Cardiology*, warns: *"With each doubling of the [statin] dose, the frequency of liver enzyme elevations [indicating liver irritation or injury] also doubles."***

New guidelines, published in 2004 by the American College of Physicians, called for statin use by all people with diabetes older than 55 and for younger diabetes patients who have any other risk factor for heart disease, such as high blood pressure or a history of smoking (*JAMA*.2004; 291: 2419-2420.). **David A. Drachman, professor of neurology at the University of Massachusetts Medical School calls statins *"Viagra for the brain."* <u>The industry is also seeking the right to sell statins over the counter.</u>**

Can honest assessment find any possible use for these dangerous drugs? **Dr. Peter Langsjoen of Tyler, Texas, suggests that** statin drugs are appropriate only as a treatment for cases of advanced **<u>Cholesterol Neurosis</u>**, created by the industry's anti-cholesterol propaganda. **In other words: If you are concerned about your cholesterol, a statin drug will relieve you of your worries.**

Statin manufacturers pay big money for creative ways to create new users. For example, one health awareness group called the Boomer Coalition supported ABC's *Academy Awards* telecast in March of 2004 with a 30-second spot flashing nostalgic images of celebrities lost to cardiovascular disease, such as actor James Coburn, baseball star Don Drysdale and comedian Redd Foxx. **While the Boomer Coalition sounds like a grass roots group of health activists, it is actually a creation of Pfizer, manufacturers of Lipitor™. *"We're always looking for creative ways to break through what we've found to be a lack of awareness and action,"* says Michael Fishman, a Pfizer spokeswoman. *"We're always looking for what people really think and what's going to make people take action,"* adding that there is a stigma about seeking treatment and many people *"wrongly assume that if they are physically fit, they aren't at risk for heart disease."* The Boomer Coalition Web site allows visitors to *"sign up and take responsibility for your heart health,"*** by providing a user name, age, e-mail address and blood pressure and cholesterol level. This is obviously just one more marketing strategy. I agree that people should take responsibility for their own health, but avoiding drugs is the best way to accomplish that goal.

Today, very few mature adults in the nation are totally drug-free, and the majority of adults are actually on multiple drugs, and now you can easily see why. The domino effect that results, and the standard treatment of ***"drugs for everything, and nothing but drugs for anything"*** often noted by Dr. Bruce West, has become an epidemic in this nation. Quite obviously, the statin drugs are a major contributor to the problem as they actually create the very conditions they profess to resolve. This is a problem that, in my opinion and that of many others, never really existed in the first place. As noted previously, just as many people who experience heart attacks and strokes have either low or normal cholesterol levels, as those whose cholesterol levels are elevated. After evaluating the facts, it should be quite obvious that the statin drugs are not the solution, but instead contributors to multiple underlying cardiovascular problems.

I find it quite interesting how the acceptable level of cholesterol has somehow dropped from 340 down to 200 (a major difference). It has also been implied that 150 might be considered even more appropriate (less than one half the original level of 340). A perfectly effective tactic to drastically broaden the market for what appears to be one of the most profitable, although potentially dangerous drugs on the market.

Another approach to expand sales was regarding **a woman doctor** who stated on the national news that women also have cardiovascular concerns that have been ignored far too long. She stressed that many women should also be taking statin drugs. I can't help but wonder how much she was paid to make such a statement, and by whom. I also noticed that following her statement more commercials began targeting women, although in the past they were focusing almost entirely on men. I am sure the fact that a woman doctor was somehow chosen to express her concern regarding women being overlooked, did not just happen by accident. The statement would obviously appear to be much more credible coming from another woman who was also a doctor (and thus must be an authority).

One can't help but notice how drug companies somehow manage to use the news media in order to promote their products in many devious ways. What appeared at the time to be the worst example of all, was a news release on the national news stating that it was discovered that anyone who is overweight or has diabetes should be taking the statin drugs, **regardless of their cholesterol level.** I believe we could easily guess where that conclusion likely came from, and the tremendous potential for opening up a whole new market. People are being continually prescribed potentially dangerous drugs for minor problems that the drugs were never approved for, such as lowering cholesterol **irrespective of the level.**

Then, just when it appeared that the promotion of statin drugs had been pushed to the very limit, along came an even more blatant attempt to do so. The following was announced by the *Associated Press* (July 13, 2004), and on the *ABC National News*:

HEART PATIENTS URGED TO SLASH CHOLESTEROL
Heart Patients Should Lower 'Bad' Cholesterol to Rock-Bottom Levels, According to New Guidelines

The Associated Press
DALLAS July 13, 2004 – Health officials are issuing a stern message to people who have recently had a heart attack: Lower your "bad cholesterol" to rock-bottom levels.
"The concept here is that lower is better with respect to cholesterol," said Dr. Steven Nissen, cardiologist at the Cleveland Clinic, who is among those who have studied the issue. "It'll be hard to get there, but we do have aggressive drugs."
New guidelines issued Monday for very high-risk heart patients call for lowering their so-called bad cholesterol, LDL, to 70. The previous guideline was 100.
Heart patients in need of drastic measures can use statin drugs including Lipitor in higher doses or combine statins, which block formation of cholesterol, with drugs that block cholesterol's uptake by the body.
Created by the National Cholesterol Education Program, the guidelines are endorsed by the American Heart Association, the American College of Cardiology and the National Heart, Lung, and Blood Institute. *A panel of the education program examined five major studies involving cholesterol-lowering medicines.*
*Dr. Scott Grundy, lead author of the guidelines, said that **as of 2001 there were about 36 million people who could benefit from drugs to lower their cholesterol. He said that it's hard to put a number on it, but the new guidelines could increase that number by "a few million"** (www.ABCNEWS.com).*

And not surprising, the following was then found in a special report from the *McAlvany Health Alert* (July 29, 2004):

"Panelists' Links to Pharmaceutical Companies Not Disclosed"
(Experts who authored new cholesterol guidelines closely tied to makers of statin drugs)

Experts on a panel for the National Cholesterol Education Program in mid-July called for the aggressive and increased use of statin medications to treat high cholesterol. However, the recent guidelines published by the panel did not list the panelists' links to drug manufacturers of statin drugs.
According to Dr. James Cleeman, the coordinator of National Cholesterol Education Program, a division of the National Heart, Lung and Blood Institute, called the

*initial omission an oversight and reassured the public that the panelists' relationships with the drug companies would be posted on the National Heart, Lung and Blood Institute's website within days. **Six out of a total of nine panelists were linked to companies that produce some of the most popular statin medications. These six panelists received grants from the pharmaceutical companies or fees for speaking or consulting.***

One of the authors, Dr. H. Bryan Brewer was recently the subject of a letter to the director of the National Institutes of health because he failed to disclose his ties to the pharmaceutical company AstraZeneca, the producer of the statin medication Crestor. Brewer authored a report in a medical journal that praised Crestor without disclosing the fact that he is a paid consultant for AstraZeneca. Dr. Sidney Wolfe wrote the letter because he feels that the public needs to be made aware of ethical conflicts of interest such as this one [Newsday.com].

As was noted in the article quoted from *Life Extension* magazine, which we previously referred to, the generic ingredients in the common cholesterol prescription drug Zocor™, costs only $8.63 to produce 100 tablets, although the cost to the consumer is actually $350.27. That is a markup of 4,059%, and a profit of $341.64! It appears that legal drugs are even more profitable than illegal drugs, and with total immunity of prosecution. We can easily see the extreme profit potential from just one class of drugs (and there are many), especially if they somehow reach their goal of 36 million (or even a few million more) as noted, since following the new guidelines. If you then consider the recommended *"drastic measures"* of using *"higher dosages or combining statins,"* and then selling them at an exorbitant profit (the sky is the limit), then guess who will be paying the tab? You likely guessed it! You and I will, either directly or indirectly. Yet, we can't forget the most critical concern of all: The proven potential danger associated with these drugs that are being so aggressively promoted, and especially at the higher recommended doses.

In summary, we learned that the statin drugs are a very profitable class of drugs, and are currently being more aggressively marketed than any other drug ever in history. Companies producing these drugs are even successful in eliciting the assistance of some federally funded agencies in convincing the public that lowering cholesterol is somehow a major national concern. This nation-wide campaign continues to escalate in spite of substantial evidence more than 30 years ago by Dr. Kilmer McCulley, M.D., that homocysteine (not cholesterol) is and always has been the major cardiovascular threat.

Because vitamins provide the only effective solution to controlling homocysteine, few people have ever heard of the real concern elevated homocysteine, or that a simple solution exists. For example, most women are also totally unaware that their birth control pills also produced by the pharmaceutical industry, actually deplete 23 important nutrients, including those necessary for controlling their homocysteine levels. Few people ever hear of health concerns that can be effectively resolved with vitamins. That is not where the real profits are, and better health would just reduce the demand for profitable drugs. Healthy people seldom go to a doctor, as that is where all the prescriptions for drugs originate.

The obvious question is: Do we really need these potentially dangerous drugs in order to maintain healthy cholesterol levels? The answer is ABSOLUTELY NOT!

CHAPTER SIX
THE IMPORTANCE OF CHOLESTEROL

Cholesterol is not actually the proverbial enemy we are led to believe, by the very industry that benefits from the tremendous profits they provide, or the statements made by the doctors on their payroll. Cholesterol actually has many uses in both the body and brain. We get only 20% of our cholesterol from the diet, and the liver produces the other 80% as the need arises. Cholesterol is necessary for producing many important hormones, as well as the bile salts in the liver. In my opinion, the low-density lipoprotein (LDL) cholesterol, considered the bad guy, actually got a bum wrap. A good analogy is a person with blood on their hands at the scene of a crime attempting to save someone's life but blamed for the crime if the person dies. Whenever there is a damaged or weakened artery wall, the potential for internal hemorrhage exists, as we could easily lose blood through a lesion in the artery wall. The LDL cholesterol then comes to the rescue and temporarily seals the artery walls reducing the potential for leakage of the vascular wall. When it is found at the scene of the crime, (the damaged arterial wall), it is automatically blamed for reducing the flow of blood, which is actually much less serious than the internal hemorrhaging that might have occurred. If and when the damage is finally dealt with, the high-density lipoprotein (HDL) cholesterol (known as the good guy) will then proceed to remove the LDL cholesterol. They are basically a team, and both have important functions.

Another function of LDL cholesterol is that of stabilizing cell membranes in the brain caused by excessive levels of alcohol. The cell membrane is made of fats, and alcohol is a solvent that destabilizes the membrane. For that very reason, when drinking excessively a person has difficulty with coherent speech and mobility. Once the membranes in the brain cells are destabilized, the cells can't effectively communicate with each other, as the cell receptors are basically unstable and out of alignment. Then comes the emergency crew, the LDL cholesterol, to hold up and stabilize the cell walls until the problem can be permanently resolved.

Another important function of cholesterol is that of sealing the cell walls to help retain water when we become dehydrated. Once the body is properly hydrated (we start drinking more water) the cholesterol is then removed.

So, as you can see, cholesterol is a valuable resource and has many important functions throughout both the body and brain.

Some important issues regarding cholesterol:

1. Approximately eighty percent of our cholesterol is actually produced by our liver, **based on the body's need**, and the remaining 20% comes from our diet.
2. **Cholesterol is in reality a noble substance, and our best friend rather than our worst enemy,** as some deliberately make it out to be.
3. **Cholesterol is necessary for producing the many different hormones that we all depend upon**.
4. Our brain contains a great deal of cholesterol, and according to Dr. Bruce West, **too low of a cholesterol level can result in dementia. He also indicated that in his opinion, 150 is definitely too low.**

So, you can stop stressing about your cholesterol! If a person's blood were tested for cholesterol when the liver was attempting to meet a potential emergency, it would obviously show up on a blood test as elevated, although it could easily fluctuate not only daily, but hourly. Our cholesterol level is thus not something we should normally concern ourselves with. In fact, just stressing about your cholesterol just before having it tested could easily raise your cholesterol levels.

Let's take just a minute and see if we can possibly find an explanation for why cholesterol seems to be found in the arteries, but not the veins. The same cholesterol that flows through the arteries also flows through the veins. So, the 64,000-dollar question is: Why does it accumulate in the artery wall and not the veins? Although I have never heard a valid explanation discussed by any doctor to date, I believe there might be a logical explanation.

As you learned, cholesterol is basically a sealant that seals potential leaks in weakened or damaged arteries. Although there is considerable pressure on the **arteries** when the heart is attempting to pump the blood throughout the body and brain, this is not the case with the veins. A good analogy would be a garden hose. Suppose we attach one end of the garden hose to a water supply under pressure (a hose bib) and turn the water on, and we just happen to have a small hole in the hose. If there were no restriction at the end of the hose (basically little or no pressure), the hole would normally go undetected. If a nozzle was placed at the end of the hose, the pressure in the hose would increase and the leak would become obvious. We can easily see why, although a sealant such as cholesterol would be a valuable resource in the arteries, it would be normally of little use in the veins, where it is not usually found.

We should be addressing the basic underlying problem: The weakened artery walls. Just some basic supplements (such as vitamin A, a good B-vitamin complex, vitamin C with bioflavonoids, and the minerals copper and zinc), can build healthy epitheal (smooth muscle) cells and strengthen the artery walls. This would also help prevent an aneurysm in the brain, as well as prevent the real cardiovascular threat (homocysteine) in the process. Prevention is so much easier than attempting to deal with a condition that has continued to progress due to a nutritional deficiency.

Absolute Proof That
Low Cholesterol Can Be More Dangerous Than Elevated Cholesterol

It should be pointed out that a reduction of cholesterol itself could actually be dangerous. Dr. Uffe Ravnskov, M.D., Ph.D., a Danish physician and author of *The Cholesterol Myths*, in an attempt to prove that lowering cholesterol in healthy but high-risk people would reduce their death rate from heart disease, states that *"The reduced rates of cardiovascular mortality were small for men and non-existent for women,"* thus proving the theory that cholesterol in our food and in our blood causes heart disease is false. In one study of elderly French women living in a nursing home, it was shown that **those with the highest cholesterol levels lived the longest** (*The Lancet*, 4/22/89). <u>**The death rate was more than five times higher for women with very low cholesterol,**</u> **and several other studies have shown similar results.** Another finding by Dr. Ravnskov is that **high cholesterol is a protective agent against cancer. Several studies have found <u>higher cancer rates in people with low cholesterol,</u>** and in one study *"there were 12 cases of breast cancer in the women taking Pravachol, compared with only one case in the untreated (control) group"*(http://www.medicalconsumers.org/page/cholesterol_skeptics.html).

The following was reported by the According to the American College of Cardiology, (http://www.chfpatients.com/heartbytes.htm#eecp_contraindications), and Dr. Mary Pickett, as follows:

December 9, 2003 - *In a study of 417 patients with chronic CHF, higher cholesterol level was linked to better survival. On average, patients with a total cholesterol level of 232 mg/dl had a 25% higher survival rate than CHFers with total cholesterol of 193 mg/dl.* ***These results agree with one earlier study that linked lower cholesterol to worse outcome in CHFers.***

This was a 2-stage study. The first stage studied the link between cholesterol level and mortality in 114 chronic CHFers treated at a CHF clinic. The link between lower cholesterol and higher mortality was then verified in a second group of 303 CHFers who had their cholesterol levels measured as part of their regular care.

Heart failure is complex. The body senses danger when the heart starts failing. The body's metabolism shifts gears completely. Hormone levels change drastically and nutrients have a different effect. Since cholesterol is the body's way of packaging and delivering fats throughout the body, low cholesterol levels may be one sign that the body has "canceled" normal operations and is reacting to a "state of emergency."

In his *Let's Talk Health* newsletter (June/July 2004), Dr. Kurt W. Donsbach, D.C., N.D., Ph.D., lists his opinions:

1. **More than half of the individuals who have coronary bypass surgery have normal or below normal cholesterol.**
2. *The immediate cause of arterial obstruction is clots, and* **cholesterol has nothing to do with clots.** *Remember* **that the same cholesterol that flows through arteries also flows through veins and much more slowly, but never causes a plaque!**
3. *Many repeat studies of any and all the statin drugs always have the same outcome –* **statin drugs lower cholesterol but do nothing to reduce mortality rates from heart disease.**
4. **Statin drugs cause serious side effects, including but not limited to: liver failure, chronic pain, global amnesia, mental function abnormalities, etc.**

Incidentally, if you are interested, the most significant cause of high blood fats is a high intake of sugar (p. 3).

And, regarding statin drugs, and the importance of cholesterol, the following article by Sally Fallon and Mary G. Enig, Ph.D., was originally posted on The Weston A Price Website (http://www.westonaprice.org/moderndiseases/statin.html):

The Dangers of Statin Drugs:
What You Haven't Been Told About Cholesterol-Lowering Medication

Hypercholesterolemia is the health issue of the 21st century. It is actually an invented disease, a "problem" that emerged when health professionals learned how to measure cholesterol levels in the blood.

Many people who feel perfectly healthy suffer from high cholesterol--in fact, feeling good is actually a symptom of high cholesterol!

Every cell membrane in our body contains cholesterol because cholesterol is what makes our cells waterproof--without cholesterol we could not have a different biochemistry on the inside and the outside of the cell.

Cholesterol is the body's repair substance.

Cholesterol is the precursor to vitamin D, necessary for numerous biochemical processes including mineral metabolism. The bile salts, required for the digestion of fat, are made of cholesterol. **Those who suffer from low cholesterol often have trouble digesting fats. Cholesterol also functions as a powerful antioxidant, thus protecting us against cancer and aging.**

Cholesterol is vital to proper neurological function. It plays a key role in the formation of memory and the uptake of hormones in the brain, including serotonin,

the body's feel-good chemical. *When cholesterol levels drop too low, the serotonin receptors cannot work.* **Cholesterol is the main organic molecule in the brain,** *constituting over half the dry weight of the cerebral cortex.*

Cholesterol regulates blood sugar levels, regulates mineral balance, and promotes healing. *The adrenal cortex also produces sex hormones, including testosterone, estrogen and progesterone,* **out of cholesterol.**

Dr. Beatrice Golomb of San Diego, California found that <u>98 percent of patients taking Lipitor</u> *and one-third of the patients taking Mevachor (a lower-dose statin)* <u>suffered from muscle problems</u>.

The Lipitor board at **www.rxlist.com** *contains more than 2,600 posts.* [Following are just a few]:

Tahoe City resident Doug Peterson developed slurred speech, balance problems and severe fatigue after three years on Lipitor. It took him five minutes to write four words, much of which was illegible. Cognitive function also declined. It was hard to convince his doctors that Lipitor could be the culprit, but when he finally stopped taking it, his coordination and memory improved.

Ed Ontiveros began having muscle problems within 30 days of taking Lipitor. He fell in the bathroom and had trouble getting up. The weakness subsided when he went off Lipitor.

Anyone suffering from myopathy, fibromyalgia, coordination problems and fatigue, needs to look at low cholesterol plus Co-Q$_{10}$ deficiency as a possible cause.

The damage is often irreversible. People who take large doses for a long time may be left with permanent nerve damage, even after they stop taking the drug.

Deaths attributed to heart failure more than doubled from 1989 to 1997. (Statins were first given pre-market approval in 1987.) Interference with production of Co-Q$_{10}$ by statin drugs is the most likely explanation. The heart is a muscle and it cannot work when deprived of Co-Q$_{10}$.

Without Co-Q$_{10}$, the cell's mitochondria are inhibited from producing energy, leading to muscle pain and weakness. The heart is especially susceptible because it uses so much energy.

Virtually all patients with heart failure are put on statin drugs, even if their cholesterol is already low. Of interest is a recent study indicating that <u>patients with chronic heart failure benefit from having high levels of cholesterol rather than low.</u>

Patients treated with statins for six months compared poorly with patients on a placebo in solving complex mazes, psychomotor skills and memory tests.

In one trial, the CARE trial, <u>breast cancer rates of those taking a statin went up 1500 percent.</u>

The medical literature contains several reports of pancreatitis in patients taking statins.

<u>*Numerous studies have linked low cholesterol with depression.*</u> *One of the most recent found that women with low cholesterol are twice as likely to suffer from depression and anxiety.*

Dr. Edward Suarez found that <u>**men who lower their cholesterol levels with medication have increased rates of suicide and violent death,**</u> *leading the researchers to theorize* **"that low cholesterol levels were causing mood disturbances."**

The True Risk Factor – Homocysteine

So as you have now learned, elevated cholesterol never has been a risk factor for heart disease, and never will be. More than 30 years ago, Dr. Kilmer S. McCulley, M.D. discovered it was instead homocysteine. A major cover-up occurred, as he was pressured not to publish his findings due to the tremendous profit potential of the statin (cholesterol lowering) drugs. He persisted and published his findings, which cost him his job and his funding. Unfortunately, the information was not acted upon, but was instead suppressed and the statin drugs are still being aggressively marketed today.

This is a prime example of what Dr. Paul Rosch, M.D. was referring to at a conference held in 2003 in Arlington, Virginia, when he indicated that half of all heart attacks occur in people with normal cholesterol levels, and stressed that: ***"Anyone who questions cholesterol usually finds his funding cut off"*** (http://www.medicalconsumers.org/page/cholesterol_skeptics.html). Fortunately, I am funding my own research.

Although the risk factor elevated homocysteine, can easily be controlled with adequate levels of the B vitamins folic acid, B_6 and B_{12} (explained later in the book), anything that can only be resolved with vitamins, but not drugs, is information that is purposely suppressed from the public. Unfortunately, many prescription medications and addictive substances deplete the very vitamins necessary for controlling your homocysteine levels. For instance:

✓ **Folic acid** – depleted by sulfa drugs, SSRI antidepressants, steroids and corticosteroids, smoking, NSAIDs (i.e. ibuprofen), mineral oil and laxatives, Histamine H_2 blockers (i.e. Tagamet™, Pepcid™, Zantac™), estrogen (and oral contraceptives), diabetic medication (especially Metformin), diuretics, decongestants (i.e. pseudoephedrine), caffeine, all cholesterol-lowering drugs, including statins and bile acid sequestrants (i.e. Questran™, Colestid™), aspirin, antiseizure medication (i.e. barbiturates), antibiotics, antacids, alcohol, food processing, heat and boiling, and physical and mental stress.

✓ **Vitamin B_6** – depleted by vasodilators (i.e. nitroglycerin), sulfa drugs, steroids and corticosteroids, smoking, sleeping pills, estrogen (and oral contraceptives), diuretics, diabetic medication, caffeine, asthma medications, antidepressants and MAO inhibitors, antibiotics, alcohol, sugar, heat (canning & roasting), and physical and mental stress. NOTE: Diuretics and cortisone also block the absorption of this vitamin.

✓ **Vitamin B_{12}** – depleted by sulfa drugs, SSRI antidepressants, smoking, sleeping pills, proton pump inhibitors (i.e. Nexium™), muscle relaxants, mineral oil and laxatives, Histamine H_2 blockers (i.e. Tagamet™, Pepcid™, Zantac™), estrogen (and oral contraceptives), diuretics, diabetic medications, all cholesterol-lowering drugs, including statins and bile acid sequestrants (i.e. Questran™, Colestid™), calcium deficiency, caffeine, antiseizure medication (i.e. barbiturates), amphetamines and diet pills, antibiotics, and alcohol. NOTE: Certain anti-gout medications, anticoagulant drugs (i.e. blood thinners such as Coumadin™), potassium supplements, medications for hypertension (high blood pressure) and Parkinson's disease, and excess cholesterol interfere with the absorption of this vitamin.

In the *Drug-Induced Nutrient Depletion Handbook, 2nd Edition* (2001/2001), **there were ninety-five different drugs listed that deplete folic acid, one hundred and eleven that depleted vitamin B_6 listed, and interestingly the same number that depleted vitamin B_{12}.** It is quite apparent that anyone taking prescription drugs could quite easily have a problem with elevated homocysteine. All three vitamins necessary for reducing homocysteine are co-factors that must all be present for proper methylation to take place. You can easily see why using prescription drugs could dramatically increase the potential for the true cardiovascular risk factor, elevated homocysteine.

Then regarding our other major concern, the depletion of the very important CoQ_{10}, caused by statin drugs, **a total of 88 drugs were shown to be responsible.** Which isn't surprising when you consider the following:

✓ **Coenzyme Q$_{10}$** – is depleted by vasodilators (i.e. nitroglycerin), diuretics, diabetic medications, all cholesterol-lowering drugs, including statins and bile acid sequestrants (i.e. Questran™, Colestid™), phenothiazines (class of antipsychotic drugs), antihypertensive (blood pressure lowering) drugs (including ACE inhibitors, beta-blockers and calcium channel blockers), antihistamines, antidepressants (especially tricyclics), and antiarrhythmics (i.e. digoxin).

We will be discussing the tremendous benefit of CoQ_{10} throughout the entire body, but especially the heart and kidneys.

Although statin drugs are unquestionably a major concern, all drugs have their associated risk factors (especially in combination), in addition to depleting many vitamins and minerals. This then results in critical nutrient deficiencies, which can potentially contribute to not only cardiovascular disease, but also all disease conditions.

According to studies of patients with dementia and other psychiatric disorders, including major depression, the homocysteine levels in their blood were found to be significantly elevated as compared with those of people in good mental health (*Stop Depression Now*, Brown, Bottiglieri & Colman, 1999, p. 137). In fact, some studies suggest that up to 50% of depressed individual exhibit significantly elevated homocysteine levels (*Life Extension* magazine, October 2006, p. 68).

The amino acid, methionine, which breaks down into homocysteine, is found in the proteins you eat (especially red meat). Ideally, homocysteine is changed right back to methionine by your body, during a process called methylation. But when that fails to happen (due to vitamin depletion from prescription drugs, for example), **your homocysteine levels soon become elevated, and immediate damage to the blood vessels can occur. Plaque will then begin to form, and the carotid and coronary arteries then thicken, restricting blood flow. The longer this continues, the higher the cardiovascular risk will be.** Studies show that **if your homocysteine is elevated *and* you already have heart disease, you are 4½ times more likely to die.**

I believe the late Robert S. Mendelsohn, M.D., author of the 1979 book *Confessions of a Medical Heretic*, sums up our healthcare in general rather well when he states that: ***"I believe that more than ninety percent of Modern Medicine could disappear from the face of the earth – doctors, hospital, drugs, and equipment – and the effect on our health would be immediate and beneficial"*** (p. 288).

I might add that I am sure Dr. Mendelsohn was not referring to the many competent surgeons who perform a great service in saving lives, especially from serious accidents. That might possibly be the ten percent he excluded, as we would obviously be in serious trouble without them. Many medical doctors would be more inclined to incorporate safer and more effective natural therapies in their practice at times if it weren't for the threat of the AMA, and the risk of losing their license to practice.

I have a tremendous amount of respect for the many doctors who place their patients' welfare above any profit potential. The doctors and scientists whose ethical standards are above reproach, and who are not willing to make false statements that they do not truly believe, no matter what the incentive possibly might be. These doctors and scientists are, in my opinion, the true heroes, whose major objective is to benefit their fellow men. Their reward may not always be financial, but is instead a clear conscience and true peace of mind.

I would suggest that anyone who has knowingly made false statements in the past, or has in any way attempted to help cover up the truth regarding the potential dangers associated with particular drugs, seriously consider their values. We must remember that money can never buy peace of mind or true happiness, and that service to our fellow man is always much more rewarding. Some people associated with the pharmaceutical industry have compromised their principles, and have basically corrupted medicine far too long. They have successfully managed to deceive the public, as well as the many doctors who have put their trust in them for decades, by creating one of the most profitable industries in the entire nation, and at the expense of millions of innocent victims (the general public).

CHAPTER SEVEN
THE SERIOUS CONSEQUENCES FROM STATIN DRUG USE -
The Resultant Depletion Of CoQ$_{10}$

As found in *the Prescription for Nutritional Healing, 3rd edition* (Balch & Balch, 2000), **the CoQ$_{10}$ depleted by statin drugs**, has been shown to be **able to lower high blood pressure** without medication or dietary changes, and **is beneficial in fighting obesity, by helping to metabolize fats and carbohydrates**. Studies have shown that **almost 50% of obese individuals have a blood serum level deficient of CoQ$_{10}$** (Dallas Clouatre, Ph.D., *AntiFat Nutrients*, 1993, p. 39).

Not only is it also **beneficial in fighting diabetes**, but also a **deficiency of CoQ$_{10}$ has even been linked to diabetes, which is a major contributor to cardiovascular disease.** It has been stated that *"In the long run, **statin drugs could predispose the patients to heart disease by lowering their CoQ$_{10}$ status, the very condition that these drugs are intended to prevent"*** (http://www.epic4health.com/index.html).

CoQ$_{10}$ plays a critical role in the production of energy in every cell in the body, aids in circulation, stimulates the immune system, and **increases tissue oxygenation.** Most importantly, *"a lack of sufficient Coenzyme Q$_{10}$ can lead to cardiovascular disease because without it, the heart does not have enough energy to circulate the blood effectively"* (Clouatre, *AntiFat Nutrients*, 1993, p. 54).

Dr. Peter Langsjoen, M.D. a specialist in congestive heart failure and other diseases of the heart muscle, noted, *"It has been pretty well documented from biopsies that the severity of heart failure correlates with the people who have the lowest levels of [Co] Q$_{10}$"* (http://www.medicalconsumers.org/pages/cholestrol_skeptics.html).

According to Jay Gordon, M.D., in an undated consumer guide to antioxidants, subtitled *"Clinical Proof That CoQ$_{10}$ Works to Save the Heart"*:

One study found 75 percent of 132 patients with heart trouble had deficiencies in CoQ$_{10}$ levels. An Italian study found that 80 percent of 1,100 patients with heart malfunction or failure improved after taking CoQ$_{10}$ supplements in oral form.

Other researchers have conducted experimental studies and examined the effects of long-term treatment with CoQ$_{10}$ on the heart muscle's ability to perform in laboratory rodents. Tests results showed improvement in the cardiac function and increased heart muscle metabolism in CoQ$_{10}$ treated subjects.

*CoQ$_{10}$ had an intriguing effect when tested on male rats fed a high sugar, low-copper diet – a diet typical of many Americans. The findings showed the diet caused severe inflammation, degeneration, and thickening of the heart muscle, as well as tissue changes that limited the body's ability to metabolize oxygen and provide energy to the heart muscle. Rats fed the high sugar, low copper diet, but supplemented with CoQ$_{10}$ showed the same decrease in mitochondria ability to produce energy, but these hearts did not degenerate. Also, **30 percent of the rats not given CoQ$_{10}$ died during the study from heart rupture. None of the CoQ$_{10}$-fed rats died even though they were on the same high sugar, low copper diet** (p. 24).*

The Depletion of CoQ$_{10}$ and Kidney Disease

Incidentally, there is even more to the story, and it's regarding kidney dysfunction. It all begins with the CoQ$_{10}$ depletion, which can then lead to reduced kidney function. A copper deficiency is often associated with kidney disease (one more problem associated with statin drug use).

According to Dr. Leslie M. Klevay, M.D.:

*There is a piece of evidence regarding **people with nephritic syndrome (kidney disease). These patients lose excessive amounts of copper in the urine.** Their risk of heart disease is also **85 times higher than that of the general population.***

Hearts of people who die of coronary heart disease are enlarged and fibrotic, they contain increased collagen and have hemorrhages. All of these pathological changes are found in animals deficient in copper.

People with coronary heart disease die suddenly.

In fact, copper deficiency was first detected in cattle who suffered from what was called "falling disease," or "quick death."

In one series of experiments, mice with supplemental copper lived six times as long as mice without a copper supplement and had no atrial thromboses, cardiac enlargement, or abnormal electrocardiograms.

*Most nutrition-minded people have heard of the nutritional substance lecithin, and how it is related to the control of plasma cholesterol. Lecithin is a substance which emulsifies fat particles. Now it turns out that **lecithin activity is related to copper.***

Lecithin activity has been related to the risk of coronary heart disease. When lecithin is low, it contributes to an increase in cholesterol (Sam Biser's Course on Curing Hopeless Health Conditions, Biser, 1993, pp. 405-405).

And in the August 2004 issue of *Life Extension* magazine, there was an article on applications for CoQ$_{10}$. An interesting concern was noted as follows:

Over the past 21 years, hundreds of studies have confirmed the safety and effectiveness of CoQ$_{10}$ supplementation for health disorders ranging from neurological aging to heart disease. Yet the US medical establishment and federal drug regulators have been hesitant to embrace these findings, reserving opinion until more large-scale trials are completed (p. 46).

Just one of the benefits of CoQ$_{10}$, mentioned in the article in *Life Extension* (August 2004), under the heading of **"CoQ$_{10}$ and Kidney Failure"** was the benefit of CoQ$_{10}$ supplementation in regard to patients with end-stage kidney disease, as follows:

*In the Journal of Nutritional and Environmental Medicine, CoQ$_{10}$ research pioneers Drs. Ram Singh and Adarsh Kumar reported the results of a very well-designed trial **indicating CoQ$_{10}$ might have a powerful role as adjunctive therapy in patients with end-stage kidney disease – in some cases even reducing or averting the need for dialysis.***

In a randomized, double-blind, placebo-controlled trial, the researchers found **CoQ₁₀** *treatment decreased progression and reversed renal dysfunction in a majority of patients with end-stage disease, many of whom were able to discontinue dialysis over the course of the 12-week trial* (p. 48).

They used a dosage of 180 mg of CoQ_{10} per day in the study. Coenzyme Q_{10} is a very complex molecule and one of the more expensive nutritional supplements on the market. It actually makes considerably more sense to avoid using drugs known to deplete CoQ_{10} in the first place.

One thing that should be quite obvious is: If CoQ_{10} is beneficial in improving a major health condition such as end-stage kidney disease, then the depletion of CoQ_{10} by drugs would unfortunately either create, or exacerbate the same problem.

The Depletion of CoQ₁₀ and The Heart

We find one more example regarding the benefits of CoQ_{10} in the same article (*Life Extension*, August 2004), under *"Cardiovascular Advances."* It was noted that, *"CoQ₁₀ has been shown to be effective against chronic inflammation of the arteries and heart muscle tissue resulting in cardiac myopathy"* and also that, **"Based on the available controlled data, CoQ₁₀ is a promising, effective, and safe approach to chronic heart failure"** (p. 49). Then, under **"Statin Update"** we find:

Evidence shows CoQ₁₀ supplementation can improve the circulatory process and prevent such irreversible and often fatal conditions as cardiomyopathy, congestive heart failure, and rhabdolmyolysis (muscle wasting induced by statin drug toxicity).

[Dr. Peter Langsjoen of East Texas University notes] **"With ever higher statin potencies and doses, and with a steadily shrinking target LDL cholesterol, the prevalence and severity of CoQ₁₀ deficiency are increasing noticeably"** (pp. 50-51).

An article in the February 2004 issue of *Life Extension* magazine introduced Dr. Langsjoen, who has become a vocal critic of statin drugs and published an article titled *"Statin-Induced Cardiomyopathy."* In an excerpt, Dr. Langsjoen describes his 17-year experience with statin drugs as follows:

I have seen a frightening increase in heart failure secondary to statin usage, "statin cardiomyopathy." *Over the past five years, statins have become more potent, are being prescribed in higher doses, and* **are being used with reckless abandon in the elderly and in patients with 'normal' cholesterol levels** (p. 14).

Dr. Langsjoen attributes these heart failure cases as being caused by *"statin-induced Coenzyme Q₁₀ depletion."*

Another resource regarding the nutrients depleted by these drugs and the associated problems they are known to create, actually come from a very credible source. The book titled: *Drug-Induced Nutrient Depletion Handbook, 2nd edition* (2001), is co-authored by four registered pharmacists (Hawkins, Krinsky, LaValle & Pelton), all with extensive backgrounds. They also have an **editorial advisory panel of <u>forty</u> M.D.s, Ph.D.s, and R.Ph.s** (registered pharmacists). It would be difficult to find a more credible source. In the introduction, the authors note:

*In the process of doing research for this book, it was amazing to uncover the large number of studies appearing in the scientific literature over the past thirty years reporting the drug-induced depletion of nutrients. Even more startling is the fact that **this information has not been communicated to the patients who are taking these drugs.** The importance* *of this book is quite simple yet powerful.* **Most health professionals are not aware of the fact that so many drugs are capable of causing nutritional deficiency-related health problems.**

It has become increasingly apparent that this information needs to get out to more people. *Physicians, nurses, chiropractors, and other health professionals should be aware of drug-induced nutrient depletions. At the same time, it is important that every individual who takes medications should have access to this information* (p. 9).

The authors noted that the CoQ_{10} is depleted by statin drugs, and the resultant **potential problems caused by this depletion by statin drugs are:** *"High blood pressure, congestive heart failure, and low energy"* (p. 509), which are known cardiovascular risk factors. Again, the very risk factors known to contribute to the life-threatening strokes and heart attacks that the statins were prescribed to prevent.

Although statin drugs are known to deplete the extremely important CoQ_{10}, they are actually not the only drugs that will do so. For example, **ALL of the 21 currently popular blood pressure medications known as beta-blockers deplete CoQ_{10}** and thus create the same basic set of symptoms that the statin drugs are known for! Also, **a total of 14 of the 18 diuretic drugs listed also deplete CoQ_{10}** and once again create (or add to) the very same set of problems that the statin (cholesterol lowering) drugs are known for. The diuretics are usually prescribed to deal with the edema (fluid retention) that results from the congestive heart failure caused by the statin drugs. The diuretics are notorious for depleting many critical vitamins and minerals, (as well as CoQ_{10}). What a catastrophe we could potentially create, and just in an attempt to resolve a problem that never really existed!

It is quite amazing that the other drugs normally prescribed for problems created by the statin drugs, actually create far more serious and varied problems than the cholesterol they were originally prescribed to resolve. We then find that the justification for increasing the dosage of statin drugs, and that more people should be placed on them, is due to the increasing the rate of strokes and heart attacks in the nation. **If the major statin drug manufacturers are successful in their deceptive and very aggressive promotional campaigns, the number of people on these drugs could quite easily double, or possibly even triple. That could easily result in a major healthcare disaster in the nation. You absolutely must become adequately informed regarding the serious consequences associated with the use of these potentially dangerous drugs! Your life (or at least your quality of life) is at stake.**

The Depletion of CoQ_{10} and The Brain

Once again, mentioned in the article in *Life Extension* (August 2004), we find under *"CoQ_{10} and the Brain"* that, *"A study conducted by **researchers at Columbia University College of Physicians and Surgeons in New York found CoQ_{10} deficiency in the brains of 17 patients with cerebellar ataxia and/or atrophy"** (p. 53).

Now, for those unfamiliar with the *term "cerebellar ataxia,"* in the *Bantam Medical Dictionary, 3rd* edition (1981/2000), we find that, ***"In cerebellar ataxia there is clumsiness of willed movements. The patient staggers when walking; he cannot pronounce words properly"*** (p. 40). Also, ***"atrophy"*** is ***"The wasting away of a normally developed organ or tissue due to degeneration of cells."*** **In this case, we are referring to the degeneration of brain cells from a CoQ_{10} deficiency.** If we then consider the problems noted, along with the reduced blood flow due to the associated vascular restriction from calcification of the arteries, we can easily see **the greatly increased potential for dementia and Alzheimer's disease.** Some people also experience lapses in short-term memory from the use of statin drugs. Then, considering the increased potential for hip fractures from the symptoms just noted, (a major concern for the elderly), we can quite easily see many potential concerns, especially regarding the elderly.

The Depletion of CoQ$_{10}$ and Muscle Weakness

Another issue is the serious muscle weakness associated with statin drugs. The elderly often already have a problem with weak muscles, and any reduced muscle function caused by statin drugs, could lead to immobility, which is a condition often responsible for many who are forced to give up their independence and move into a nursing home prematurely. The question is: Just how many people might currently be in nursing homes for that very reason? Also, with the established more aggressive guidelines, just how much more might we be increasing that potential? The amount of the very valuable CoQ$_{10}$ depleted is in direct relationship to the dosage. In other words, **the more potent the drug (such as Crestor™) and the higher the prescribed dosage (like doubling the dosage, as many doctors are now doing), the more serious the associated problems you should expect.** The elderly tend to react more rapidly to any drug, so they would normally experience even more dramatic reactions to the increased dosage than others.

Another potential problem is regarding the smooth muscles surrounding the vascular system, which are responsible for both constricting and dilating (expanding or contracting) of the arteries. This is one way the body can regulate the blood flow, by diverting the blood to the various areas of the body, such as the brain or muscles, based on demand. If they lose their strength and elasticity, supplying oxygen where it is needed the most, would likely be less effective.

Sometimes we fail to consider just how many functions in our body depend upon muscles and their proper tone and efficiency. For example, our breathing, and thus adequate oxygen intake requires muscle action. Even the peristaltic action in the intestinal tract for proper elimination is important to assure the effective removal of toxins. Also, the muscle tone in the eye muscles that control our vision for close up reading and distant vision could be influenced. The obvious question is: Could the weakening of muscles also influence our vision?

As you can easily see, the statin drugs could quite easily have far-reaching influences that we have yet failed to consider. The potential for damage by drugs in general, from their nutrient depletion and domino effect, to their interactions with other drugs, is like playing Russian roulette with your life.

Dr. Julian M. Whitaker, M.D., author, founder and director of the Whitaker Wellness Institute Medical Clinic in Newport Beach, California, feels so strongly regarding the dangers of statin drugs, he petitioned the FDA to mandate that the following warning be included in the package inserts of all statin drugs (as is already being done in several other countries), with a big black "WARNING" box surrounding the text:

> <u>*Warning:*</u> *HMG CoA reductase inhibitors (statin drugs) block the endogenous biosynthesis of an essential cofactor, Coenzyme Q$_{10}$, required for energy production. A deficiency of Coenzyme Q$_{10}$ is associated with impairment of myocardial function, with liver dysfunction and with myopathies (including cardiomyopathy and congestive heart failure). All patients taking HMG CoA reductase inhibitors should therefore be advised to take 100 to 200 mg per day of supplemental Coenzyme Q$_{10}$* (Life Extension *magazine, February 2004, pp. 14-17).*

Dr. Whitaker's meticulously documented petition was filed on **May 24, 2002**. However, according to *Life Extension* magazine, as of February 2004 the FDA has ignored it. The result is that **millions of statin drug users are still needlessly being subjected to lethal side effects.**

The failure of the FDA to amend the drug package insert to recommend that statin users supplement with CoQ$_{10}$ is a medical travesty. Since the underlying science is irrefutable, this is a

blatant example of large drug companies influencing the FDA into <u>not</u> taking actions that would save lives.

What is truly ironic, according to the article in *Life Extension* magazine (February 2004), **is that from 1985 to 1994, the FDA made a concerted effort to completely <u>outlaw</u> CoQ$_{10}$.** One of the FDA's arguments was that because CoQ$_{10}$ is sold as a prescription drug in Japan, it should not be freely available to Americans as a dietary supplement.

Dr. Jere Goyan, M.D., FDA commissioner from 1979 to 1981, noted that during that era, the FDA exerted totalitarian authority over what Americans were allowed to read about dietary supplements and drugs. According to the FDA at that time, any advertising claim that even implied that a supplement provided a health benefit automatically turned that supplement into an illegal *"unapproved new drug."*

In response to growing reports that drug companies are engaged in all kinds of nefarious behavior that results in consumers being prescribed dangerous drugs, Dr. **Goyan was quoted in the *Detroit Free Press* on November 5, 2003 as stating: *"We as patients have got to raise the questions ourselves and take care of our own selves"*** (*Life Extension* magazine, February 2004).

Considering the FDA's historically rigid position that American consumers are too stupid to make their own health care choices and therefore need the FDA to *"**protect**"* them, **this statement by a former FDA commissioner that people have to *"take care of their own selves"* is a revolutionary admission.** Too bad so many innocent people had to die because the FDA denied them access to the findings from scientific journals about the disease-prevention benefits of dietary supplements.

Statin Drugs and The Depletion of Vitamin K

As we have seen, the depletion of the critical nutrient CoQ$_{10}$ by the statin drugs is well established and undisputed. It turns out though, **that the statin drugs can also deplete the less-known vitamin K.** In the March 2004 issue of the *Life Extension* magazine, we learn:

> *Several conditions, however, can <u>set the stage for vitamin K deficiency,</u> including:*
> - *A poor or restricted diet*
> - *Crohn's disease, ulcerative colitis, or other ailments that interfere with nutrient absorption*
> - *Liver disease that interferes with vitamin K storage*
> - ***Certain drugs,*** *including broad-spectrum antibiotics,* ***cholesterol-lowering agents,*** *mineral oil,* ***aspirin, and blood thinners.***
>
> ***More subtle deficits may increase the risk of osteoporosis, arteriosclerosis,*** *and other ailments* (p. 66).

Although vitamin K has always been considered important for the proper clotting of blood, research has uncovered many other uses for vitamin K in the body. We also find that, ***"Vitamin K helps keep bones strong and slows the calcification of tissues.*** *It also can destroy certain types of cancer cells, protect the skin, and* ***may prove useful in the fight against Alzheimer's disease, diabetes, and aging"*** (*Life Extension*, March 2004, p. 66). So as you can see, **vitamin K actually has many potential uses throughout the body**.

Now we will evaluate what part vitamin K might play regarding cardiovascular health (our major focus), and the proposed objective of the statin (cholesterol lowering) drugs. *Life Extension* (March 2004) goes on to tell us that, ***"Vitamin K also helps keep calcium out of the linings of arteries and other body tissues, where it can be dangerous"*** (p. 67). **As a result of vitamin K deficiency, *"Over time, [the arteries] tend to thicken and stiffen as the body deposits calcium into the artery walls. This condition, known as arteriosclerosis, is a risk factor for heart disease and stroke"*** (p. 67). This is just one more way the statin drugs are actually responsible for creating the very same risk factors for heart disease and stroke that they are supposed to resolve!

That is not the only potential problem in regards to vitamin K depletion. If we look a little further, we find that, ***"Studies suggests that vitamin K may help combat cancer,"*** and that *"preliminary reports suggest that vitamin K may one day be used to 'instruct' cancer cells to stop their dangerous, unregulated growth,"* and finally that:

> ***Relatively large amounts of vitamin K are found in the pancreas,*** *the organ that manufactures the insulin that regulates blood sugar. In a study with laboratory animals, Japanese researchers found that a* ***deficiency of vitamin K interferes with insulin release and glucose regulation in ways similar to diabetes*** (*Life Extension*, March 2004, p. 67).

Anything that can negatively influence insulin release and glucose regulation also increases the risk for cardiovascular disease.

Reasons Why Some People Experience Side Effects From Statin Drugs Much Sooner Than Others

1. **One determining factor is which statin drug (such as Lipitor™, Zocor™, or Crestor™) that a person might be taking,** as some are stronger than others.

2. **The dose the doctor prescribes is another factor.** More aggressive measures, and higher prescribed dosages now being recommended by the **experts,** is a major concern and will just make the current problem even worse. **The higher the dosage, the more CoQ$_{10}$ is depleted.** That basically means that **everyone on a higher dosage should not only expect <u>worse</u> reactions, but would likely experience them much <u>sooner</u> also.**

There is a limit as to how much coenzyme the body can actually produce, and it is extremely critical for efficient energy production of every single cell in the body. The heart, brain, kidneys, and liver are the organs where the most serious reactions are normally experienced. CoQ$_{10}$ is a very complex molecule, and thus one of the most difficult for the body to synthesize. In order for the body to produce CoQ$_{10}$, it requires a 17-step process involving seven different vitamins, and numerous minerals. There are also many different ways that the complex process of synthesizing CoQ$_{10}$ can be interrupted. Due to the depletion of both vitamins and minerals by prescription drugs, we could easily see why those resorting to prescription drugs for solutions would likely be CoQ$_{10}$ deficient. Also as previously noted, 88 different drugs are known to deplete CoQ$_{10}$.

3. **Age is also an issue,** as approximately 75% of the people over 50 years of age are already low in CoQ$_{10}$, before statin drugs begin their dangerous depletion. There are many reasons that might likely be true. **Our ability to effectively digest and assimilate food is normally reduced as we age, as is our liver function,** which is responsible for converting foods into vitamins, minerals, and amino acids, for our use, as well as removing toxins. The liver actually has many important functions, which normally become less efficient as we age.

4. **Our liver** is very much like an extremely complex and efficient laboratory and detoxification center. This miracle in our body was created to help provide for our body's many needs, by Our Creator whose only concern is our health, rather than any personal profit potential. It appears that the **statin (cholesterol lowering) drugs**, and the antidepressants known as **Selective Serotonin Reuptake Inhibitors** (SSRIs) such as Prozac™, Paxil™, Zoloft™, etc, **might very well be two of the worst classes of drugs on the market.** Unfortunately, they are also some of the most widely promoted and abused. **The exact same P450 enzyme in the liver responsible for detoxifying alcohol, also attempts to metabolize and eliminate both the statin drugs, and the SSRI antidepressants.** If there

were any potential beneficial from the use of these drugs, why would the liver be attempting to eliminate them in the first place?

5. **Another factor** regarding how long it might take for people to experience major problems when taking statin drugs is **how many other drugs a person might actually be taking in addition to the statin drugs.** Most people are fully aware of the damage to the liver caused by alcohol, but fail to realize that **prescription drugs are inorganic chemicals and thus also considered as toxins by the liver, and are actually taking their toll on the liver.**

6. Then there is another potential problem that I will be addressing in my forthcoming book on weight loss. Our body stores toxins that the liver often can't effectively eliminate at any one time. When this problem exists, the excess toxins are stored in the fat tissue. The more drugs you have been taking, the more drug residues will be found in your fat tissue. Approximately 60% of the people in the nation today are currently overweight, and many are attempting to lose weight. **The very worst time to be placing more people on statin drugs, or increasing the dosage for those already on the drugs, is when they are also following the surgeon general's advice to start losing weight.** As the fat tissue is removed, the toxins will be released, and guess whose job that will be to resolve? You guessed it – your liver. For that very reason, as we are already placing an added burden on the liver during fat removal, we certainly don't need another burden such as statin drugs. Also, a deficiency of CoQ_{10} (caused by the statin drugs) results in reduced metabolism, which is a major contributor to obesity! And, with the added detoxification load from the toxins released with the fat tissue, more of the statin drugs would likely get around your liver and more of the valuable CoQ_{10} would also be depleted. What a terrible waste of such a valuable resource. **This would basically sabotage your weight loss efforts, as well as precipitating the serious problems associated with the statin drugs' CoQ_{10} depletion.**

I don't know of a better way to describe prescription medications, other than they are really scary and extremely unpredictable. The more we learn about them, the more obvious that will become. They are the primary contributors to our rapidly escalating national healthcare crisis. We must realize the damage we are doing to our bodies, by our increasing dependence on such potentially dangerous drugs as the only solution. A lifetime of drugs is not, and never will be a viable solution to any health concern. The only way we can resolve any health issue is by addressing the basic underlying problem, followed by providing the natural organic nutrients our body can immediately recognize and utilize to effectively heal itself. Unfortunately, that process will not be very effective if you are also taking drugs known to deplete the very vitamins and minerals necessary for healing to take place. That would just be counterproductive, and basically tend to undermine the important healing process.

CHAPTER EIGHT
A FEW OF NATURE'S MIRACLES

One Recent Discovery – The Mangosteen Extract

Now that we've learned from many prominent and very knowledgeable medical doctors that medications are not a viable solution and should thus be avoided, it would be helpful if we learned of some natural options that are available. As you are likely aware at this point, my objective is to show you how you can finally become totally free from the curse of a lifetime dependency on prescription and over-the-counter medications.

I will now introduce you to three relatively new discoveries of mine. We will begin with mangosteen juice, which consists of the mangosteen fruit along with the rind, (which contains most of the medicinal benefit). Although there are other companies that now sell the mangosteen juice, XanGo™ was the first product to be introduced in the United States. It is sold by the MLM company XanGo™, in Utah, and is only available through its distributors. As it is not yet that well known, I felt it might be best to first introduce you to the mangosteen fruit itself, and give you a little background on it.

The whole mangosteen appears to have a fairly broad range of benefits. One important issue is that the mangosteen doesn't seem to interact with medications. It is the 43 active compounds called xanthones found mostly in the pericarp (rind) that are attributed to its surprising medicinal benefit. It is basically a very broad-range adaptogen (containing multiple benefits), similar to some herbs. I consider it to be at least one of Our Creator's masterpieces.

Together, Dr. David Morton, Ph.D., a professor at the University of Utah, and Dr. Fredrick Templeman, M.D., a family practitioner, recently conducted research and clinical studies on the benefits of the entire mangosteen fruit. Dr. Morton began basically researching the research, while Dr. Templeman began conducting clinical studies using XanGo™ with his patients. Dr. Morton soon discovered that decades of research had already been conducted on the mangosteen and its many different xanthones. He found that many major universities throughout the world had conducted studies on the various benefits of the xanthones found in the mangosteen.

Dr. David Morton's brother Joe discovered the mangosteen while working on a project in Thailand, and was responsible for bringing it to the U.S. in the form of a juice, after first filing several patents on the processing and combining of both the fruit and rind. And once Dr. Templeman began trying the mangosteen with his patients, he soon found it to be more effective in resolving a broad range of conditions than many of the drugs he had been prescribing in his practice for over 20 years. Thus he was finally able to eliminate many medications he had been prescribing for years, just by replacing them with this healthy juice. As I noted, an important factor is the lack of interaction of the mangosteen with the medications his patients were currently taking. This just makes their withdrawal (my primary objective), that much easier.

I do have one advantage that Dr. Templeman currently doesn't, and that is decades of research using natural supplements for disease prevention. Dr. Templeman was instead trained in the use of drugs as a solution, as most traditionally trained doctors were. In Dr. Templeman's own words:

Until the arrival of mangosteen in North America, I had steadfastly refused to endorse food supplements (whole plant preparations, not extracts, vitamins, minerals or micronutrients), because I remained unconvinced that any of them deserved to be promoted at the expense of standard pharmacology (*Mangosteen The X-Factor*, 2003, p. 1).

He also noted that:

When I was approached to personally investigate the benefits of mangosteen, I brought all of my scientific skepticism with me. At the outset of the investigations, I fully expected that I would finish by concluding that it was "just another food supplement." I only agreed to participate because a scientist friend of mine, whose judgment I respect, was ecstatic about what he had found when he examined the scientific evidence backing up the folk medicine claims made about the mangosteen.

My position today on the question of supplements has changed. I am now convinced that mangosteen will, without a doubt, be the most successful food supplement ever (p. 2).

This is an area Dr. Templeman is currently working on, since learning just how valuable natural substances can be in resolving health issues. I met with Dr. Templeman in Salt Lake City, just before he was about to leave for Madras, India to learn more about Ayruvedic medicine. Incidentally, I made several trips to both Madras and Calcutta, India, beginning in 1951 as a young merchant seaman. I also met with Dr. Morton, who was about to leave for Peru. It just so happens that I also traveled to Peru, although that was only about 8 years ago. I traveled down the Amazon from Iquitos Peru to Columbia and then Brazil. I was able to travel by canoe up several tributaries and visit different native villages and talk to some of their healers through an interpreter. A lot of our herbs come from the Amazon, and in Iquitos Peru I discovered several blocks of nothing but herbal shops in a large outdoor market. I also visited a leper colony in Columbia, which included a large hospital for the lepers, and it was a very humbling experience. Just seeing all those lepers, and the result of such a terribly destructive disease, is a reminder of just how fortunate we really are. It would be a good experience for anyone suffering from self-pity, as would a trip to India (an experience I never forgot).

After returning back up the Amazon to Iquitos Peru, I proceeded to Cuzco Peru by plane. That was basically going from sea level to 11,000 feet elevation, and finally by train to a village close to Machu Picchu. The only access to the village is by train, which actually gains elevation by traversing the rugged terrain by continually reversing direction; something I had never experienced prior to that adventure. The train actually goes just as fast in reverse as it does when traveling forward, which was quite an experience in and of itself.

At 6:00 am the following morning, I took the bus from the village up a steep winding road with many switchbacks to the ruins at the base of the mountain. After touring the ruins I headed up the mountain called Machu Picchu, by myself (a big mistake). It is much more of an obstacle course than a regular hiking trail, where I normally hike at home. Traversing the mountain involves negotiating both trails and some steps about 3 feet high, and then under one long cliff overhang, approximately 4 feet high, and through a couple caves. One cliff ascent was via logs lashed together forming a ladder. I actually arrived at the top in less than half the time considered as normal, which I felt pretty good about (especially at 65). Incidentally, that is about 13,000 feet elevation.

Surprisingly, it was the descent that turned out to be the greatest challenge of all! I soon discovered there was more than one trail leading to the top (something I hadn't considered). At times, when going through the jungle, I wasn't really sure which fork in the trail to take in order to get back. Thus, I spent several hours non-stop through the rather challenging obstacle course, at times re-tracing the same trail. Needless to say, it was a pleasant sight, finally arriving at the ruins below, after over five hours. Fortunately, I had made many 12-mile hikes non-stop on some pretty steep mountain trails at home, although the major differences were the altitude, and I knew which trail to follow. Luckily, I learned about coca leaves, and found that when drank as a tea, it actually helps adapt to high altitudes, and really does make a difference. I later discovered that both the maca root and the goji seem to have similar properties. They both apparently cause the red blood cells to release oxygen to the cells more efficiently via an enzyme called 23BPG. This tends to make better use of the available oxygen. Interestingly, all three (maca, goji, and the coca plant) grow at high altitudes and under harsh conditions.

Now that our little expedition to Peru is over, we'll get back to business and Dr. Templeman's discoveries. I hope you will forgive the temporary diversion, but discussing medications can be rather depressing at times, and possibly a little diversion might be good therapy. If it's not for you, it certainly was for me, and you have my apology.

Following are some of Dr. Templeman's conclusions after approximately 18 months of implementing mangosteen in his clinical practice with his patients, as reported in the *Health Journal* (2004, vol. 44, no. 2). Although some of the words are Dr. Templeman's, the emphases' (bold print) are mine.

Medical Doctor Finds Mangosteen Juice Effective for Patient Care

Dr. Templeman is a primary care physician with 20 years experience. He is board certified in both the United States and Canada.

"I have been using a Mangosteen functional beverage with my patients long enough to draw valid clinical conclusions about its effectiveness in many medical conditions. Initially, I used it as a fallback product only when the regular medicines I prescribed proved ineffectual. I now use it as a first-line therapy in a wide range of conditions because it has, in my experience, proven to be as efficacious or more efficacious than the prescription medicine I used to prescribe for numerous disease states.

"My logic for using Mangosteen extract rather than a drug is relatively simple. All drugs are potentially dangerous. There is no safe drug."

"I use mangosteen extract as a first-line therapy in the following conditions:

* **Acid dyspepsia** or *gastritis*
* *Mild to* **moderate anxiety**
* **Fatigue** or *low energy states*
* **Mild depression** or *dysthymia*
* *Mild to moderate* **asthma**
* **Irritable bowel disease**
* **Gastro-esophageal reflux disease** [GERD]
* *Otitis externa*
* *Recurrent* **urinary tract infection**
* **Non-arthritis muscle or joint pain**

* **Diverticulitis**
* **Arthritis**
* **Fibromyalgia**
* **Hiatal hernia**
* **Sleep disorders**
* **Allergic rhinitis**
* **Seborrhea**
* **Eczema**
* **Neurodermatitis**

"I am well aware that many conditions are unsatisfactorily treated with prescription drugs. Whether doctors are prepared to admit this to their patients or not, they know it to be true.
"I cannot express the relief I feel, as a physician, knowing that there is a safe, efficacious, natural alternative I can use in the conditions I have listed. It may be helpful for those reading this piece to also have a list of some of the prescriptions and over the counter drugs that I have discontinued in

my patients when the Mangosteen extract has equaled or outperformed them:

- *Nexium, Prevacid Aciphex and other proton pump inhibitors*
- *Zantac, Pepcid and other H_2 blockers*
- *Allegra, Zyrtec, Claritin, Clarinex and other antihistamines*
- *Singulair*
- *Prednisone*
- *Litrisone, Topicort, Cutivate, Iprolene and other topical corticosteroids used for skin conditions (eczema, psoriasis, seborrhea)*
- *Valium, Xanax, and other minor tranquilizers*
- *Tegretol, Neurontin and other anti-epileptic drugs when used for chronic pain relief*
- *Anusol and other hemorrhoid preparations*
- ***Prozac, Zoloft, Paxil, Lexapro and other antidepressants when used for dysthymia and anxiety states***
- *Vicodin, Percocet, Duragesic patches, Methadone and other narcotics used for chronic pain control*
- ***Celebrex, Vioxx, Bextra,*** *Naproxen, Arthrotec,* ***Ibuprofen and other anti-inflammatories*** *used for musculo-skeletal pain and inflammation control or menstrual pain*
- *Ultram, Talwin, and other non-opioid pain preparations*
- *Midrin, Fioricet, Imitrex, Amerge, Maxalt, Zomig and other migraine headache preparations*
- ***Lipitor, Zocor, Pravachol and other lipid-lowering agents.***
- *Valtrex for herpes infections*
- ***Aricept, Cognex and other Alzheimer's preparations***

"My purpose in setting out these lists is to allow patients to evaluate for themselves whether pharmaceuticals or phytoceuticals should be used to treat their conditions. The basic question I ask is this: ***'Why would anyone even use a drug to obtain some effect that can be found in a food?'"***

We have not seen food-drug interactions with this product.
You'll be surprised with the benefits it can provide in chronic illness at doses of one or two ounces before meals, ideally three times daily. For prevention, one ounce a day is adequate (pp. 1-2).

Another Discovery - Noni Juice

Noni is an evergreen tree that typically grows and thrives in tropical, volcanic regions such as Tahiti and Hawaii, and is capable of bearing fruit year round. Its juice has been used as a healing and medicinal plant by ancient cultures for more than 2,000 years. Noni contains over 140 important vitamins, minerals and other nutrients, as well as other unknown positive substances that have yet to be identified. Noni also contains a powerful phytonutrient called Damancanthal, which Japanese researchers have found to have a very beneficial effect on pre-cancerous cells. **It has the ability to actually open the cell wall, allowing more nutrients to be absorbed into our cells, as well as more waste material to be removed from weak or damaged cells, thus increasing cellular activity, nutritional intake, and overall cellular health. No matter what nutrient you combine with noni, it increases the power, availability, absorption, and overall effects of all other nutrients.**

Scopoletin is another powerful ingredient found in noni, which is known to bind with serotonin. **Scopoletin also acts as an antifungal (which assists in fighting candida), an antihistamine, an anti-viral, and an anti-inflammatory, as well as reducing high blood pressure by dilating blood vessels.** Although noni juice is naturally acidic, (with an extremely low pH of 3.4 to 3.8), it has a pH balancing (or neutralizing) effect on the body.

Dr. R. Lindsey Duncan, president and CEO of Genesis Today™, has found the following medicinal effects of noni on the human body to be astounding:

*On external skin conditions, diluted with water as a sinus rinse and an eye rinse, as well as a host of internal problems ranging from digestive issues, allergies, hormonal imbalances, circulatory problems, **support of major organs such as heart, brain, lung, kidneys, pancreas, liver, and intestines. It offers powerful nervous system support, it helps with depression and exhaustion, obesity, candida, parasites, and much more.***

As reported by some 50 doctors monitoring approximately 10,000 patients, the following health complaints can be helped by 100% pure noni:

* High Blood Pressure	* Arthritis	* Circulatory Problems
* Hormonal Imbalances	* Diabetes	* Digestive Disorders
* Intestinal Parasites	* Stomach Ulcers	* Immune Disorders
* Inflammatory Conditions	* Allergies	* Aging Problems
* Lung Conditions	* Infections	* Heart Problems
* Emotional Disorders	* Depression	* Bowel Conditions
* Nervous System Disorders	* Fatigue	* Headaches
* Pain (emotional & physical)	* Insomnia	* Kidney & Bladder
* All Skin Conditions	* Obesity	* Candida
		…. and many more

A Third Discovery – The Chinese Wolfberry, or Goji Berry Juice

Dr. Victor Marcial-Vega, M.D., whom I met several years ago at a health conference in Palm Springs, has been studying the before- and after-effects of various treatments on the blood, with thousands of his patients. He discovered that when the blood is too acidic, the red blood cells tend to clump together, and there is normally a higher level of bacteria in the blood as well.

Dr. Marcial-Vega discovered that in only 24 to 36 hours after drinking Goji juice, the blood became more alkaline, and the red blood cells had separated, making oxygen delivery to the cells more efficient. Some of his research was published in the August 2006 issue of *Breakthroughs In Health* magazine (vol. 1, issue 1), as follows:

He noticed that as the alkalinity changed, so did the reversal of all illnesses, including cancer, high blood pressure, diabetes, chronic renal failure, obesity, high cholesterol, arthritis and other illnesses associated with physical or mental discomforts, including attention deficit disorder, anxiety and depression.

He found that 90 percent of the patients had reversed their acidity to alkalinity just by ingesting goji juice.

He also observed high cholesterol levels decreased a minimum of 50 points in four weeks in 67 percent of the patients; high blood pressure dropped in 80 percent of the patients, and 50 percent of these patients decreased or eliminated their high blood pressure medications. Dr. Marcial-Vega also observed that 85 percent of his obese patients had a significant decrease in their weight, while their lean body mass remained the same or increased. "That means they did not lose muscle," he says. "So now we see that the alkaline-acidity thing we are talking about makes a difference."

"Most of the patients that are acidic have a low temperature, meaning low energy. When you are ill, your energy is low. When you are acidic, the energy is low."

"Blood sugar levels decrease in 64 percent of the patients with diabetes, and more than half of them decreased or eliminated their medications" (p. 13).

The ancient Himalayan healers were also aware thousands of years ago that people were much healthier, stronger, had more endurance, and even lived longer when they consumed goji. A well-known story is told of Li Qing Yuen, a Chinese man born in 1678, who lived to be 252 years old! His life span has even been verified by scholars, who found that *"each day he consumed a 'soup' made of the Goji berry."* Rather than containing xanthones, as the mangosteen does, the *lycium barbarum* strain of goji berry derives its benefits from five different polysaccharides (named LBP1, LBP2, LBP3, LBP4, and LBP1-5), and is explained, as follows:

It was discovered that certain types of polysaccharides could cause profound and beneficial changes in the human body.

Bioactive polysaccharides, also called proteoglycans, are a family of complex carbohydrates bound to proteins. They are produced by some plants as an extremely effective defense mechanism against attack by viruses, bacteria, fungi, soil-borne parasites, cell mutations, toxic pollutants and environmental free radicals.

There are many types of bioactive polysaccharides, and they all seem to differ in their properties, health benefits and degrees of activity.

These polysaccharide-producing species include those that must attempt to survive under great stresses, such as temperature extremes, high altitude or wildly unpredictable precipitation. No plant on Earth grows under more stressful conditions than does goji. It was not surprising, therefore, when scientists found the little, red berry to be a treasure trove of highly bioactive polysaccharides.

LBP polysaccharides proved to be glycoconjugates, meaning that they are exceptional sources of the essential cell sugars – rhamnose, xylose, glucose, manose, arabinose and galactose – that are necessary for proper immune function and intercellular communication. In fact, goji may be the richest source of glyconutrients yet found.

*Research strongly suggests that goji's unique polysaccharides work in the body by serving as directors and carriers of the instructions that cells use to communicate with each other (*Breakthroughs In Health*, August 2006, Vol. 1, issue 1, pp. 45-46).*

Other benefits of goji, as listed in the Genesis Today™ materials, written by Dr. Lindsay Duncan, N.D., C.N., are as follows:

- *The accumulation of sticky lipid peroxides in the blood can lead to cardiovascular disease, heart attack, atherosclerosis and stroke. Goji increases levels of an important blood enzyme that inhibits the formation of dangerous lipid peroxides.*
- *Goji is known as the "longevity fruit."Goji is a renowned blood builder and rejuvenator. In one study, the berry caused the blood of older people to revert to a markedly younger state.*
- *Goji stimulates the release by the pituitary gland of hGH (human growth hormone) the youth hormone. The benefits of hGH are extensive and include reduction of body fat, better sleep, improved memory, accelerated healing, restored libido and a more youthful appearance.*
- *Goji has been historically used in Asia for the natural treatment of insomnia.*
- *Goji has also been used in a number of recent clinical trials for treatment of bone marrow deficiency conditions (low production of red blood cells, white blood cells and platelets).*
- *For ages, Goji has been the yin tonic of choice to restore hormonal balance.*
- *Goji polysaccharides enhance and balance the activity of all classes of immune cells.*
- *Goji has long been used in the treatment of atrophic gastritis, a weakening of digestion caused by reduced activity of stomach cells.*
- *Goji is the premier "brain tonic" in Asia. It contains betaine, which is converted in the body into choline, a substance that enhances memory and recall ability.*
- *Exposure to chemicals, pollutants and free radicals can cause DNA damage and breakage, leading to genetic mutations, cancer, and even death. Goji's betaine and polysaccharides can restore and repair damaged DNA.*
- *Goji has long been known to be a kidney supertonic, supporting ultimate kidney health and function.*
- *Goji contains cyperone, a sesquiterpene that benefits the heart and blood pressure. Its anthocyanins help to maintain the strength and integrity of coronary arteries.*
- *Goji is one of Asia's premier adaptogens. Goji increases exercise tolerance, stamina and endurance. It helps to eliminate fatigue, especially when recovering from illness.*
- *A 1998 research study indicated that high blood pressure could be managed by the polysaccharides in Goji.*

- *Goji contains beta-sitosterol, which has been shown to lower cholesterol levels. Its antioxidants keep cholesterol from oxidizing and forming arterial plaques.*
- *Goji has been used in China for the treatment of adult-onset diabetes for many years. Its polysaccharides have been shown to help balance blood sugar and insulin response.*
- *Goji has been used historically in Asia as a premier sexual tonic.*
- *As an adaptogen goji helps the body to adapt and to cope with stress. It provides the energy reserves to help with any type of difficulty, both mental and physical.*
- *In Asia, goji is known as the "happy berry." It has been historically used in China to uplift and elevate. It is said that constant consumption brings about a cheerful attitude.*
- *Goji can help to restore the balance of the important anti-inflammatory SOD enzyme.*
- *Goji is especially good for diseases of the liver, as it exerts liver protection. The liver is the body's primary detoxification organ.*
- *Goji polysaccharides are shown to reduce body weight by enhancing the conversion of food into energy instead of fat.*
- *Goji contains a cerebroside that has been shown to protect liver cells, even from highly toxic chlorinated hydrocarbons.*

Dr. Duncan was one of several speakers at a recent health conference I attended in Seattle, and claimed that in his opinion, of the three juices we've just discussed, goji was his favorite, followed by noni, and then mangosteen, although he did feel that the Acai juice, garlic, algae, spirulina, and chlorella are all beneficial as well. From my research, I pretty much agree. I personally would add the alfalfa, often referred to as the "king of herbs." Although inexpensive, alfalfa contains a treasure trove of important nutrients including chlorophyll and, as usual, in a natural form. It's quite amazing what a broad range of benefits these very amazing juices seem to have and something the ancients were very aware of thousands of years ago.

On a CD titled "Goji – Listen To What Doctors Are Saying", are discussions by different doctors relating their experiences using goji with their patients, as well as themselves. Many of the benefits associated with goji, which they discovered, were basically the same as those that Dr. Marcial-Vega and Dr. Duncan also discussed. I'll just mention a few that weren't discussed, as follows:

➢ Dr. Matthew Silver mentioned that his periodontal disease, difficulty breathing, difficulty sleeping, afternoon fatigue, and even prostate problems, all resolved after taking goji. It also helped his patients resolve chronic fatigue, depression, and one woman no longer experienced the many symptoms associated with years of chlorine poisoning, from an over-chlorinated pool.

➢ Dr. Peter Lazarnick found that his wife experienced total relief from suffering with years of hot flashes, (as did her friend Tara, after sharing her experience).

➢ Dr. Carlos Orozco, from Mexico City, told of one 42-year-old woman who had been plagued with migraines for years, but is now migraine-free. He told of another patient who had breast cancer that migrated to her liver. After a few months, her liver was totally cancer-free, and the size of the tumor in her breast was greatly reduced. He also discussed an 80-year-old lady, whose severe emphysema had completely resolved in only three weeks.

➢ Dr. David Bridgman from Queensland, Australia, experienced some outstanding results from goji with his patients. First, he was a runner and soon discovered an improvement in his fitness level, as well as a considerable drop in his heart rate when running. That would likely indicate an increase in oxygen efficiency. He also recognized an increase in hemoglobin and white blood cell levels. He used a biometric testing device, which measures the stored energy in various organs, and found considerable improvement in 90% of his patients. Although the ideal level is 50, he claimed that the majority of his patients' initial reading was 20 to 30, but soon normalized at the optimal level of 50.

As he normally recommends the blood type diet for his patients, he decided to see if goji might not be beneficial for all blood types, which is true with some herbs. After testing each one, he discovered that goji was actually beneficial for all blood types. An important issue for anyone following the blood type diet, and are familiar with the importance of eliminating certain foods, in order to recognize the most benefit. In his book *Eat Right For Your Type* (1996), Dr. Peter D. D'Adamo, N.D. discusses the importance of following a diet based on your blood type.

By far, the most dramatic results he experienced were regarding two different individuals who were scheduled for lung transplants. Neither patient required the transplant! A quite amazing discovery! The condition they were both diagnosed with is considered a fatal lung disease called "Bronchiectasis [which] *is an abnormal stretching and enlarging of the respiratory passages caused by mucus blockage.*" The American Lung Association gives the following explanation:

> *When the body is unable to get rid of mucus, mucus becomes stuck and accumulates in the airways. The blockage and accompanying infection cause inflammation, leading to the weakening and widening of the passages. The weakened passages can become scarred and deformed, allowing more mucus and bacteria to accumulate, resulting in a cycle of infection and blocked airways.*
>
> *Bronchiectasis patients are often given antibiotics for infection and bronchodilator medicines to open passages.*
>
> Lung   transplants   are   [sometimes]   *an   option   for   severe   cases* (http://www.lungusa.org/site/pp.asp?c=dvLUK9O0E&b=35009).

➤ Dr. F.G. Nicley told of one patient who was on oxygen 24/7, and was able to get off his oxygen just by consuming two ounces of goji twice daily. He also tells of one lady who had an elevated blood pressure level of 158/98, and was taking two medications to control her blood pressure. She was able to get off both medications, after her blood pressure normalized. Dr. Nicley states that in his 45 years of practicing medicine, he never encountered anything that paralleled the many benefits of goji.

➤ Dr. Eddie Rettstatt is a chiropractor that uses the bioenergic synchronization technique in his practice. He said his wife suffered with severe allergies for years. She often couldn't' go outside without suffering a severe allergic reaction. After taking goji a few months, she was totally allergy-free. He mentions other patients with swelling of hands and feet, psoriasis, and headaches that were resolved with goji. The most outstanding was a 67-year-old gentleman who suffered neck and back injuries from a fall. The problem was, his doctor said that as he had two prior triple-bypass surgeries, and also had considerable restriction in his carotid arteries, the knee he needed surgery on would in his opinion be too risky. Surprisingly, in only a few months of drinking goji, (he didn't specifically how long or the amount), but the blockage in his carotid arteries went from 43% flow to an amazing 73%, an unbelievable reduction. I'm not aware of any therapy (not even IV chelation) that could possibly remove plaque that rapidly. That benefit, combined with the improvement in the red blood cells in only 36 hours or less, (that Dr. Victor Marcial-Vega alluded to), should definitely help the circulation, and reduce the risk of blood clots as well. Two things that many could definitely benefit from, (especially anyone who had prior bypass surgery).

One reason why goji is my favorite is its potential for promoting longevity, which has been my primary focus for the past several years, and the reason I established the Longevity Research Center. In order to achieve longevity, we must learn how to avoid all life-threatening diseases. It all comes down to establishing a clean environment (by detoxification), along with a healthy pH, and then providing our body with the necessary nutrients, which should ideally come from natural sources. Only from an unhealthy environment in the body can disease establish and exist. Although most disease can be cured using the natural approach, our focus should always be on prevention. It's far easier to prevent disease, than it is to resolve it, and then repair the damage to the body they inflict.

I always set my goals rather high, and am constantly searching for answers. I believe I am aware of many solutions that even most natural practitioners are unaware of. It seems as though I have changed very little physically, (at least the past 20 years), and possibly even improved in some areas. I would consider that it might just be wishful thinking, if it wasn't for the recent comments from three different individuals. Recently, a lady who works at a local refuse disposal site where I have gone at least once monthly for the past 15 years, said *"You have been coming here for years, and never seem to change!"* Since then, a stone mason who worked here on a project over 9 years ago, came up to do some repairs. His first comment was *"You actually look younger than you did when I was working here."* And finally, I ran into a drywall contractor who was working on the same project, who said *"You seem to keep getting younger!"* None of them actually knew each other, and unless they were all wrong, possibly it's not just my imagination. I know that I actually have more endurance than I did 50 years ago when I first began my quest, although I was 30 pounds heavier back then. My retention and recall are definitely much better, as is my overall health, and at 75 I am totally drug-free. I figure that if Li Qing Yuen lived to be 252 by eating healthy, and consuming goji berries daily, that is something I should do as well, although I personally would prefer the goji juice.

The ORAC Scale

The Oxygen Radical Absorbance Capacity (ORAC) measurement is a standardized test adopted by the US Department of Agriculture to measure the Total Antioxidant Potency of foods and nutritional supplements. It provides us with a very precise way of determining the Free Radical destroying or neutralizing power of a particular food, supplement or compound. For example, raspberries have 1,220 ORAC units per 100 grams, while blueberries have 2,400, which is considerably higher than most fruits. However, Goji actually outdoes them all by far, with an amazing ORAC rating of 25,300! Dr. Duncan warns us that ORAC value has been used as a marketing tool by some manufacturers, and warns that *"Some goji, noni, and mangosteen blends are spiked to alter the ORAC value and make it higher. Pure, undiluted goji berries, noni fruit, and mangosteen fruit are the most medicinally beneficial."*

Hertz Measurement

This is another energy unit, named for the German physicist Heinrich Rudolf Hertz, who proved in 1887 that energy is transmitted through a vacuum by electromagnetic waves. According to the Hertz measurement, mangosteen measures 2,300 and goji measures 6,000.

The Bovis Energy Scale

Dr. Sandy Boice, Ph.D. explains:

Energy equates life. Fruits are designed to take the sun's life-giving energy and store it like a battery. Because of where goji grows, so close to the sun at such a high altitude, it is storing more of the sun's life-giving energy than any other fruit.

And we have some ways of measuring that. My favorite is called the Bovis Energy Scale, a scale for rating life energy. The human body is commonly 6,500. Some other functional beverages come in at 5,000 or 10,000, and one comes in at 17,000. But to help you understand the life-giving energy that specially prepared goji juice can deliver to your body, it comes in at 355,000, beyond anything else imaginable (*Breakthroughs In Health*, 2006, Vol. 1, Issue 1, pp. 60-61).

BOVIS ENERGY RATINGS:

Humans	6,500
Noni	17,000
Mangosteen	53,000
GOJI	**355,000**

Now that we've evaluated three of nature's miraculous resources with their many amazing benefits, you can easily see that all three juices have tremendous value individually, but could you imagine their potential collectively? You can also see some additional reasons why goji is my personal favorite: The outstanding ORAC scale, the Hertz measurement, and the truly amazing Bovis energy rating.

We will next determine how we can best evaluate the many products on the market in which they can be found. Both price and potency are important issues to consider.

How You Can Do Your Own Evaluations

My primary objective is to show you ways in which you can decide for yourself what products would provide the most benefit for your investment. It might be through an MLM company, and then again it might not. Learn how to evaluate, and then you can be the judge. If a product is only available through a multi-level marketing ("MLM") company, you will obviously have to get it through a distributor, and normally be required to sign up and pay to get it at the distributor price. If you don't know a distributor, the company should be able to assist you in finding one in your area. Sometimes a product is first announced through a MLM company (as XanGo™ was) and then later becomes available through other sources.

I might also suggest shopping around to find the best source of mangosteen, Chinese wolfberry (goji) juice, or Noni, if you would like to try them. First of all, check the ingredients so you will know exactly what you are paying for. I have found bottles of so-called mangosteen that were mostly water and reconstituted mangosteen. Even XanGo™ contains 8 other juices to enhance the flavor. Also check the sequence of the ingredients, as they are listed by highest quantity first, followed by lesser quantity. Although whole fruit mangosteen is the first entry in XanGo™, for instance, and thus the highest quantity, the next four entries are: apple fruit juice, pear fruit juice, grape fruit juice, and pear fruit puree. Although they do enhance the flavor, they also contain sugar, are relatively inexpensive, and in my opinion not nearly as beneficial as the mangosteen itself, or the remainder of the juices. The last five juices (smallest quantities) listed are: blueberry fruit juice, raspberry fruit juice, strawberry fruit juice, cranberry fruit juice, and cherry fruit juice. Of all the added juices, the blueberry is not only the highest on the ORAC scale, but also in my opinion the most beneficial, (other than the mangosteen). If you are not sure of the benefits of each juice, check them out on the Internet. It's to your advantage to learn how to do your own evaluation as much as possible.

The more juices added to the basic product, and the cheaper the juices added, the lower the cost to produce, and also the less benefit you will likely experience. You would likely be required to drink more XanGo™ (or any other product) for instance, to experience the benefit you are looking for, due to the dilution by other juices. The added juices do provide some benefit (some more than others), and they are normally added to enhance the flavor, as some people will not drink any juice, no matter how beneficial, if it doesn't taste good. However, the added juices can be counterproductive in treating conditions like diabetes, cancer, and candidiasis, in which sugar should be avoided. And, the two major diseases of greatest concern in the nation today, (diseases that most people die prematurely from), are cancer and diabetes. Cancer thrives on sugar, and excess sugar is the primary contributor to diabetes. So, doesn't it make more sense to use the juice with the benefits you are looking for, without any of the added sugar that we should be avoiding?

How the fruit is processed is also an important issue in order to assure the phytochemicals and enzymes in the original fruit remain intact. In order to receive the most benefit from any product for your investment, be sure and read the labels and do a little research. You will soon discover that there is often a major difference between the content of the primary ingredient, as well as the quality of different products, based on processing. As companies are continually producing new products in an attempt to corner as much of the market as possible, I will just show you some examples, and explain how you can learn to evaluate them for yourself. Unless you are well informed, you could quite easily pay twice as much for one product as you might for a comparable product, due not only to the processing or dilution, but also how good they are at marketing, so learn to become an informed consumer. Doing a little homework is well worth the effort, especially if you plan to consume it for a few years.

Although the XanGo™ seems to provide a fairly broad range of benefits, it does seem to take fairly high doses to resolve some of the most serious health conditions. Two ounces, three times a day, is recommended for resolving major health issues, which is why many people drink the juice. At six ounces a day, and only 25.35 ounces in a bottle, one bottle would last slightly over four days, and for a couple, it would last only half that long.

It appears from Dr. Templeman's experience, that the mangosteen has a great deal of potential for resolving many different health issues, and if you compare the cost with that of many medications, (which only suppress symptoms), it's still much more cost effective. Unfortunately, your insurance is not about to compensate you for your XanGo™, or any other juice for that matter, no matter how beneficial it might be. I believe we all owe a debt of gratitude to both Dr. Templeman and Dr. Morton, for evaluating and documenting the many benefits of mangosteen.

At least if you're like me, and avoiding disease and maintaining optimum health is a high priority, and the reason you are taking supplements, your top priority is likely not the taste, but experiencing optimum benefit. You will find that some companies who dilute the primary juice with the benefit you are looking for (such as mangosteen or goji) with other much cheaper juices tend to focus a great deal on how good they taste. At least if I were looking for taste, I would likely opt for a pineapple malt, although that's something I only do about once or twice a year.

There is absolutely no reason why you can't buy your own apple or grape juice (or any other juice for that matter) and mix your own if you like. You can usually find a large 64-ounce bottle of either apple or grape juice for less than two dollars. If you purchase the 100% undiluted juice you at least know exactly how much of the beneficial juice you are getting. I recently learned of a company that produces all three juices in a pure undiluted form, from a friend who owns a health food store. The good news is, you can likely find it at your local health food store, and are not required to pay a fee and sign up with some MLM company just for the privilege of acquiring their highly diluted juice. It might be OK for someone interested in multi-level marketing, but I believe the majority of people are like me, and have other priorities in life.

Personally, I can't in good conscience promote anything that I don't truly believe in myself, and was quite amazed when I discovered just how little of the mangosteen, goji, or noni are in many products, which normally just tend to focus on how good they taste, (something we can all do with a little creativity). Although some people do seem to experience considerable benefit from some of the diluted products, fairly high dosages are normally required to get real results; something many can't afford on an ongoing basis, (at least unless they are making up for it by making a profit "doing the business"). From my experiences over the years, it appears that the people who normally make a good income doing an MLM business, are often the husband/wife teams, whose lives are basically dedicated to the business. They are the ones companies tend to use as examples to recruit new distributors. Although some make money doing the business, in my opinion the majority of their products tend to be overpriced, (even at distributor prices). That seems to be especially true regarding some of the "highly diluted" juices.

The undiluted noni, goji, and mangosteen, which I recently learned about, are produced by a company called Genesis™ Today, owned and operated by the very knowledgeable and highly respected Dr. Lindsay Duncan, N.D., C.N., whose mentor for years was the highly respected nutritionist Bernard Jensen. Dr. Duncan tends to focus on quality, which Dr. Gary Young of Young Living™ also does with his quality essential oils. Dr. Young does produce a product called Berry Young Juice™, which contains goji juice. Of all the diluted juices I researched, his is in my opinion the best. According to his chemist, the Berry Young Juice™ actually contains 53% goji. It also contains the more beneficial juices such as blueberry, as well as lemon and orange essential oils.

Another product called Himalayan Goji juice, formulated by Dr. Earl Mindell and marketed by the MLM company FreeLife™ International, appears to contain considerably less reconstituted goji juice, combined with grape juice concentrate, pear juice concentrate, apple juice concentrate, pear puree, and natural flavor. As you can easily see, the added juices are some of the least expensive to produce.

Although Dr. Young's formulation is "much more expensive to produce," and should in my opinion, be much more beneficial than Dr. Mindell's formulation, it's still not 100% goji, and is only sold through MLM, so you are required to purchase it through a distributor. I met Dr. Young several years ago, and recently met Dr. Mindell. Although Dr. Young's primary focus appeared to be on the quality of products, (especially essential oils), Dr. Mindell's focus seemed instead to be more on marketing, something he is apparently very successful at. According to Dr. Mindell, he lives in Beverly Hills, not far from Larry King. Definitely a high rent district!

In Summary – Additional Considerations

Just keep in mind that each of the three nature's miracles that we just discussed, have their own particular benefits, although some are at times very similar. Also keep in mind that the dilution (if any), the dosage, and how long a person might be taking any of the juices, are all important factors. Our bio-individuality, as well as our diet and supplements, (or medications), come into play as well. So basically, no two people would likely experience the same benefits from the same dosage of the very same juice. Our age and overall health, (and especially the condition of our liver), are determining factors as well.

I don't know about you, but optimum health and longevity are my goals. Thus I plan to take advantage of the benefits of all three, and in the pure undiluted form, in order to assure the best overall results. Each juice has its very own phytochemicals (plant based nutrients), and thus unique benefits we can benefit from. Also, keep in mind that not everyone would necessarily agree on which juice they might consider as the most beneficial. As I plan to use all three, it doesn't really matter. Hopefully you now have sufficient information necessary for drawing your own (informed) conclusion.

ANOTHER VALUABLE RESOURCE – CELTIC SEA SALT

Although we normally think of salt as the kind of table salt that most people consume, all forms of salt are not the same. The white refined table salt that is cheap and convenient, and is consequently added to most, if not all processed foods. It consists solely of sodium chloride with a little aluminum added so it will flow more freely, and in some cases iodine is also added. Aluminum is not only a carcinogen, but is also suspected of creating problems in the brain (possibly contributing to Alzheimer's disease).

Celtic Sea Salt, (which I have used the past 15 years), has no added ingredients, is slightly damp, and light gray in color, as it contains many minerals. The salt ionizes with the clay in the marshes in an area in northern France, known as Brittany, where the pristine seawater is free of pollution. Any future reference I make to sea salt will be referring to the Celtic Sea salt, imported only by the *Grain and Salt Society*, available at any health food store or by mail order. I might add that I do not sell salt, and am not in any way associated with the *Grain and Salt Society* that imports and sells it. However, I use it myself, because it is much healthier than common table salt and contains so many important minerals. Many of these minerals are important to assure that our neurons can function effectively, and unfortunately are missing from the common table salt most people use.

Celtic sea salt contains at least 84 known minerals, all natural and in an ionized easily assimilatable form, which makes them effective at much lower doses than most minerals normally found in supplements. **In nature, trace elements are found in trace (minute) amounts, and that is why they are referred to as trace minerals. These trace minerals, found in trace amounts in nature, are also found in this salt. Dr. Jacques de Langre, Ph.D., author of the book *Seasalt's Hidden Powers* (1992) stresses this important issue when he states that *"macro-nutrients* as well as *trace elements should never be taken carelessly in any quantity"* (p. 21).**

The salt, as found in nature, is critical for our health, and is an important issue that many doctors are totally unaware of, as many often recommend that their patients avoid salt. In common table salt the potassium is removed, and sodium by itself causes water retention. Sodium and potassium work together synergistically to get the nutrients into each cell and the toxins out. This very critical process is referred to as the sodium- potassium pump. Although the Celtic sea salt also contains the trace element organic iodine, important for healthy thyroid function, the common iodized table salt actually contains an excessive level of inorganic iodine instead. And even though a trace amount of iodine is important for producing the thyroid hormone, an excessive level of iodine can actually suppress the normal thyroid function. There are some things that the body needs only in trace amounts, and iodine is one of them.

A major difference between table salt and Celtic sea salt is that any excess table salt is not always adequately excreted. It can solidify and harden in the kidneys, and thus can contribute to some kidney problems, although Celtic sea salt won't. Quoting Dr. de Langre (*Seasalt's Hidden Powers*, 1992), *"Unrefined Celtic Salt has the opposite effect: its sodium drains out rapidly, keeping the kidneys at peak function, as well as promoting flexibility in the articulations"* (p. 87). Healthy kidneys and joints sounds like a much better option to me.

Celtic sea salt also helps prevent over-acidity. Although the regular processed table salt that most people consume daily is actually acidic, Celtic sea salt is instead alkaline. Incidentally, cancer thrives in an acidic environment, as it contributes to the depletion of available oxygen.

You have just learned two little-known, but very beneficial resources that can assist you with your efforts toward a drug-free approach to maintain your health. We will now be looking at three true-life personal experiences, and discover just how easy it is to eliminate the need for several prescription medications, and normally do so in only one or two months.

CHAPTER NINE
AL'S STORY –
A Body-Builder's (Seemingly Mysterious) Muscle Loss

If anyone should be considered as a poster boy, regarding the dangers associated with statin (cholesterol lowering) medications, I believe a friend of mine named Al would have definitely made a prime candidate. Al, a retired professor, had been a professional body-builder since his teens, and even claims he once worked out with Arnold Schwarzneger. I met Al a several years ago at the spa where we both work out. We had never really discussed any health issues, until one day after discovering that I was a doctor, he voiced a major health concern, and wondered if I had any idea what his problem might possibly be. He indicated that he had been experiencing increasing difficulty working out, excruciating muscle pain, and extreme fatigue. He had also been experiencing more difficulty remembering things, although he had a good memory in the past. He said, *"Dave, I feel like I'm checking out,"* indicating that he basically felt like his days were numbered. I noticed he looked extremely fatigued after a workout, and usually sat and rested about a half-hour after completing his workout.

Some of my observations were: Although I only worked out approximately one-half hour, twice a week, I discovered that Al normally worked out four times a week, for at least one hour. Although I did work out when I was younger, I was never a serious weight lifter or body-builder, like Al was. I saw a picture of Al at 60 years of age, and he was in terrific shape, with solid muscle and no visible fat, and he actually looked about half his age.

The mystery seemed to be that only 15 years later, at 75, something obviously went wrong. Al's muscles were almost entirely gone, as if he had liposuction and someone accidentally removed the muscle tissue instead of the fat, and then he all of a sudden grew fat tissue mostly around the midsection. On the surface, this major transition made absolutely no sense. For instance, at the time I was 71 years old, and Al was 75. Although he was in terrific shape only 15 years prior, he seemed to have suddenly lost it all, and for no apparent reason. I personally am in much better condition now than I was 50 years ago, and also 30 pounds lighter. That is when I first learned the importance of a healthy diet, and adequate supplementation, along with exercise (something I had failed to maintain). My current weight, as well as my muscle-to-fat ratio is approximately the same as it was when in my late teens and early twenties. Even though I only work out about one-forth as many hours a week as Al did, I currently have even more strength and endurance than I did fifty years ago. I also noticed that I was doing considerably more weight than Al was, which didn't seem at all logical. Nothing seemed to add up, as Al was much more knowledgeable than I in exercise physiology, and optimum muscle building exercise strategy, from years of bodybuilding experience. According to Al, although his diet, supplementation, and exercise routine had basically remained the same, his physique had somehow made a dramatic metamorphosis, and unfortunately in the wrong direction.

So, when Al voiced his concerns regarding his rapid and seemingly unexplainable deterioration and fatigue, I suggested we get together and see if we could possibly identify his problem. I asked him to bring with him a list of any the medications, and supplements that he might be taking. It didn't take long to identify the basic underlying problem, which would have a much more dramatic influence on Al than it would with the average individual who exercises very little. As usual, the problem was associated with his medications.

One thing that seemed quite obvious, Al had been rapidly trading muscle tissue for fat. Fortunately, this process can be stopped, just by discontinuing the medications responsible for creating the problem, and then restoring the important nutrients they had been depleting, although actually getting back to where he could have and should have been, would be rather difficult. Al had not only lost a considerable amount of muscle, but he had also gained 18 pounds (mostly fat tissue). Although his first prescribed medication, the blood thinner Coumadin™, was likely responsible for some of his disturbing side effects, the cholesterol lowering drug Zocor™ was a major contributor to the problem. That is especially true when combined with the beta-blocker medication Atenolol, which his doctor also prescribed for high blood pressure. Of primary concern is Zocor's depletion of CoQ_{10}, a major energy molecule for all muscles in the body (including the heart), as well as the mitochondria in the brain. As it turns out, the blood pressure medication Atenolol also depletes CoQ_{10}! I might add that both deplete several other important nutrients as well.

To make matters even worse, after about 7 months Al's doctor somehow decided to double his dosage of Zocor™ from 20 mg to 40 mg. Then, after another 7 months (the magic number), he decided Al's already doubled dosage should again be doubled to 80 mg (now 4 times the original dosage). For some unknown reason, his doctor chose not to discuss what his cholesterol level actually was. The same applied to his blood pressure reading when the blood pressure medication was prescribed. Al indicated that his blood pressure had typically run lower than normal his entire life.

Then, to add insult to injury, Al's doctor somehow felt it necessary to prescribe another cholesterol lowering drug called Colestid™. Al indicated that he only took a few doses, as his stomach was soon in such a state of chaos that he had difficulty keeping anything down. He said he also found it extremely difficult to swallow his vitamins. Every muscle in the body (including those in the throat important for swallowing) became weakened. What a terrible disservice some doctors are doing to their patients.

So that you can better see the damage for yourself, following are the four medications Al was on, with an evaluation of each: The **side effects** in bold print are those Al had been experiencing.

Drug #1: Atenolol = generic name / Tenormin™

Beta-blocker, used to lower blood pressure, lower heart rate, reduce chest pain (angina), and reduce the risk of recurrent heart attacks.

❖ **Nutrients depleted: Magnesium, phosphorus, potassium, sodium, zinc, and Coenzyme Q_{10}.**

You may notice a tingling feeling on your scalp when you first begin to take this medication.

Common side effects include: **Breathing difficulty and/or wheezing, cold hands and feet, mental depression, shortness of breath, slow heartbeat (especially less than 50 beats per minute), swelling of ankles, feet, and/or lower legs,** decreased sexual ability, **dizziness or lightheadedness,** drowsiness (slight), trouble in sleeping, vertigo, **unusual tiredness or weakness, weight gain.**

Rare side effects include: Back pain or joint pain, chest pain, **confusion (especially in elderly patients),** dark urine, dizziness or lightheadedness when getting up from a lying or sitting position, fever and sore throat, **hallucinations (seeing, hearing, or feeling things that are not there), irregular heartbeat,** red, scaling, or crusted skin, skin rash, **unusual bleeding and bruising,** yellow eyes or skin.

Other side effects may include: **Anxiety and/or nervousness,** changes in taste, constipation, diarrhea, dry or sore eyes, frequent urination, itching of skin, nausea or vomiting, nightmares and vivid dreams, **numbness and/or tingling of fingers and/or toes,** numbness and/or tingling of skin, (especially scalp), stomach discomfort.

After you have been taking a beta-blocker for a while, it may cause unpleasant or even harmful effects if you stop taking it too suddenly. After you stop taking this medicine or while you are gradually reducing the amount you are taking, you may experience chest pain, fast or irregular heartbeat, general feeling of discomfort or illness or weakness, headache, shortness of breath (sudden), sweating or trembling.

If you have a history of severe congestive heart failure, Tenormin should be used with caution. Tenormin should not be stopped suddenly. It can cause increased chest pain and heart attack. Dosage should be gradually reduced.

If you suffer from asthma, seasonal allergies, or other bronchial conditions, coronary artery disease or kidney disease, this medication should be used with caution.

This medication may mask the symptoms of low blood sugar or alter blood sugar levels. Diabetics should use with caution.

Possible interactions:

- Heart medication such as nifedipine (Procardia, Adalat), reserpine (Serpasil), verapamil (Calan, Verelan, Isoptin), diltiazem (Cardizem, Dilacor XR), clonidine (Catapres), digoxin (Lanoxin), doxazosin (Cardura), guanadrel (Hylorel), prazosin (Minipress), or terazosin (Hytrin)
- Diabetes medication such as insulin, glyburide (Micronase, Glynase, Diabeta), glipizide (Glucotrol), chlorpropamide (Diabinese), or metformin (Glucophage);
- Nonsteroidal anti-inflammatory drugs (NSAID) such as ibuprofen (Motrin, Advil, others), naproxen (Aleve, Anaprox, Naprosyn, others), ketoprofen (Orudis, Orudis KT, Oruvail), and others
- Respiratory medication such as Albuterol (Ventolin, Proventil, Volmax, others), bitolterol (Tornalate), metaproterenol (Alupent, Metaprel), pirbuterol (Maxair), terbutaline (Brethaire, Brethine, Bricanyl), or theophylline (Theo-Dur, Theochron, Theolair, others)
- **Stomach medication cimetidine (Tagamet, Tagamet HB); or**
- **Prescription or over-the-counter cough medicines, cold medicines, or diet pills.**
- Ampicillin (omnipen, others)
- **Calcium-containing antacids (Tums)**
- Calcium-blocking blood pressure drugs such as Calan and Cardizem
- Certain other blood pressure drugs such as reserpine (Diupres)
- Epinephrine (EpiPen)
- Indomethacin (Indocin)
- Insulin
- Oral diabetes drugs such as Micronase
- Quinidine (Quinidex)

MY OBSERVATION: The three items underlined above are typical medications commonly used to treat the potential side effects associated with both the statins, Zocor™ and Colestipol, which Al was also taking.

Drug #2: Colestid™ / generic name = Colestipol

A bile acid sequestrant (cholesterol-lowering non-statin drug).

❖ **Nutrients depleted: Vitamin A and beta carotene, vitamin B$_{12}$, vitamin C, folic acid, vitamin D, vitamin E, vitamin K, calcium, iron, magnesium, phosphorus, zinc, and Coenzyme Q$_{10}$.**

Long-term use of Colestipol may be connected to increased bleeding, from a lack of vitamin K.

Most common side effects may include: Constipation, worsening of hemorrhoids.

Less common or rare side effects may include: **Abdominal bloating or distention/cramping/pain, aches and pains in arms and legs, angina (crushing chest pain), anxiety, arthritis,** backache, belching, bleeding hemorrhoids, blood in stool, bone pain, chest pain, diarrhea, **dizziness,** drowsiness, **fatigue,** gas, headache, **heartburn,** hives, **indigestion,** insomnia, **joint pain,** light-headedness, loose stools, loss of appetite, migraine, **muscle pain,** nausea, **rapid heartbeat**, rash, **shortness of breath,** sinus headache, skin inflammation, **swelling of hands or feet,** vertigo, vomiting, **weakness.**

MY OBSERVATIONS:
      Rapid heartbeat is listed as a side effect, which would increase the blood pressure. Al was prescribed the beta-blocker Atenolol for this condition, to slow down the heart!
      Both heartburn and indigestion are listed as side effects. There is a risk when taking medication for indigestion or heartburn, while also taking the beta-blocker Atenolol. Al's prescribed Zocor™ also lists heartburn as a common side effect.
       The side effects underlined above are symptoms Al began to experience shortly after being placed on Colestipol.

If Colestid is taken with certain other drugs, the effects of either drug could be increased, decreased, or altered. **It is especially important to check with your doctor before combining Colestid with the following:**

- **Anticoagulants (blood thinners) – The effects of the anticoagulant may be altered**

- Digitalis glycosides (heart medicine)
- Diuretics (water pills) *(MY NOTE:* **Swelling of hands or feet** *were listed as possible side effects associated with Atenolol)*
- Penicillin G, taken by mouth, or
- Propranolol, taken by mouth, or
- Tetracyclines (medicine for infection), taken by mouth, or
- Thyroid hormones or
- Vancomycin, taken by mouth—Colestipol may cause these medicines to be less effective; these medicines should be taken 4 to 5 hours apart from Colestipol

Tell your doctor your medical history, especially if you suffer from: constipation, hemorrhoids, diabetes, phenylketonuria (PKU), low thyroid hormone levels (hypothyroidism), stomach/intestinal disease, gall bladder disease, kidney disease, liver disease, unusual bleeding or bruising, any allergies.

Drug #3: Zocor™ / generic name = Simvastatin

An HMG CoA reductase inhibitor (statin cholesterol-lowering drug) that blocks the production of cholesterol (a type of fat) in the body.

❖ **Nutrients depleted: Vitamin A, vitamin B$_{12}$, folic acid, vitamin D, vitamin E, vitamin K, Coenzyme Q$_{10}$, calcium, magnesium, iron, phosphorus, and zinc.**

Common side effects may include: Constipation, diarrhea, gas, headache, nausea, stomach pain, <u>**heartburn.**</u>

Less common side effects may include: Fever, **muscle aches, unusual tiredness or weakness, severe stomach pain**, insomnia, <u>**upper respiratory infections, weight gain.**</u>

MY OBSERVATION: See "possible interactions" regarding Atenolol, the beta-blocker. Medications to treat the side effects underlined above are risky while taking Atenolol.

Tell your doctor if you have or have ever had liver, kidney, or heart disease; a severe infection; low blood pressure; or seizures.

<u>**Since Zocor may cause damage to muscle tissue,** be sure to tell your doctor of any unexplained muscle tenderness, weakness,</u> or pain right away, especially if you also have a fever or feel sick.

MY OBSERVATION: The warning Al never saw was the potential for damage to the muscle tissue. Obviously not what a body-builder would consider if he was alerted to the potential risk. Apparently the weight gain listed would be associated with an increase of fat tissue (not muscle).

Possible interactions:

- Cyclosporine (Sandimmune, Neoral)
- Gemfibrozil (Lopid), clofibrate (Atromid-S), or fenofibrate (Tricor)
- Niacin (Nicolar, Nicobid, Slo-Niacin, others)
- Erythromycin (E-Mycin, E.E.S., Ery-Tab, others) or clarithromycin (Biaxin)
- **Cholestyramine (Questran) or colestipol (Colestid)** *(MY NOTE: Also prescribed – a potential risk)*
- An antifungal medication such as itraconazole (Sporanox), fluconazole (Diflucan), or ketoconazole (Nizoral)
- Nefazodone (Serzone)
- **Warfarin (Coumadin)** *(MY NOTE: Also prescribed – another potential risk!)*
- Digoxin (Lanoxin, Lanoxicaps)
- A protease inhibitor such as amprenavir (Agenerase), indinavir (Crixivan), nelfinavir (Viracept), ritonavir (Norvir), lopinavir-ritonavir (Kaletra), or saquinavir (Invirase, Fortovase)
- Amiodarone (Cordarone, Pacer one)
- Verapamil (Calan, Covera-HS, Isoptin, Verelan)

Alcohol increases the side effects caused by simvastatin.

If you are having surgery, including dental surgery, tell the doctor or dentist that you are taking simvastatin.

Plan to avoid unnecessary or prolonged exposure to sunlight and to wear protective clothing, sunglasses, and sunscreen. Simvastatin may make your skin sensitive to sunlight.

Drug #4: Coumadin™ / generic name = Warfarin

An anticoagulant (blood thinner).

❖ **Nutrients depleted: Vitamin B^{12}, C and K.**

Blocks the absorption of vitamin K. *(MY OBSERVATION: Both Colestipol and Zocor™ also deplete vitamin K)*

More common side effects may include: Hemorrhage: Signs of severe bleeding resulting in the loss of large amounts of blood depend upon the location and extent of bleeding. **Symptoms include: chest, abdomen, joint, muscle, or other pain; difficult breathing or swallowing; dizziness;** headache; low blood pressure; numbness and tingling; **paralysis; shortness of breath**; unexplained shock; **unexplained swelling; weakness.**

Less common side effects may include: **Abdominal pain and cramping, allergic reactions,** diarrhea, **fatigue,** feeling cold and chills, feeling of illness, fever, **fluid retention and swelling,** gas and bloating, **hepatitis,** hives, intolerance to cold, itching, lethargy, <u>liver damage,</u> loss of hair, nausea, <u>**necrosis (gangrene),**</u> **pain,** purple toes, rash, severe or long-lasting inflammation of the skin, taste changes, vomiting, **weight gain,** yellowed skin and eyes.

(MY NOTE: Although the liver damage and gangrene underlined were not experienced by Al, they are extremely dangerous conditions I called your attention to.)

Possible interactions:

- Amiodarone (e.g., Cordarone)
- **Cimetidine (e.g., Tagamet)**
- Metronidazole (e.g., Flagyl)
- **Omeprazole (e.g., Prilosec)**
- Zafirlukast (e.g., Accolate)—Effects of anticoagulants may be increased because of slower removal from the body

MY OBSERVATION: Tagamet and Prilosec (both available over-the-counter) are often taken to relieve the side effect of indigestion and heartburn associated with the statin drugs Colestipol and Zocor™. This could create an undesirable drug interaction.

- Anabolic steroids (nandrolone [e.g., Anabolin], oxandrolone [e.g., Anavar], oxymetholone [e.g., Anadrol], stanozolol [e.g., Winstrol]) o
- Androgens (male hormones)
- Antifungals, azole (e.g., Diflucan)
- Antithyroid agents (medicine for overactive thyroid)
- Aspirin or other salicylates, including bismuth subsalicylate (e.g., Pepto-Bismol)
- Cephalosporins (medicine for infection)
- Cinchophen
- Clofibrate (e.g., Abitrate, Atromid-S)
- Danazol (e.g., Danocrine)
- Dextrothyroxine
- Diflunisal

- Disulfiram (e.g., Antabuse)
- Fluvoxamine (e.g., Luvox)
- Inflammation or pain medicine (except narcotics)
- Lepirudin (e.g., Refludan)
- Medications causing low platelet count
- Paroxetine (e.g., Paxil)
- Propafenone (e.g., Rythmol)
- Quinidine (e.g., Quinidex)
- Sertraline (e.g., Zoloft)
- Sulfapyridine
- Sulfasalazine (e.g., Azulfidine)
- Thyroid hormones
- Ticlopidine (e.g., Ticlid)
- Zileuton (e.g., Zyflo)—These medications may increase the effects of anticoagulants and may increase the chance of bleeding

- Carbenicillin by injection (e.g., Geopen)
- Dipyridamole (e.g., Persantine)
- Divalproex (e.g., Depakote)
- Moxalactam (e.g., Moxam)
- Pentoxifylline (e.g., Trantal)
- Plicamycin (e.g., Mithracin)
- Sulfinpyrazone (e.g., Anturane)
- Thrombolytic agents (medicine for blood clots)
- Ticarcillin (e.g., Ticar)
- Valproic acid (e.g., Depakene)—Using any of these medicines together with anticoagulants may increase the chance of bleeding

- Alcohol (with chronic use)
- Barbiturates or
- Carbamazepine (e.g., Tegretol)
- Corticosteroids (cortisone-like medicine)
- Glutethimide (e.g., Doriden)
- Griseofulvin (e.g., Fulvicin)
- Phenylbutazone (e.g., Butazolidin)
- Phenytoin (e.g., Dilantin)
- Primidone (e.g., Mysoline)
- Rifampin (e.g., Rifadin)—Effects of anticoagulants may be decreased because of faster removal from the body

- Vitamin K (e.g., AquaMEPHYTON)—Vitamin K helps produce some important blood clotting factors and may decrease the effects of anticoagulants if used at the same time

The presence of other medical problems may affect the use of anticoagulants. Many medical problems and treatments will affect the way your body responds to this medicine. **Make sure you tell your doctor if you have *any* other medical problems, or if you have recently had any of the following conditions or medical procedures, especially Aneurysm (swelling in a blood vessel) especially in the head or chest, or bleeding in the brain**

MY OBSERVATION: Taking Coumadin, which blocks the absorption of vitamin K, along with the other two statin drugs that are also known to deplete vitamin K, could additionally increase the risk of a stroke from an aneurysm. A vitamin K deficiency also causes a calcification (hardening) of the arteries, leading to another cardiovascular risk factor. Vitamin K is important for escorting calcium to the bones where it is needed.

- Blood disorders or diseases, especially thrombocytopenia (low platelet count), polycythemia (high red blood cell count), or leukemia
- Bruising, excessive
- Cancer of the internal organs, especially of the abdomen
- Childbirth, recent
- Diabetes mellitus (sugar diabetes)
- Diverticulitis
- Falls or blows to the body or head
- Heart infection
- Hemophilia or other bleeding problems
- **Hypertension (high blood pressure)** *(MY NOTE: Atenolol also prescribed is a potential risk)*
- Inflammation of blood vessels
- Intestinal problems, especially conditions that may affect the absorption of food or vitamins
- Liver disease
- Pregnancy, terminated
- Spinal anesthetics or spinal puncture
- Surgery, major, especially of the head or eye, or dental surgery
- Toxemia of pregnancy
- Ulcers, active, of the stomach, lung, or urinary tract
- Vitamin K deficiency
- Wounds, open, surgical or from an ulcer—These conditions may increase the chance of bleeding

MY OBSERVATION: As you can easily see, Coumadin™ is extremely risky, as it can interact with so many different medications and conditions.

Now let's see if we can play Crime Scene Investigators (CSI) and attempt to identify and convict the responsible parties. The first thing that comes to mind is: How can a couple medications that so many in the nation are currently taking, create so much chaos and turn muscle into fat in less than two years, while also depleting energy levels in the process? And we can't forget that we also have a retired professor, who has mysteriously become the proverbial "Absent-minded Professor". On the surface, it sounds more like fiction than fact, but Al can easily verify its authenticity, as I can just from observation.

CoQ$_{10}$ just happens to be the key player in the mystery. The basic problem stems from the increasing CoQ$_{10}$ depletion, from two different sources, especially along with eventually quadrupling the dosage of the biggest thief of cellular energy of all (Zocor™), which is by far our most likely suspect. But, we are also dealing with an accomplice who has the same basic objective of stealing CoQ$_{10}$, while at the same time lowering the heart rate (double jeopardy). That is just one more way of stealing Al's energy. If you then consider that a dedicated body-builder normally combines aerobic exercise with a rigorous weight-training routine during every workout, you definitely have a seriously incompatible combination, when combined with Al's medications.

A warm-up with aerobic exercise usually comes first. One primary objective of aerobic exercise is to increase the heart rate. But we can easily see who was attempting to undermine Al's success in that respect: Mr. Beta-blocker. His job is to keep Al's blood pressure lower by reducing his heart rate, and to stop it from increasing to meet the need of an increased demand for oxygen. Two major sources of energy for the hundreds of mitochondria (energy sites) for each cell are oxygen and CoQ_{10}, along with the third major source glucose. So the combination of Zocor™ and Atenolol are busy stealing two of our three resources. Our accomplice, Mr. Beta-blocker, will then ensure that sufficient oxygen will not be available, thus the glucose is not efficiently metabolized. This basically leads to two problems: (1) The production of lactic acid, and (2) Carbon monoxide instead of carbon dioxide. The lactic acid from anaerobic (oxygen deficient) metabolism not only causes muscle pain, but it can only be metabolized in the liver with the assistance of (guess who?), oxygen. If sufficient oxygen is unavailable for the conversion of lactic acid, this can contribute to a very unhealthy condition known as acidosis (low pH). This unhealthy condition then leads to oxygen depletion, as an acidic condition results in the reduction of available oxygen. You might temporarily side step the oxygen deficiency issue, but there is no way around the problem.

We still have the carbon monoxide issue to deal with. Normal respiration with sufficient oxygen is not a problem, as carbon dioxide is easily expelled in the lungs so the red blood cells can effectively pick up more oxygen. The problem is, carbon monoxide is much more tenacious than carbon dioxide. As a result, fewer red blood cells will be able to pick up and deliver an adequate supply of oxygen. Thus anaerobic (oxygen deficient) respiration (energy production) is obviously less efficient.

Another major concern is: We are also creating a perfect environment for cancer to thrive. Most people who contract cancer have a pH of 4.5 to 5.0 (very acidic). Cancer also thrives in an anaerobic environment, which are basically the two conditions being created by Al's medications. One more contributor to cancer is free radicals, and the harder we work out or exercise in general, the more free radicals will be produced. In addition to the primary function of CoQ_{10} of energy production, it also serves as a very effective antioxidant. So as we can see, we are contributing to cancer by allowing the free radicals to damage DNA unchecked. A person can often have cancer for ten years or more before it is detected.

I can't help but question the necessity of Al's doctor prescribing the blood pressure medication. The primary reason for my conclusion is: According to Al, his blood pressure had typically run low his entire life. Many who check their own blood pressure at home find that it invariably tests higher than normal when going to the doctor (the White Coat syndrome). Possibly doctors might consider wearing a different color jacket. All too often, doctors' recommendations are based on a new idea that the once acceptable blood pressure level should now be lowered. Unfortunately, this is an all too common occurrence in medicine today, especially regarding the recommended levels of both blood pressure and cholesterol (obviously a very successful marketing strategy).

According to Al, his doctor never discussed his blood pressure or cholesterol levels when he was originally placed on the medication, or when the dosages were arbitrarily doubled. They could easily have been borderline, which might have been perfectly acceptable the day before the announcement. The companies who produce the drugs have learned effective ways to influence the announcements made on the National News, regarding the now lower acceptable levels of blood pressure and cholesterol. Each time the determination is somehow made that they should be lowered (by authorities willing to make a statement for a price), most doctors immediately respond accordingly.

Considering that Al had been an avid body-builder for years, it makes absolutely no sense to prescribe a beta-blocker to lower his heart rate, if that was really a concern (which I doubt). I know beyond a doubt that his cholesterol level wasn't, and never will be a problem. In most cases, the blood pressure can be controlled without medication, especially when the patient is not diabetic, which was the case with Al. If medication was somehow necessary for lowering blood pressure, there are options other than beta-blockers available. Anyone who is physically active, or exercises on a regular basis such as Al, does not belong on a beta-blocker! I can't begin to stress that importance enough. Beta-blockers not only reduce the available oxygen, but also the level of the energy molecule CoQ_{10}, (as does Zocor™), thus you are creating an unhealthy and potentially dangerous environment, especially when combined with exercise. I believe we now have sufficient evidence to prove our case, and convict the responsible parties.

So, we will now call our star witness (the victim) to come forward and allow him to describe his experiences, in his own words, and how he managed to resolve the problem:

During the time I was on these prescription drugs, I began to experience a number of disturbing side effects, which included:

1. *Dizziness and difficulty in maintaining balance*
2. *Increased loss of short-term memory*
3. *Extreme tiredness*
4. *Constipation*
5. *Insomnia*
6. *Lack of appetite*
7. *Extreme upset stomach*
8. *Shortness of breath **
9. *Heavy pressure in chest **
10. *Lack of energy **
11. *Dramatic loss of strength **
12. *Extreme muscle soreness **

* Numbers 8 – 12 were felt especially during physical exercise.

It was becoming more difficult each day to maintain normal exercise routines due to these side effects. There was a continual lowering of weights used and repetitions of the exercises at each workout. This resulted in a dramatic decrease in muscle strength and size.

On 5 November 2004, I stopped taking all of the drugs that had been prescribed for me by my primary care physician.

The change in my overall health since abandoning my prescription drug therapy has been nothing short of remarkable. Within days, I began to feel the many positive changes that were beginning to occur in my body. Up to this date, all of the bad side effects that I experienced while on drug therapy have vanished. My short-term memory loss has greatly improved and getting better. My workout routines have improved beyond my expectations. I go through my exercise routines with great vigor and intensity. I no longer suffer with intense muscle pain and my muscle mass has increased and it is apparent by the weights used and repetitions completed that my muscle strength has returned to a normal level (and beyond).

I truly feel that I was never a candidate for any sort of prescription drug therapy. I have led a healthy and active life with only a few physical problems. It was only when I started taking prescription drugs that my body responded in a very negative way.

Unfortunately, Al learned the hard way, that you can easily spend the better part of a lifetime building muscle, and suddenly experience a rapid deterioration of that hard-earned muscle. Unfortunately, although exercise is important to our health, it can be catabolic (destructive to muscle tissue), when adequate supplies of CoQ_{10} and oxygen are insufficient or missing.

There is also an additional possibility we still haven't addressed. Statin drugs can easily lead to dangerously low levels of cholesterol, which is important for healthy cells as well as many hormones, including testosterone for building muscle. When testosterone levels decrease in a man, muscle is gradually replaced by fat tissue.

As we can easily see, there is a good explanation for the rapid loss of muscle tissue, along with the seemingly unexplainable increase in fat tissue. As we learned, the verdict is in, and the apparent mystery finally solved, with the two guilty parties being Mr. Cholesterol-Stomper Zocor™ (for a non-disease!), along with his accomplice Mr. Beta-Blocker Atenolol. Although Al had to learn the hard way – hopefully you won't! However, for anyone desiring to replace muscle tissue with fat, we now have a perfect solution. Just keep in mind that along with your statin drugs and beta-blockers, it will require a considerable amount of effort on your part. In order to experience the most effective conversion from muscle to fat, you must exercise, exercise, exercise!

The Basic Problem – Standard Medical Protocol

I considered calling Al's primary care physician to the stand, but I already know what his response would likely have been: *"I just adhered to standard protocol along with following the most recent recommendations."* Every single person I encountered who had been taking statin medications, recently indicated that their doctor recommended doubling the dosage, irrespective of their current cholesterol level, (two were already dangerously low). Most had no idea what their level was at the time the recommendation was made.

So How Did Al's Doctor Respond To His Discovery?

Incidentally, Al felt this was a major issue his doctor should be aware of, so he gave him a copy of the part of my book focusing on the cholesterol issue and the dangers associated with the medications that he had been prescribed. He also explained how much improvement he had made after stopping his medications.

At the next appointment, his doctor basically skirted the whole issue. When he asked his doctor if he read the information, his response was ***"I don't have time to read that stuff."*** Apparently his doctor got burned out from all the required reading while in medical school. Unfortunately, a lot of his effort was wasted on inaccurate information. Even though Al had described his terrible experiences from taking the medications, and how much better he has done since he stopped, his doctor apparently didn't think it was worth his time to investigate. The research had already been done, and validated by many credible sources. Most importantly, he had positive proof from Al's experience, to validate what he could have, and should have read. As a result, many of his patients will likely experience similar results from their medications, but unfortunately never really understand why. So, that's Al's story. Now what is yours?

I believe you now understand the wisdom in becoming better informed, and taking more responsibility for your own healthcare. Some doctors even go so far as to chastise their patients for not following their orders and for taking matters into their own hands, even though they definitely benefited from doing so. I would recommend under those circumstances that you go doctor shopping. Make sure you know where he or she stands on issues that are important to you.

Would You Prefer to Become Drug-Free?

If you are you like so many people in the nation apprehensive about stopping your medication? Read on, and I believe you will likely change your mind. It is essential that you become better informed regarding the potential dangers they possess, especially from long-term use and in combination. You will soon discover that in nearly every case, the potential for damage to our health far outweighs any benefit you might experience. It's often said that knowledge is power, and that is especially true in regard to your health. Although I was well aware of the many problems associated with the prescription, and over-the-counter medications currently on the market, even I was totally amazed at what we eventually uncovered. As Paul Harvey often enunciated: "You will now learn the rest of the story" (or possibly the whole story).

CHAPTER TEN
MARY LOU'S STORY

Following is Mary Lou's true story, which chronicles the events that led to the prescribing of the nine medications she was eventually taking. It apparently began many years ago, shortly after she was placed on the newly announced and aggressively promoted wonder drug, Prozac™, for temporary depression, which she actually remained on for 16 years! One thing that made her unique is that she had been an alcoholic most of her adult life. I did a great deal of research on the causes of, and solutions to both addictions and depression, and I believe I can explain the basic underlying problems that contributed to Mary Lou's addiction to alcohol.

First, let's take a look at some serious concerns that Dr. Ann Blake Tracy discovered after ten years of research and clinical study of depression and antidepressants, and wrote about in her book *Prozac – Panacea or Pandora* (1991/1994). Dr. Tracy noticed that:

> **Patients on Prozac consistently report developing an overwhelming compulsion to consume alcohol.** *These reports are coming even from those who have never previously used alcohol. Patients, who are recovering alcoholics, with their addictions under control for many years, report that they return to alcoholism while using Prozac.*

> *America already has an estimated 10 – 15 million alcoholics. To increase that number with a reaction from prescription drugs which causes a compulsion to drink is a tragedy! What a sad state of affairs that a drug which is actually being promoted as a treatment for alcoholism has the potential to create alcohol craving behavior. What a self-defeating and terribly frustrating scenario for those who are working so hard to overcome alcoholism* (pp. 124-125).

Dr. Tracy discovered that many people, who rarely drank or never drank before Prozac™, were consuming excessive amounts of alcohol after starting the use of the drug. She also found that it is rare for a reformed alcoholic, after using Prozac™, to be able to stay away from alcohol because, as they describe it:

> *"The overwhelming drive to drink becomes too overpowering."*

> *"I've been a reformed alcoholic for twelve years, but while on Prozac I started craving alcohol again!"*

> *"Although it was completely out of character for me, the compulsion to drink was so strong after starting on Prozac that it became impossible for me to drive past a bar."*

Another problem associated with long-term use of Prozac™, is the development of diabetes, which Mary Lou didn't have before being placed on the medication, but she now has thanks to the long-term use of Prozac™. As a person progresses from hypoglycemia to diabetes, the ability to effectively metabolize both alcohol and sugar decreases, and this basically compounds the problem. Dr. Janice Keller Phelps, M.D., author of *The Hidden Addiction and How To Get Free* (1986), and a recovering alcoholic herself, claims that diabetics are much more prone to become alcoholics. In her opinion, from both clinical studies and personal experience, the problem stems from inability to effectively metabolize sugars. And as the ability to properly metabolize sugar and alcohol decreases, the addiction basically worsens.

Mary Lou just happens to be dealing with a genetic problem also. She is one-half Native American, and Native Americans don't deal well with alcohol. Their ancestors were not exposed to alcohol, until the White Man, who had been consuming it for centuries, introduced it to them. Our liver goes through two phases in the detoxification of alcohol. In Phase I, alcohol is converted to the metabolite Acetaldehyde, which takes place fairly rapidly with Native Americans. It is the critical Phase II that takes considerably longer than normal to complete. And it is during Phase II that the acetaldehyde is converted to acetic acid and water (both benign substances).

From research, it was discovered that when the very toxic acetaldehyde remains in the body for an extended period of time, it is sometimes metabolized through an alternate pathway into a less toxic but very addictive substance known as **t**e**t**ra**h**ydro**i**so**q**uinolone (THIQ). This substance was discovered during autopsies, and found in the brains of some transient alcoholics. When THIQ was injected into a monkey who would normally not touch alcohol, it would suddenly consume alcohol at every opportunity.

Another genetic predisposition that Native Americans have is a tendency toward hypothyroidism, and two of the most common symptoms associated with the condition are depression and mood swings. Any stressor, be it physical or emotional, suppresses the thyroid function. In most people, once the stressor is removed, the thyroid will rebound and return to normal. With those of Native American and Irish descent especially, the suppressed thyroid condition can remain (often for decades). And as a result of the reduced metabolism, they often remain depressed. This also means that all 3,000 enzymes in the body are functioning less efficiently. Also, toxins (which include prescription medications and alcohol) are not metabolized or removed nearly as efficiently as they normally would be.

If a person is also taking Prozac™ (as Mary Lou was), which is highly protein-binding, and thus very difficult to metabolize, an already bad problem now becomes even worse. The very same P450 enzyme in the liver that metabolizes Prozac™ (as well as other medications) also detoxifies alcohol. The enzyme action in the liver is also suppressed due to the reduced metabolism. It's actually a miracle that Mary Lou is still alive, as a counselor at a local rehabilitation center also indicated. That is especially true once we evaluate the eight additional medications that her doctor had also placed her on. One thing I discovered that makes overcoming any addiction extremely difficult, is that addictive substances such as alcohol, sugar, or tobacco, all deplete important nutrients necessary for reducing the cravings for other addictive substances. So, in order to eliminate the cravings that often result in continued substance abuse, all addictive substances must be eliminated, and supplements should be taken to restore the deficiency created.

The problem in Mary Lou's case was not only the antidepressant Prozac™ that basically stimulates tremendous cravings for all addictive substances, but also the eight other medications her doctor had also placed her on. Every one of her medications was not only creating many undesirable symptoms, but they were also depleting many vitamins and minerals that are important in sufficient quantity to help eliminate addictions. If we also take into consideration the reduced metabolism, which she had been dealing with for years, she would be getting a considerably higher dosage of all her medications. Thus she would experience an even greater depletion of vitamins and minerals than others would normally experience, on the very same dosage.

The greatest travesty of all is: She needed absolutely none of the medications she had been placed on by her doctor in the first place. If the thyroid condition, stimulated by a stressful event, had been properly diagnosed and treated (actually very easy to accomplish), the prescription for Prozac™, as well as the years of cravings for alcohol that followed, would never have happened. The other medications she was later placed on, were also totally unnecessary, and made absolutely no sense.

If we just do a little detective work, I believe we can trace the trail that led to the prescriptions for the additional medications Mary Lou had been placed on. First, let's take a look at the drugs she had been taking prior to their elimination. The **side effects in bold** are not necessarily the worst, but are those that Mary Lou identified as the ones she had been experiencing. We will now evaluate the very first drug she was prescribed (Prozac™).

69

Drug #1: Prozac™ or Sarafem™ / generic name = Fluoxetine

Selective Serotonin Reuptake Inhibitor (SSRI) antidepressant.

❖ **Nutrients depleted:** Vitamin B_1, vitamin B_2, vitamin B_3, vitamin B_6, vitamin B_{12}, folic acid, vitamin C, vitamin D, Coenzyme Q_{10}, calcium, magnesium, manganese, selenium, sodium, zinc, and glutathione.

More common side effects may include: Abnormal dreams, abnormal vision, **anxiety,** diarrhea, **diminished sex drive, dizziness, dry mouth,** flu-like symptoms, flushing, gas, **headache, inability to sit still, insomnia,** itching, loss of appetite, **nausea, nervousness,** rash or hives, **restlessness,** sinusitis, sleepiness, **sore throat**, sweating, tremors, upset stomach, vomiting, **weakness,** yawning.

Less common side effects may include: **Abnormal taste,** agitation, **bleeding problems,** chills, **confusion,** ear pain, **emotional instability,** fever, frequent urination, **high blood pressure, increased appetite,** loss of memory, palpitations, **ringing in the ears, sleep disorders, weight gain.**

Rare side effects may include: Breast enlargement or pain; convulsions (seizures); fast or irregular heartbeat; purple or red spots on skin; symptoms of hypoglycemia (low blood sugar), including anxiety or nervousness, chills, cold sweats, confusion, cool pale skin, difficulty in concentration, drowsiness, excessive hunger, fast heartbeat, headache, shakiness or unsteady walk, or unusual tiredness or weakness; symptoms of hyponatremia (low blood sodium), including confusion, convulsions (seizures), drowsiness, dryness of mouth, increased thirst, lack of energy; symptoms of serotonin syndrome, including diarrhea, fever, increased sweating, mood or behavior changes, overactive reflexes, racing heartbeat, restlessness, shivering or shaking; talking, feeling, and acting with excitement and activity you cannot control; trouble in breathing; unusual or incomplete body or facial movements; unusual secretion of milk, in females.

In children and adolescents, less common side effects may also include: Agitation, excessive menstrual bleeding, frequent urination, hyperactivity, mania or hypomania (inappropriate feelings of elation and/or rapid thoughts), nosebleeds, personality changes (sometimes extreme), rage, suicidal thoughts, and thirst.

While you are taking fluoxetine you may need to be monitored for worsening symptoms of **depression and/or suicidal thoughts especially at the start of therapy or when doses are changed.** Your doctor may want you to monitor for the following symptoms: **anxiety, panic attacks, difficulty sleeping, irritability, hostility, impulsivity, severe restlessness, and mania** (mental and/or physical hyperactivity). These symptoms may be associated with development of **worsening symptoms of depression and/or suicidal thoughts or actions.**

After you stop taking fluoxetine, your body may need time to adjust. The length of time this takes depends on the amount of medicine you were using and how long you used it. During this period of time, check with your doctor if you notice any of the following side effects:

Anxiety; **dizziness;** feeling that body or **surroundings are turning**; general feeling of discomfort or illness; **headache;** nausea; **sweating;** unusual tiredness or weakness.

A wide variety of other very rare reactions have been reported during Prozac therapy. If you develop any new or unexplained symptoms, tell your doctor without delay.

Make sure you tell your doctor if you have any other medical problems, especially:

- Brain disease or mental retardation or
- Seizures, history of—The chance of having seizures may be increased

- **Diabetes—The amount of insulin or oral antidiabetic medicine that you need to take may change**

- Kidney disease or
- Liver disease—Higher blood levels of fluoxetine may occur, increasing the chance of side effects

- Parkinson's disease—May become worse

- Weight loss—Fluoxetine may cause weight loss. This weight loss is usually small, but if a large weight loss occurs, it may be harmful in some patients

Prozac can occasionally cause decreased appetite and weight loss, especially in depressed people who are already underweight and in those with bulimia. If you notice changes in your weight or appetite, tell your doctor.

Do not take this medication if you are recovering from a heart attack or if you have liver disease or diabetes.

If you are taking any prescription or nonprescription drugs, notify your doctor before taking Prozac. *(MY NOTE: Although Mary Lou wasn't taking other medications when Prozac™ was first prescribed, several were added later).*

Do not drink alcohol while taking this medication. *(MY NOTE: Something Mary Lou was doing, and one craving caused by Prozac™.)*

If Prozac is taken with certain other drugs, the effects of either could be increased, decreased, or altered. **It is especially important to check with your doctor before combining Prozac with the following:**

- Carbamazepine (Tegretol)
- Clozapine (Clozaril)
- Diazepam (Valium)
- Drugs that impair brain function, such as sleep aids and narcotic painkillers
- Flecainide (Tambocor)
- Haloperidol (Haldol)
- Pimozide (Orap)
- St Johns Wort
- Vinblastine (Velban)
- Warfarin (Coumadin)

Although certain medicines should not be used together at all, in other cases two different medicines may be used together even if an interaction might occur. In these cases, your doctor may want to change the dose, or other precautions may be necessary. When you are taking fluoxetine, it is especially important that your health care professional know if you are taking any of the following:

- Alprazolam (e.g., Xanax)—Higher blood levels of alprazolam may occur and its effects may be increased

- Anticoagulants (blood thinners) or
- Digitalis glycosides (heart medicine)—Higher or lower blood levels of these medicines or fluoxetine may occur, increasing the chance of unwanted effects. Your doctor may need to see you more often, especially when you first start or when you stop taking fluoxetine. Your doctor also may need to change the dose of either medicine

- Astemizole (e.g., Hismanal)—Higher blood levels of astemizole may occur, which increases the chance of having a very serious change in the rhythm of your heartbeat

- Buspirone (e.g., BuSpar) or
- Bromocriptine (e.g., Parlodel) or
- Dextromethorphan (cough medicine) or
- Levodopa (e.g., Sinemet) or
- **Lithium (e.g., Eskalith)** *(MY NOTE: A medication Mary Lou was taking!)*
- Meperidine (e.g., Demerol) or
- Nefazodone (e.g., Serzone) or
- Pentazocine (e.g., Talwin) or
- Selective serotonin reuptake inhibitors, other (citalopram [Celexa], fluvoxamine [e.g., Luvox], paroxetine [e.g., Paxil], sertraline [e.g., Zoloft]) or
- Street drugs (LSD, MDMA [e.g., ecstasy], marijuana) or
- Sumatriptan (e.g., Imitrex) or
- Tramadol (e.g., Ultram) or
- **Trazodone (e.g., Desyrel)** *(MY NOTE: Another medication Mary Lou was placed on!)*
- Tryptophan or
- Venlafaxine (e.g., Effexor)—Using these medicines with fluoxetine or within 5 weeks of stopping fluoxetine may increase the chance of developing a rare, but very serious, unwanted effect known as the serotonin syndrome. This syndrome may cause confusion, diarrhea, fever, poor coordination, restlessness, shivering, sweating, talking or acting with excitement you cannot control, trembling or shaking, or twitching. If you develop these symptoms contact your doctor as soon as possible. Taking tramadol with fluoxetine increases the chance of having convulsions (seizures). Also, taking tryptophan with fluoxetine may result in increased agitation or restlessness and intestinal or stomach problems

- Moclobemide (e.g., Manerex)—The risk of developing serious unwanted effects, including the serotonin syndrome, is increased. Use of moclobemide with fluoxetine is not recommended. Also, it is recommended that 7 days be allowed between stopping treatment with moclobemide and starting treatment with fluoxetine, and it is recommended that 5 weeks be allowed between stopping treatment with fluoxetine and starting treatment with moclobemide

- Phenytoin (e.g., Dilantin) or

- Tricyclic antidepressants (amitriptyline [e.g., Elavil], amoxapine [e.g., Asendin], clomipramine [e.g., Anafranil], desipramine [e.g., Pertofrane], doxepin [e.g., Sinequan], imipramine [e.g., Tofranil], nortriptyline [e.g., Aventyl], protriptyline [e.g., Vivactil], trimipramine [e.g., Surmontil])—Higher blood levels of these medicines may occur, which increases the chance of having serious side effects. Your doctor may want to see you more often and may need to change the doses of your medicines. Also, taking amitriptyline, clomipramine, or imipramine with fluoxetine may increase the chance of developing the serotonin syndrome

- Monoamine oxidase (MAO) inhibitor activity (isocarboxazid [e.g., Marplan], phenelzine [e.g., Nardil], procarbazine [e.g., Matulane], selegiline [e.g., Eldepryl], tranylcypromine [e.g., Parnate])— *Do not take fluoxetine while you are taking or within 2 weeks of taking an MAO inhibitor.* If you do, you may develop confusion, agitation, restlessness, stomach or intestinal problems, sudden high body temperature, extremely high blood pressure, and severe convulsions. At least 14 days should be allowed between stopping treatment with an MAO inhibitor and starting treatment with fluoxetine. If you have been taking fluoxetine, at least 5 weeks should be allowed between stopping treatment with fluoxetine and starting treatment with an MAO inhibitor

Quite possibly, Mary Lou was experiencing one of the potential side effects associated with Prozac™ (**depression**). The very condition Prozac™ was prescribed for. As usual, although Prozac™ obviously wasn't doing the job he was hired for, Mary Lou's doctor somehow felt it advisable to keep him on the payroll anyhow. If he did absolutely nothing, it wouldn't be so bad, but unfortunately that doesn't appear to be the case. Prozac™ is more like the enemy within. You will soon learn exactly what Prozac™ was likely busy doing behind the scenes, some things Prozac™ is well known for.

We now come to another antidepressant called Desyrel™, to see if he can do a better job. Although it is a well-known fact that Prozac™ and Desyrel™ might not get along too well together, it appears to be a risk worth taking, so Desyrel™ was brought on board. So, let's see what Desyrel™ is capable of doing for Mary Lou. Then after evaluating the other antidepressant Desyrel™, we will look at the remaining seven of the total of nine medications Mary Lou was taking. Following our evaluation of each, we will do a little detective work. You will soon learn how failing to accurately identify and properly treat the source of her temporary depression, eventually led to nine different medications (all inappropriate). So read on and discover what the underlying problem actually was and what the appropriate solution should have been.

Drug #2: Trazodone = generic name / Desyrel™

Antidepressant.

❖ **Nutrients depleted: Vitamin B$_6$, vitamin C, vitamin D, Coenzyme Q$_{10}$, and sodium.**

More common side effects may include: Abdominal or stomach disorder, **aches or pains in muscles** and bones, anger or hostility, **blurred vision**, brief loss of consciousness, **confusion,** constipation, decreased appetite, diarrhea, **dizziness or light-headedness, drowsiness, dry mouth, excitement,** fainting, fast or **fluttery heartbeat, fatigue, fluid retention** and swelling, **headache, inability to fall or stay asleep,** low blood pressure, nasal or **sinus congestion, nausea, nervousness,** nightmares or vivid dreams, **tremors,** uncoordinated movements, vomiting, **weight gain** or loss.

Less common or rare side effects may include: Allergic reactions, **anemia, bad taste in mouth,** blood in the urine, chest pain, delayed urine flow, **decreased concentration, decreased sex drive,** disorientation, excess salivation, gas, **general feeling of illness,** hallucinations or delusions, <u>**high blood pressure,**</u> impaired memory, impaired speech, impotence, increased appetite, increased sex drive, menstrual problems, more frequent urination, muscle twitches, **numbness,** red, tired, itchy eyes, restlessness, **ringing in the ears, shortness of breath,** sweating or clammy skin**, tingling or pins and needles**.

Desyrel may cause you to become drowsy or less alert and may affect your judgment. Therefore, you should not drive or operate dangerous machinery or participate in any hazardous activity that requires full mental alertness until you know how this drug affects you.

Desyrel has been associated with priapism, a persistent, painful erection of the penis. Men who experience prolonged or inappropriate erections should stop taking this drug and consult their doctor.

Tell your doctor if you are being treated with electroshock therapy and if you have or have ever had:

- Cancer
- A heart attack or irregular heart beat
- **High blood pressure**
- Human immunodeficiency virus (HIV) or acquired immunodeficiency syndrome (AIDs)
- Low white blood cell count
- **Thoughts of suicide**
- Heart disease

Notify your doctor or dentist that you are taking this drug if you have a medical emergency, and before you have surgery or dental treatment. Your doctor will ask you to stop using the drug if you are going to have elective surgery.

If Desyrel is taken with certain other drugs, the effects of either could be increased, decreased, or altered. It is especially important to check with your doctor before combining Desyrel with the following:

- Antidepressant drugs known as MAO inhibitors, including Nardil and Parnate
- Barbiturates such as Seconal
- Central nervous system depressants such as Demerol and Halcion
- Chlorpromazine (Thorazine)
- Drugs for high blood pressure such as Catapres and Wytensin
- **Other antidepressants, especially SSRIs such as <u>Prozac</u> and Norpramin**
- Anticoagulants ('blood thinners') such as Warfarin (Coumadin)
- Antifungal medications such as fluconazole (Diflucan), itraconazole (Sporanox), and ketoconazole (Nizoral)
- Cimetidine (Tagamet)
- Clarithromycin (Biaxin, Prevpac)
- Cyclosporine (Neoral, Sandimmune)
- Canazol (Danocrine)

- Delaviridine (Rescriptor)
- Dexamethasone (Decadron)
- Digoxin (Digitek, Lanoxin, Lanoxicaps)
- Diltiazem (Cardizem, Dilacor, Tiazac)
- Erythromycin (E.E.S., E-Mycin, Erythrocin)
- HIV protease inhibitors such as indinavir (Crixivan), nelfinavir (Viracept), ritonavir (Norvir), and saquinavir (Fortovase, Invirase)
- Isoniazid (INH, Nydrazid)
- Medications for allergies, cough or colds
- **Medications for <u>anxiety</u>, <u>high blood pressure</u>,** irregular heartbeat, mental illness or pain
- Medication for seizures such as carbamazepine (Tegretol), ethosuximide (Zarontin), phenobarbital (Luminal, Solfoton), and phenytoin (Dilantin)
- Metronidazole (Flagyl)
- Muscle relaxants
- Nefazodone
- Oral contraceptives (birth control pills)
- Rifabutin (Mycobutin)
- Rifampin (Rifadin, Rimactane)
- Sedatives
- Sleeping pills or tranquilizers
- Troleandomycin (TAO)
- Verapamil (Calan, Isoptin, Verelan)
- Zafirlukast (Accolate)
- St John's Wort

Also, tell your doctor or pharmacist if you are taking the following medications, called MAO inhibitors, or if you have stopped taking them within the past two weeks: isocarboxazid (Marplan), phenelzine (Nardil), selegiline (Eldepryl, Carbex), or tranylcypromine (Parnate).

<u>Drug #3: Zocor™ / generic name = simvastatin</u>

Blocks the production of cholesterol (a type of fat) in the body.

- ❖ **Nutrients depleted: Vitamin A, vitamin B_{12}, folic acid, vitamin D, vitamin E, vitamin K, Coenzyme Q_{10}, calcium, magnesium, iron, phosphorus, and zinc.**

Common side effects: constipation, diarrhea, gas, **headache, nausea,** stomach pain, **heartburn.**

Less common side effects: fever, **muscle aches,** unusual **tiredness or weakness,** severe stomach pain, **insomnia, upper respiratory infections, weight gain.**

Since Zocor may cause damage to muscle tissue, be sure to tell your doctor of any unexplained muscle tenderness, weakness, or pain right away, especially if you also have a fever or feel sick.

Possible interactions:

- Cyclosporine (Sandimmune, Neoral)

- Gemfibrozil (Lopid), clofibrate (Atromid-S), or fenofibrate (Tricor)
- Niacin (Nicolar, Nicobid, Slo-Niacin, others)
- Erythromycin (E-Mycin, E.E.S., Ery-Tab, others) or clarithromycin (Biaxin)
- Cholestyramine (Questran) or colestipol (Colestid)
- An antifungal medication such as itraconazole (Sporanox), fluconazole (Diflucan), or ketoconazole (Nizoral)
- Nefazodone (Serzone)
- Digoxin (Lanoxin, Lanoxicaps)
- Warfarin (Coumadin)
- A protease inhibitor such as amprenavir (Agenerase), indinavir (Crixivan), nelfinavir (Viracept), ritonavir (Norvir), lopinavir-ritonavir (Kaletra), or saquinavir (Invirase, Fortovase)
- Amiodarone (Cordarone, Pacer one)
- Verapamil (Calan, Covera-HS, Isoptin, Verelan).

Drug #4: Eskalith™ / generic name = Lithium carbonate

Lithium is used to treat manic episodes of manic-depressive illness. Lithium reduces chemicals in the body that cause excitation or mania.

❖ **Nutrients depleted: Inositol, choline and sodium.**

Side effects that may occur when you start taking lithium include: Abdominal discomfort, anorexia, diarrhea, **drowsiness,** frequent urination, **hand tremor, headache, thirst, nausea, upset stomach.**

Other side effects may include: Abdominal pain, acne, blackout spells, **blurry vision,** cavities, **changes in taste perception,** coma, **confusion, dehydration, dizziness,** dry hair, **dry mouth,** ear noises, eye pain, fainting, **fatigue,** flu or cold with fever, gas, **hair loss,** hallucinations, increased salivation, **indigestion,** involuntary tongue movements, involuntary urination or bowel movements, irregular heartbeat, itching, loss of appetite, low blood pressure, menstrual problems, **muscle aches,** muscle rigidity, muscle twitching, **painful joints, poor memory,** psoriasis worsening, rash on hands and feet, restlessness, **ringing in ears,** seizures, sexual dysfunction, shakiness, shortness of breath, skin problems, **sleepiness, slowed thinking, slurred speech,** startle response, swelling, **thinning hair,** thyroid problems (coldness and dry, puffy skin), **tightness in chest, vision problems,** vomiting, **weakness, weight gain,** weight loss.

If the Eskalith dosage is too low, you will derive no benefit; **if it is too high, you could suffer lithium poisoning.** You and your doctor will need to work together to find the correct dosage. Initially, this means frequent blood tests to find out how much of the drug is actually circulating in your bloodstream. As long as you take Eskalith, you will need to watch for side effects.

Signs of lithium poisoning include vomiting, unsteady walking, diarrhea, drowsiness, tremor, and weakness. Signs of mild toxicity include drowsiness, sluggishness, unsteadiness, tremor, muscle twitching, vomiting or diarrhea.

Contact your doctor at the first sign of toxicity or lithium poisoning. Because more severe cases can cause lasting brain damage or death, serious lithium poisoning usually requires aggressive treatment with hemodialysis.

While taking Eskalith, you should drink 10 to 12 glasses of water or fluid a day.

To minimize the risk of harmful side effects, eat a balanced diet that includes some salt and lots of liquids. If you have been sweating a great deal or have had diarrhea, make sure you get extra liquids and salt.

If you develop an infection with a fever, you may need to cut back on your Eskalith dosage or even quit taking it temporarily. While you are ill, keep in close touch with your doctor.

Eskalith may affect your judgment or coordination. Do not drive, climb, or perform hazardous tasks until you find out how this drug affects you.

You should be careful in hot weather to avoid activities that cause you to sweat heavily. Also avoid drinking large amounts of coffee, tea, or cola, which can cause dehydration through increased urination. Do not make a major change in your eating habits or go on a weight loss diet without consulting your doctor. **The loss of water and salt from your body could lead to lithium poisoning.**

MY NOTE: Mary Lou was also taking an ACE inhibitor and a diuretic. Both cause a loss of water, increasing the risk for lithium poisoning, which can be extremely dangerous (and even life threatening).

Your doctor will prescribe Eskalith with extra caution if you have a heart or kidney problem, brain or spinal cord disease, or a weak, run-down, or **dehydrated condition.**

Also make sure your doctor is aware of any medical problems you may have, including **diabetes,** epilepsy, **thyroid problems**, Parkinson's disease, and difficulty urinating.

If Eskalith is taken with certain other drugs, the effects of either could be increased, decreased, or altered. It is especially important to check with your doctor before combining Eskalith with the following:

- **ACE-inhibitor blood pressure drugs such as Capoten or Vasotec**
- Acetazolamide (Diamox)
- Amphetamines such as Dexedrine
- **Antidepressant drugs that boost serotonin levels, including Paxil, <u>Prozac</u>, and Zoloft**
- Bicarbonate of soda
- Caffeine (No-Doz)
- Calcium-blocking blood pressure drugs such as Calan and Cardizem
- Carbamazepine (Tegretol)
- **Diuretics such as Lasix or HydroDIURIL**
- Iodine-containing preparations such as potassium iodide (Quadrinal)
- Major tranquilizers such as Haldol and Thorazine
- Methyldopa (Aldomet)
- Metronidazole (Flagyl)
- **Non-steroidal anti-inflammatory drugs such as Advil,** Celebrex, Feldene, Indocin, and Vioxx
- Phenytoin (Dilantin)

- Sodium bicarbonate
- Tetracyclines such as Achromycin V and Sumycin
- Theophylline (Theo-Dur, Quibron, others)

Drug #5: Hydrochlorothiazide = generic name

A thiazide diuretic (water pill), used to lower blood pressure and to decrease edema (swelling).

❖ **Nutrients depleted: Vitamin B_1, vitamin B_2, vitamin B_6, vitamin B_{12}, folic acid, vitamin C, vitamin D, Coenzyme Q_{10}, calcium, magnesium, manganese, phosphorus, potassium, sodium and zinc.**

Side effects may include: Abdominal cramping, diarrhea, **dizziness upon standing up, headache,** loss of appetite, low blood pressure, **low potassium** (leading to symptoms such as **dry mouth, excessive thirst,** weak or irregular heartbeat, **muscle pain** or cramps), stomach irritation, **stomach upset, weakness.**

Less common or rare side effects may include: **Anemia,** blood disorders, **changes in blood sugar,** constipation, **difficulty breathing, dizziness,** fever, fluid in the lung, **hair loss,** high levels of sugar in the urine, hives, hypersensitivity reactions, impotence, inflammation of the lung, inflammation of the pancreas, inflammation of the salivary glands, kidney failure, muscle spasms, **nausea,** rash, reddish or purplish spots on the skin, restlessness, sensitivity to light, skin disorders including Stevens-Johnson syndrome (blisters in the mouth and eyes), skin peeling, **tingling or pins and needles,** vertigo, **vision changes,** vomiting, weight gain, yellow eyes and skin.

Diuretics can cause your body to lose too much potassium. Signs of an excessively low potassium level include muscle weakness and rapid or irregular heartbeat. To boost your potassium level, your doctor may recommend eating potassium-rich foods or taking a potassium supplement.

If you have bronchial asthma or a history of allergies, you may be at greater risk for an allergic reaction to this medication.

Dehydration, excessive sweating, severe diarrhea or vomiting could deplete your body's fluids and cause your blood pressure to become too low. Be careful when exercising and in hot weather.

Possible interactions:

- Barbiturates such as phenobarbital
- Cholestyramine (Questran)
- Colestipol (Colestid)
- Corticosteroids such as prednisone and ACTH
- Digoxin (Lanoxin)
- Drugs to treat diabetes such as insulin or Micronase
- **Lithium (Lithonate)**
- Narcotics such as Percocet
- **Non-steroidal anti-inflammatory drugs** such as Naprosyn

- Norepinephrine (Levophed)
- **Other high blood pressure medications** such as Aldomet
- Skeletal muscle relaxants, such as tubocurarine

Hydrochlorothiazide may increase the effects of other drugs that cause drowsiness, including sedatives (used to treat insomnia), pain relievers, seizure medicines, **antidepressants,** alcohol, antihistamines, anxiety medicines, and muscle relaxants. Tell your doctor about all medicines that you are taking, and do not take any medicine without first talking to your doctor.

Make sure you tell your doctor if you have any other medical problems, especially:

- **diabetes**
- gout
- a collagen vascular disease such as systemic lupus erythematosus
- pancreatitis
- kidney disease
- liver disease
- **high levels of cholesterol** or triglycerides (types of fat) in your blood

Drug #6: Lisinopril = generic name / Prinivil™

ACE inhibitor used to treat hypertension (high blood pressure).

❖ **Nutrients depleted: Vitamin B_{12}, magnesium, phosphorus, sodium, zinc, and Coenzyme Q_{10}.**

More common side effects may include: Chest pain, **cough,** diarrhea, **dizziness, headache,** low blood pressure.

Less common or rare side effects may include: Abdominal pain, **anemia,** arm pain, **arthritis, asthma,** back pain, blood clot in lungs, **blurred vision, breast pain, bronchitis, changes in sense of taste,** chills, common cold, **confusion,** constipation, coughing up blood, cramps in stomach/intestines, **decreased sex drive, dehydration, diabetes,** dizziness on standing, double vision, **dry mouth,** fainting, **fatigue, feeling of illness,** fever, flu, **fluid retention, flushing,** gas, gout, **hair loss,** heart attack, **heartburn,** hepatitis, **hip pain,** hives, **inability to sleep** or sleeping too much, **incoordination, indigestion,** inflamed stomach, intolerance of light, irregular heartbeat, **irritability, joint pain,** kidney trouble or failure, **knee pain,** laryngitis, leg pain, little or no urine, lung cancer, lung inflammation, **memory impairment, muscle pain** or cramps, **nasal congestion** or inflammation, **nausea, neck pain, nervousness, nosebleed, numbness or tingling, painful breathing,** painful urination, pelvic pain, **pneumonia, prickling** or burning **sensation, rapid or fluttery heartbeat,** rash, reddening of skin, **respiratory infection, ringing in ears,** runny nose, sensitivity to light, skin infections or eruptions, **shoulder pain,** sinus inflammation, sleepiness, **sore throat,** spasm, stroke, sweating, swelling of face or arms and legs, **taste disturbances,** thigh pain, **tremor, urinary tract infection,** vertigo, virus infection, vision changes, vomiting, **weakness, weight** loss or **gain, wheezing,** yellow eyes and skin.

If you have congestive heart failure or other heart problems, a kidney disorder, or a connective tissue disease such as lupus, you should use this drug with caution.

If you are taking lisinopril, a complete assessment of your kidney function should be done and kidney function should continue to be monitored. Lisinopril is used with great caution after a heart attack if the patient also has kidney problems.

This drug also should be used with caution if you are on dialysis. There have been reports of extreme allergic reactions during dialysis in people taking ACE inhibitor medications such as lisinopril.

If you are taking high doses of a diuretic (water pill) and lisinopril, you may develop excessively low blood pressure. This problem is also more likely if you are being treated for heart failure.

Lisinopril may cause some people to become dizzy, light-headed, or faint, especially if they have heart failure or are taking a water pill at the same time.

Avoid salt substitutes that contain potassium. Limit your consumption of potassium-rich foods such as bananas, prunes, raisins, orange juice, and whole and skim milk. Ask your doctor for advice on how much of these foods to consume.

Excessive sweating, dehydration, severe diarrhea, or vomiting could cause you to lose too much water and cause your blood pressure to drop dangerously.

Possible interactions:

- A potassium supplement such as K-Dur, Klor-Con, and others
- **Salt substitutes** that contain potassium
- Any of the diuretics (water pills) triamterene (Dyrenium, Maxzide, Dyazide), spironolactone (Aldactone), or amiloride (Midamor)
- **Any other diuretic (water pill) such as hydrochlorothiazide (HCTZ,** HydroDiuril, others), furosemide (Lasix), bumetanide (Bumex), indapamide (Lozol), and others.
- **Lithium** (Lithobid, **Eskalith,** others)
- Indomethacin (Indocin)

Drug #7: Intal™ / generic name = Cromolyn Sodium inhalation

An anti-inflammatory inhalant, used as preventative treatment for asthma.

❖ **Nutrients depleted: Folic acid, vitamin C, calcium, iron, and magnesium.**

More common side effects may include: **Cough, nasal congestion** or irritation, **nausea,** sneezing, **throat irritation, wheezing.**

Less common or rare side effects may include: Angioedema (**swelling of** face around **lips,** tongue, and throat, swollen arms and legs), **bad taste in mouth,** burning in chest, difficulty swallowing, **dizziness,** ear problems, **headache,** hives, joint swelling and pain, **nosebleed,** painful urination or frequent urination, postnasal drip, rash, severe allergic reaction, swollen glands, swollen throat, teary eyes, **tightness in throat.**

Drug #8: Alupent™ / generic name = Metaproterenol

Bronchodilator, used to treat asthma, bronchitis, and emphysema.

❖ **Nutrients depleted: Vitamin B$_6$, vitamin C, vitamin D, potassium, and essential fatty acids.**

Side effects may include: **Bad taste in mouth, cough, dizziness, headache, <u>high blood pressure,</u> nausea, nervousness, rapid or throbbing heartbeat,** stomach and intestinal upset, **throat irritation, tremors,** vomiting, <u>**worsening or aggravation of asthma**</u>.

Rare side effects may include: **Chest** pain or **discomfort,** muscle cramps or twitching.

Before taking this medication, tell your doctor if you have

- heart disease
- **high blood pressure**
- epilepsy or another seizure disorder
- **diabetes**
- an overactive thyroid (hyperthyroidism)
- liver disease
- kidney disease

Unless you are directed to do so by your doctor, do not take this medication if you have an irregular, rapid heart rate.

Alupent can cause significant changes in blood pressure.
(MY NOTE: Something Mary Lou was taking medication to control!)

If Alupent is taken with certain other drugs, the effects of either could be increased, decreased, or altered. It is especially important to check with your doctor before combining Alupent with the following:

- Beta-adrenergic blocking agents (acebutolol [e.g., Sectral], atenolol [e.g., Tenormin], betaxolol [e.g., Kerlone], carteolol [e.g., Cartrol], labetalol [e.g., Normodyne], metoprolol [e.g., Lopressor], nadolol [e.g., Corgard], oxprenolol [e.g., Trasicor], penbutolol [e.g., Levatol], pindolol [e.g., Visken], propranolol [e.g., Inderal], sotalol [e.g., Sotacor], timolol [e.g., Blocadren])—These medicines may make your condition worse and prevent the adrenergic bronchodilators from working properly
- Disopyramide
- Quinidine
- Phenothiazines, or
- Procainamide—These medicines may increase the risk of heart problems
- MAO inhibitors (antidepressant drugs such as Nardil and Parnate)
- **Bronchodilators such as Ventolin and Proventil inhalers**
- Tricyclic antidepressants such as Elavil and Tofranil

Drug #9: Proventil ™ / generic name = Albuterol (oral)

Used to treat bronchospasms, associated with asthma.

❖ **Nutrients depleted:** Vitamin B$_6$, vitamin C, vitamin D, potassium, and essential fatty acids.

More common side effects may include: Aggression, **agitation,** allergic reaction, **anxiety,** back pain, **chest pain or discomfort,** chills and fever, coordination problems, **cough,** decreased appetite, **depression,** difficulty speaking, <u>diabetes</u>, diarrhea, **dizziness** or light-headedness, drowsiness, **dry mouth and throat,** excitement, **fluid retention and swelling,** flushing, general bodily discomfort, **headache,** heart palpitations or **rapid heartbeat, heartburn,** hives, increased appetite, <u>**increased blood pressure,**</u> **difficulty or labored breathing, indigestion,** muscle cramps or spasm, **nasal inflammation, nausea, nervousness,** nightmares, **nosebleed, rapid heartbeat,** rash, **respiratory infection** or disorder, restlessness, **ringing in the ears, shakiness, sleeplessness,** slowed movement, stomachache, **stuffy nose,** sweating, swelling of mouth and throat, taste sensation on inhalation, **throat irritation**, tooth discoloration, **tremors, unusual taste,** urinary problems, vomiting, **weakness, wheezing.**

Rare side effects may include: **Chest discomfort** or pain; **drowsiness or weakness;** irregular heartbeat; **irritation of throat** or mouth; muscle cramps or twitching ; **nausea** and/or vomiting; **restlessness; trouble in sleeping; dizziness,** severe; **feeling of choking,** irritation, or swelling in throat; flushing or redness of skin; hives; increased shortness of breath; skin rash; **swelling of** face, **lips,** or eyelids; **tightness in chest or wheezing, troubled breathing.**

Possible interactions:

- Amphetamines or
- Appetite suppressants (diet pills) or
- **Medicine for** colds, **sinus problems,** or **hay fever** or other allergies (including nose drops or sprays) or
- **Other medicines for asthma or other breathing problems—The chance for side effects may be increased**

- Beta-adrenergic blocking agents taken orally or by injection (acebutolol [e.g., Sectral], atenolol [e.g., Tenormin], betaxolol [e.g., Kerlone], bisoprolol [e.g., Zebeta], carteolol [e.g., Cartrol], labetalol [e.g., Normodyne], metoprolol [e.g., Lopressor, Toprol XL], nadolol [e.g., Corgard], oxprenolol [e.g., Trasicor], penbutolol [e.g., Levatol], pindolol [e.g., Visken], propranolol [e.g., Inderal], sotalol [e.g., Sotacor], timolol [e.g., Blocadren])—These medicines may prevent the adrenergic bronchodilators from working properly
- Beta-adrenergic blocking agents used in the eye (betaxolol [e.g., Betoptic], levobunolol [e.g., Betagan], metipranolol [e.g., OptiPranolol], timolol [e.g., Timoptic]—Enough of these medicines may be absorbed from the eye into the bloodstream to prevent the adrenergic bronchodilators from working properly

- Cocaine—Unwanted effects of both medicines on the heart may be increased

- Digitalis medicines (e.g., Lanoxin) or

- Quinidine (e.g., Quinaglute Dura-Tabs, Quinidex)—The risk of heart rhythm problems may be increased

- Monoamine oxidase (MAO) inhibitor activity (isocarboxazid [e.g., Marplan], phenelzine [e.g., Nardil], procarbazine [e.g., Matulane], selegiline [e.g., Eldepryl], tranylcypromine [e.g., Parnate])—Taking adrenergic bronchodilators while you are taking or within 2 weeks of taking monoamine oxidase (MAO) inhibitors may dramatically increase the effects of MAO inhibitors

- Thyroid hormones—The effect of this medicine may be increased

- Tricyclic antidepressants (amitriptyline [e.g., Elavil], amoxapine [e.g., Asendin], clomipramine [e.g., Anafranil], desipramine [e.g., Norpramin], doxepin [e.g., Sinequan], imipramine [e.g., Tofranil], nortriptyline [e.g., Aventyl, Pamelor], protriptyline [e.g., Vivactil], trimipramine [e.g., Surmontil])—The effects of these medicines on the heart and blood vessels may be increased

Make sure you tell your doctor if you have any other medical problems, especially:

- Convulsions (seizures)—These medicines may make this condition worse

- **Diabetes mellitus (sugar diabetes)**—These medicines may increase blood sugar, which could change the amount of insulin or other diabetes medicine you need

- Enlarged prostate—Ephedrine may make the condition worse

- Gastrointestinal narrowing—Use of the extended-release dosage form of albuterol may result in a blockage in the intestines.

- Glaucoma—Ephedrine or epinephrine may make the condition worse

- **High blood pressure or**
- Overactive thyroid—Use of ephedrine or epinephrine may cause severe high blood pressure and other side effects may also be increased

- Parkinson's disease—Epinephrine may make stiffness and trembling worse

- Psychiatric problems—Epinephrine may make problems worse

- Reduced blood flow to the brain—Epinephrine further decreases blood flow, which could make the problem worse Reduced blood flow to the heart or
- Heart rhythm problems—These medicines may make these conditions worse

Why Was Mary Lou Placed On All Those Medications?

We will begin with the very first drug (Prozac™) that not only started the cravings for alcohol, leading to Mary Lou's addiction, but also kept her addiction going. In addition, it also started the nutrient-depletion process, and it appears that Prozac™ should win an award for nutrient depletion. With a total of sixteen nutrients depleted, it should definitely be at the top of the class. If you consider that it also includes mostly the very important ones, it would likely be a candidate for first prize!

Mary Lou eventually developed both the bipolar condition and diabetes (both common side effects associated with Prozac™). For the bipolar condition, she was placed on a potentially dangerous form of lithium (lithium carbonate). Two primary issues of concern are: (1) Both lithium and Prozac™ are known to suppress the thyroid, and (2) both contribute to diabetes (which she also developed), basically double jeopardy. If you want to see just how dangerous, I suggest you read the chapter on Bipolar Disorder and Lithium Therapy, later in this book.

Two primary issues of concern are: (1) Both lithium and Prozac™ are known to suppress the thyroid, and (2) both contribute to diabetes (basically double jeopardy). You will discover that there are some even worse potential side effects associated with lithium carbonate than with Prozac™, such as permanent kidney scarring, other kidney damage, liver disorders, coma, and even death. There are many others, but these are just some of the more serious ones. A rather scary drug I would say, and just to deal with **one** of the side effects of Prozac™. As Dr. Ann Blake Tracy tells us, Prozac™ is actually a stimulant, although lithium is a well-known suppressant. That being true, they would basically tend to cancel each other out! Why not just stop taking both (something Mary Lou eventually did)! It would certainly make more sense, and eliminate the potential of a great deal of unnecessary side effects, as well as the depletion of many important nutrients.

Incidentally, that is not the end of the antidepressant story. Not only the bipolar disorder, but also **depression, is a potential side effect of Prozac™**. Apparently that was a problem in Mary Lou's case also, as her doctor somehow deemed it necessary to place her on **another** antidepressant called Desyrel™! You will also find a warning of potential interactions when combining either lithium or Desyrel™ with Prozac™, which her doctor apparently overlooked, or just ignored. That could easily pose a major threat for a serious drug interaction, especially if alcohol was also consumed (one more contra-indication). Although Prozac™ is known to produce cravings for alcohol, doctors all too often ignore that concern, in spite of the warning against drinking alcohol while on Prozac™! According to Dr. Tracy, Prozac™ potentiates alcohol ten times, thus one drink basically equates to drinking ten, which greatly increases the potential risk from drinking alcohol. One can't help but wonder just how much time was invested in evaluation before such a potentially dangerous combination of medications was prescribed, and especially for someone known to have an alcohol addiction.

Now that we covered the drugs Mary Lou had been placed on for depression, we will look at those prescribed for cardiovascular concerns. We will begin by evaluating the cholesterol-lowering drug Zocor™. There are many excuses used to justify prescribing this class of drugs. One such excuse is high blood pressure, which just happens to be one potential side effect associated with both of her antidepressants. Another is diabetes, which both Prozac™ and lithium carbonate are known to contribute to, (and something Mary Lou developed). I might add that during this time, Mary Lou was still dealing with an unresolved hypothyroid condition. Two common conditions associated with low thyroid function are depression (thus the Prozac™ solution), and elevated cholesterol (and thus Zocor™).

So, Mary Lou definitely qualified for, and was prescribed Zocor™, which then lead to a whole series of cardiovascular problems. The very first normally experienced, is elevated blood pressure. So then, blood pressure medication was in order. Actually, not one but two medications were prescribed to deal with the problem. One was the ACE inhibitor Lisinopril, and the other was the diuretic (water pill) hydrochlorothiazide. We have another serious concern regarding possible interactions when combining the ACE inhibitor (blood pressure medication) and the diuretic hydrochlorothiazide, **(especially when combined with lithium).** Mary Lou was unfortunately prescribed all three. Lithium is well known for the excessive excretion of both water and sodium through the kidneys, thus greatly increasing the risk of dehydration. Not only can a diuretic contribute to dehydration, but one potential side effect of the ACE inhibitor is dehydration also. Under the circumstances, why in the world would any doctor in his or her right mind, possibly prescribe a diuretic that not only removes water (increasing the risk for dehydration), but also wastes many important vitamins and minerals in the process?

I asked Mary Lou if she knew why her doctor chose to include the diuretic with her ACE inhibitor. She said her doctor indicated it was common practice to do so, (but most people are normally not also taking lithium). I can't help but wonder how many doctors actually take the time to evaluate the potential for interaction when new medications are added. Obviously in Mary Lou's case, that consideration was apparently just an oversight, although this appears to be a common problem, rather than just an exception. (How about your doctor?)

This finally brings us to one more class of drugs, those prescribed to treat asthma. Actually, not one but three of them were prescribed for Mary Lou! My first thought was: What in the world could possibly create such a serious case of asthma that would require the use of three different medications to control? As we are now fully aware, no drug created could possibly resolve any condition (that's not what drugs do), so a lifetime of controlling the symptoms is the only option.

From past experience, I suspected that her other medications might possibly be contributing to the problem, and was I right! It appeared that every single one of her other medications in it's own way, could very well to be contributing to the problem. Following are the six culprits (her other medications) and the potential side effects associated with each that would lead to breathing difficulties:

1. Prozac™: Trouble in breathing.
2. Lithium: Tightness in chest.
3. Desyrel™: Chest pain and shortness of breath.
4. Zocor™: Upper respiratory infection
5. Lisinopril: **Asthma,** bronchitis, and painful breathing.
6. Hydrochlorothiazide: Difficulty breathing, fluid in the lung, inflammation of the lung.

We also find some additional issues regarding all three asthma medications. First, **two of three list high blood pressure as possible side effects.** Then, **the drug Alupent™ lists worsening or aggravation of asthma as one possibility.** And, both Albuterol and Intal™ list allergic reaction as a potential side effect. The problem is, allergic reactions are known to stimulate the production of histamine. Elevated histamine in turn, results in a constriction of the bronchial tubes in the lungs, and can thus contribute to asthma.

Albuterol appears to be the worst of the three medications Mary Lou was taking for asthma for. It is not only one of the two that can contribute to hypertension, but following you will find twenty <u>major concerns</u> of the total of at least 67 potential side effects associated with Albuterol use (those in bold print appear to be the most serious):

* **Depression**
* **Aggression**
* Agitation
* Allergic reaction
* Anxiety
* Coordination problems
* **Diabetes**
* Drowsiness
* Excitement
* Fluid retention and swelling
* Heart palpitations
* **Increased blood pressure**
* **Increased difficulty breathing**
* **Irritability**
* Nervousness
* Overactivity
* Rapid heartbeat
* Respiratory infection or disorder
* Restlessness
* Sleeplessness

Mary Lou was basically in disbelief as she reviewed the potential side effects associated with each drug she had been taking. As she began identifying each one that applied to her, it was such a relief knowing it was actually the side effects from her medications that were responsible for the symptoms she had been suffering from for so many years. Once the problem had been identified, the solution was quite obvious. When she discovered that Zocor™ was totally unnecessary, and the basic contributor to the elevated blood pressure she was taking medications for, as well as many other problems such as fatigue, it was the very first to go. Her next focus was the Prozac™ that had contributed to the bipolar disorder and diabetes, as well as the issue that both Prozac™ and lithium contributed to her already low thyroid condition. And finally, because the fluoride in Prozac™ not only suppresses the thyroid function but is also an enzyme inhibitor, that means she would not only be more prone toward depression, but she would also experience more side effects from all her medications (which she did). Then, we can't overlook the issue of the continual cravings for all addictive substances, (but especially alcohol), being stimulated by Prozac™.

It soon became apparent that the underlying cause of her addiction and the many symptoms she had experienced for years, were actually caused by her medications (and the depletion of nutrients they caused). Needless to say, armed with that knowledge, she was super-motivated to get off her medications, and as soon as possible. And in only two months, Mary Lou was totally drug-free!

My Recommendations:

Due to her sixteen years of Prozac™ use, I recommended she follow a more conservative withdrawal program. I had her immediately stop her cholesterol medication (which absolutely no one needs). This immediately brought her blood pressure into the normal range again. I then suggested that she stop drinking fruit juices, and reduce her intake of sugar and starches, and then begin the following:

1. Drink two ounces of mangosteen juice, three times daily.
2. Drink ten 8-ounce glasses of water daily.
3. Take one teaspoon of Celtic sea salt (coarse crystals) daily.
4. Take two high-potency coenzyme vitamin B-complex capsules daily.
5. Take two 200-mcg capsules of chromium picolinate, twice daily.
6. Take four 1,000 IU soft gel flax seed oil daily.
7. Take a multi-mineral, containing calcium, magnesium, and zinc.

An Explanation of Recommended Supplements

The mangosteen is a broad-spectrum adaptogen with a wide range of benefits, such as reducing sugar cravings, stabilizing the blood sugar, and mood elevation. Dr. Templeman discovered that in his practice, he was able to replace twenty-two medications with the mangosteen juice. I might add that at the time of Mary Lou's withdraw, I had not yet learned about the amazing benefits of goji juice or noni, also broad-spectrum adaptogens, although I'm quite certain that any of these three juices would have proven extremely beneficial in this case.

The water and Celtic sea salt combined provide an alternate source of energy for the brain, reducing the need for carbohydrates. Celtic sea salt also contains the natural form of the trace mineral lithium.

A vitamin or mineral deficiency (caused by Mary Lou's NINE prescription medications) can lead to many disorders, including both mental and behavioral. The coenzyme form of B-complex vitamins is the most effective, as the conversion in the liver is bypassed.

The chromium picolinate reduces the insulin resistance. The flax seed oil helps restore the insulin and serotonin receptors.

I also recommended she request that her doctor replace her thyroid hormone Synthroid™ (which seldom works) with the natural Armour™ thyroid (which seldom fails).

In 60 days, all nine of her medications had been successfully eliminated, and she indicated that she hadn't felt so good in years. It's quite obvious that Mary Lou (like so many others) definitely didn't need any of the medications she had been taking for so many years (sixteen years on Prozac™!). We can also see that the majority of her medications were to treat side effects associated with the drugs she was already taking. Drugs basically create the need for more drugs, (a domino effect).

Nutrient Depletion Contributes To The Domino Effect

We will now evaluate the nutrients depleted by Mary Lou's nine medications. In order to truly understand the significance of the nutrients depleted, the REFERENCE GUIDE TO SUPPLEMENTS provided at the end of this book will help you to determine the benefits of each. Once you discover the tremendous benefit of each nutrient depleted, you can better appreciate the important part each plays in your overall health, and why it should be an absolute top priority to begin eliminating your dependence on the medications responsible for creating this unnecessary depletion. The potential for a serious deficiency basically increases with each drug's contribution to the problem, as well as the many unpleasant side effects associated with each.

Following are the nutrients being depleted by the nine medications Mary Lou had been taking, followed by the number of drugs responsible for depleting each. Those in **bold** are considered some of the most important and widely used. The nutrients that appear most likely to lead to depression when deficient are identified with an asterisk.

Vitamins Depleted:
Vitamin A – 1
Vitamin B$_1$ – 2
Vitamin B$_2$ – 2
* Vitamin B$_3$ – 1
* **Vitamin B$_6$ – 5**
* **Vitamin B$_{12}$ – 4**
Vitamin C – 6
Vitamin D – 6
Vitamin E – 1
Vitamin K – 1
Choline – 1
* **Folic Acid – 4**
* Inositol – 1

Minerals Depleted:
* **Calcium – 4**
* Iron – 2
* **Magnesium – 5**
Manganese – 2
Phosphorus – 3
* **Potassium – 3**
Selenium – 1
* **Sodium - 5**
Zinc – 4

Other Depletions:
Choline – 1
* **Coenzyme Q$_{10}$ – 5**
Essential Fatty Acids – 2
Glutathione – 1

Although Mary Lou is just one example, many others are on even more medications. So, what is your story? And most importantly, will it have a happy ending? Just remember, you (not your doctor) are in charge of, and responsible for your health! That is not only your responsibility, but also your right, and something you must never forget. Those who took the initiative, and made the decision to end their lifetime dependency on medications, were amazed to discover it was not only possible, but also surprisingly easy. For Mary Lou, it was a pleasant experience to finally be free from the many side effects associated with the medications she had unnecessarily been taking. It was a real eye-opener to Mary Lou, when she discovered that following her doctor's advice for so long was the basic underlying cause of the many unexplained conditions she had been experiencing all those years.

Next we will be evaluating solutions to several common conditions, using natural therapies.

CHAPTER ELEVEN
LOWERING EXCESSIVELY ELEVATED CHOLESTEROL LEVELS WITHOUT DRUGS

If you noticed, we are addressing ways we can lower **"Excessively Elevated"** cholesterol only. Cholesterol has many important functions in the body, and too low cholesterol can actually be an even greater risk than when it's elevated.

Many decisions that doctors make on a daily basis are the result of findings announced through government agencies that are supposedly the authority. One such example is the announcement a few years ago that the acceptable cholesterol level should be lowered. It was determined that more people should also be placed on medication for lowering their cholesterol, and many should have their dosage increased as well. The criterion for determining those who qualified was extremely broad: Anyone who had diabetes, was considered obese, or had any cardiovascular risks, would qualify. That obviously just happens to include by far the majority of adults in the nation today. As might be expected, **the majority of "experts" on the panel that made that determination were being paid by the companies that were producing the extremely profitable statin (cholesterol lowering) drugs.**

The majority of your doctor's decisions are also influenced either directly or indirectly, by the companies that produce the medications they are writing an excessive amount of prescriptions for. Even Dr. Templeman, who was very candid about his experiences prior to discovering the value of mangosteen, indicated that he often wrote about 40 prescriptions a day. He seems to be very conscientious, and was convinced at the time, that there was no other viable option than the medications he had prescribed for twenty years, (the result of traditional medical training).

An extremely important issue to remember is: **By lowering your cholesterol <u>naturally</u>, you will <u>not</u> force your cholesterol below the level required by your body to maintain your health,** which is contrary to statin drugs that basically suppress the body's natural regulatory system. **Statin drugs can easily reduce your cholesterol to dangerously low levels!**

We will now identify many different options for maintaining healthy cholesterol levels. Just keep in mind that although I am providing you with many different options, they are just that (**options**). I'm sure there are others, and trying all is not necessary. I just want you to be aware that if your cholesterol level is somehow a concern, rather than stress about it (which will just raise your cholesterol), you have many resources available, thus dangerous statin drugs are totally unnecessary.

Also keep in mind that just because someone **"arbitrarily"** concluded that half the cholesterol level once considered as normal is somehow now ideal, **does not make it a fact!** You must consider the source, and the financial ties. If you do, the motivation to make such statements will be obvious. I have yet to meet anyone who has been on cholesterol-lowering medications for any length of time, (especially at higher doses), who is not terribly tired. I might add that I have never had my cholesterol tested, and never plan to. I have always eaten as many eggs as I choose, and will continue to do so. And as I noted, at 75 I have never been healthier. Also remember that LDL cholesterol is not actually the bad guy, but instead serves many important functions in the body and brain, and that elevated cholesterol is a **"contrived disease"**, created by man.

Following are a few natural options:
1. **Strengthen Your Thyroid. A low thyroid condition will often result in elevated cholesterol.** In fact, elevated cholesterol was once used as an indicator that a hypothyroid (low thyroid) condition might exist. Also, **an underactive thyroid gland inhibits the absorption of B vitamins, thus causing the true risk factor homocysteine to become elevated.** Once the thyroid condition has been resolved, your cholesterol level will normally stabilize, and your homocysteine levels will normalize also.

I believe I can possibly help explain this phenomenon. **When the thyroid is underactive, our metabolism and thus our body temperature lowers accordingly.** Dr. E. Denis Wilson, M.D., author of the book *Wilson's Syndrome – The Miracle of Feeling Well* (1996), discovered in lab tests that enzymes are extremely sensitive to temperature variations. **When our body temperature is just one degree below the normal 98.6°, our enzyme action becomes much less efficient.** As we have approximately 3,000 enzymes and 7,000 enzyme actions (some do double duty), it can easily influence every system throughout the body. One is the liver's ability to efficiently metabolize excess cholesterol. There is much more detailed information in the chapter in the Hypothyroidism, later in this book.

2. **Vitalzyme™.** According to Dr. William Wong, N.D., **the natural protolytic (protein digesting) enzyme, Vitalzyme™ has been found to reduce cholesterol levels by 21% in only 3 weeks.** He attributes the action to the fat digesting enzyme (lipase) in the formula. Although the protein-digesting enzyme (protease) also found in the formula won't likely have an influence on cholesterol, it will remove the fibrin in the arteries that can contribute to the restriction of blood flow. This can help prevent the clotting that often results in heart attacks or strokes, our primary objective.

3. **Niacin (vitamin B$_3$) is proven to lower cholesterol and to improve circulation.** Niacin also **assists in the metabolism of both carbohydrates and fats, and cholesterol is a fat.** High doses of the non-flushing form of niacin are highly effective in removing cholesterol, although regarding some people, long-term use can sometimes result in liver inflammation. If so, the problem can be easily eliminated simply by discontinuing its use. Niacin is commonly depleted by alcohol, antibiotics, caffeine, and SSRI antidepressants, as well as stress.

4. **The omega-3 fatty acid DHA, derived from fish oil, not only helps thin the blood, but also lowers both the blood pressure and cholesterol levels,** all important for our overall cardiovascular health, although it can easily be depleted by both estrogen and oral contraceptives.

5. **Large doses of vitamins C** lowers cholesterol levels and prevents oxidization of cholesterol, as well as lowering high blood pressure. It also aids in the production of anti-stress hormones. Vitamin C is commonly depleted by sugar, alcohol, caffeine, antidepressants, oral contraceptives, but especially smoking. An increased level of vitamin C assists in the conversion of cholesterol to bile acids, which promotes the digestion of fats, and the removal of excess cholesterol.

6. **The hormone melatonin** prevents the oxidation of cholesterol, and also assists in maintaining healthy cholesterol levels. It should be taken at night, 30 minutes before retiring, as it is also beneficial as a sleep aid. 3 mg should be adequate.

7. **Pregnenolone, another important hormone,** is used by the body to produce progesterone and is actually synthesized from cholesterol. Progesterone is instrumental in preventing excessively elevated estrogen levels, and assisting in the **production of adequate levels of thyroid, which helps stimulate metabolism.** As the level of pregnenolone drops, the level of other important hormones will also drop (as pregnenolone is a precursor to the other hormones), and **it all begins with adequate cholesterol.** Also as we learned, when the thyroid function is normalized, the cholesterol level normally stabilizes also.

8. **Chromium Picolinate** lowers total cholesterol levels and improves HDL-to-LDL ratio, as well as controlling blood glucose levels. High quantities of sugar in the diet can cause a loss of chromium from the body.

9. **Vanadium** is a little-known mineral that works in conjunction with the mineral chromium in reducing insulin resistance and regulating blood sugar. **Vanadium is also helpful in controlling cholesterol, and preventing cardiovascular blockage.**

10. **Guggul.** Documentation shows that **the herb known as guggul outperforms prescription pharmaceuticals in the reduction of total cholesterol, lowering triglycerides and increasing the HDL level.** As stated in the July 2003 *Health Sense* Nutritional Supplement, Published by the American Council on Collaborative Medicine, Inc. (ACCM), in one study, 20 patients with high cholesterol were given guggul two times a day for 16 weeks, resulting in cholesterol levels that dropped 22%, triglycerides down 27% and HDL up by 36%. Another study showed it reduced the tendency of blood to clot by 30-

40% in patients with coronary heart disease and helped prevent or correct atherosclerosis by removing plaque. As you can easily see, Guggul is a valuable resource in resolving multiple cardiovascular issues.

11. **Flax Seed Oil.** An article in the October 2002 issue of the *Health Alert* newsletter stated that **if you have abnormally high cholesterol levels, take at least one tablespoon of raw flax oil daily. This may be one of the most profound ways to normalize cholesterol.** A flax oil study was reported in an editorial in the medical journal *Circulation*, February 16, 9999, showing that **people consuming flax oil daily enjoyed a 70% reduction in deaths from heart disease compared to those not getting the oil.** Incidentally, flax oil is inexpensive and readily available, and is often beneficial in resolving depression also.

12. **Policosanol**. The American Council on Collaborative Medicine published the following information (*ACCM Health Sense*, July 2003):

Policosanol Inhibits Cholesterol Synthesis

A waxy long-chain alcohol derived from Caribbean sugar cane, policosanol is not considered a sugar molecule, thus is safe for diabetics. ***One of the newest discoveries for controlling cholesterol, 14 separate studies show policosanol not only lowers total cholesterol by significant margins, but reduces LDL up to 29% while increasing HDL by 8-15%.***

Research shows it is also considered equally as effective as statin drugs (such as Lipitor™) for normalizing cholesterol levels, thus avoids common side effects like muscle atrophy and liver dysfunction (p. 1).

13. **Fiber also appears to be helpful in the removal of cholesterol from the intestine before it can be re-absorbed into the bloodstream.** Although, the question we must ask ourselves is: Would our body possibly be attempting to save the cholesterol at times for a very good reason? Remember, as we have shown, **cholesterol has many important uses throughout both the body and brain.** It is thought that when there is a deficiency of cholesterol during high demand, cholesterol is sometimes acquired by the catabolization (removal) of cholesterol from the brain. That could possibly explain why **excessively low levels of cholesterol can sometimes lead to dementia,** as indicated by Dr. Bruce West, from his experience with patients.

14. **Alpha lipoic acid (ALA). This universal antioxidant recycles and enhances the activity of vitamin C and E, as well as the very important CoQ$_{10}$. It also enhances the conversion of glucose (a form of sugar) into energy and reduces insulin resistance, which is a definite plus for diabetics. And, it prevents the oxidation of LDL (low density) cholesterol, as well as lowering total cholesterol.**

15. **Garlic** lowers cholesterol, triglycerides levels, and blood pressure, as well as protecting against cardiovascular disease. Available in tasteless and odorless forms. For best results, take 2 capsules, 3 times daily.

16. **Cayenne**, either as a supplement in capsule form or in a tincture, reduces cholesterol and triglycerides levels, acts as a natural blood thinner, improves circulation, and benefits the heart, as well as the entire cardiovascular system.

17. **Turmeric.** Another valuable natural resource is **the herb normally used as a spice known as turmeric.** The active ingredient **curcumin** is perfectly safe and, as you will soon discover, it has several important benefits in the body. In the February 2004 issue of *Life Extension* magazine, we find:

New research shows that turmeric – and its main bioactive compound, curcumin – has the power to block inflammation, stop cancer, kill infectious microbes, and improve heart health.

*Some of the most intriguing new research on curcumin's potential benefits involves its apparent **ability to improve cardiovascular health.***

*Researchers in Egypt noted that **curcumin protected rats from oxidative stress injury following experimentally induced stroke.***

They noted that when curcumin was administered at the highest levels, injury-related oxidants, believed to be responsible for the majority of I/R damage, were significantly reduced.

*Scientists have shown that **curcumin prevents lipid peroxidation and the oxidation of cellular and subcellular membranes that are associated with atherosclerosis.***

*Still more intriguing than its ability to limit peroxidation is the finding that **curcumin raises HDL ("good") cholesterol levels, even as it reduces LDL levels.** In a small study of human volunteers, researchers reported **a highly significant 29% increase in HDL among subjects who consumed one-half gram (500 mg) of curcumin per day for seven days. Subjects also experienced a** decrease in total serum cholesterol of more than 11%, and a decrease in serum lipid peroxides of 33%.*

Curcumin appears to prevent certain cancers, inhibit cardiovascular disease, and quell inflammation, and may even offer protection against Alzheimer's disease (pp. 83-88).

18. **Lecithin** emulsifies cholesterol and other fats and helps keep them in a liquid state, it helps reduce the viscosity (thickness) of the blood, reducing the risk of heart attacks and strokes. Lecithin is available in both granules and capsules. The granules are the most cost effective. Two tablespoons daily should be adequate.

19. **Avoid stress.** Just stressing about your cholesterol level can quite easily increase your cholesterol level. From research, it was discovered that during finals students' cholesterol levels became elevated, and the same applied to accountants during the tax season (the result of stress). If you are going to your doctor to have your cholesterol level tested, and stressed about the possible result, your cholesterol could also be elevated, although it might actually be normal under ordinary circumstances.

Our body uses cholesterol to produce hormones, and when we are under stress, the need for stress hormone production would increase. The liver would be required to produce more cholesterol, to basically meet the increased demand. Stress hormones are also notorious for suppressing the thyroid, and thus the metabolism. This then results in a lower body temperature. Cholesterol is a fat, and the lower the body temperature, the more solid it will become. The fats in our body are very temperature sensitive, and just one degree can be critical regarding how soluble a fat such as cholesterol will be. In a solid or semi-solid state, cholesterol would tend to remain in the bloodstream much longer. It would thus be more prone to increase the viscosity (thickness) of the blood, and possibly accumulate in the existing plaque in the arteries.

Although cholesterol is an important component of our cell walls, it must be in a liquid state in order to be effectively utilized, which could easily explain the connection between low thyroid (lower body temperatures) and elevated cholesterol.

20. **Avoid Chloride (or chlorine).** According to Dr. Sherry A. Rogers, in *Detoxify or Die* (2002), chlorine contributes to arterial damage, and in her own words she states that *"Chlorine drills holes in arterial walls"* (p. 21), which indicates that it leads to elevated cholesterol (needed to repair the damage of the drilled holes). Another problem regarding chlorine is that it initiates the production of free radicals, which in turn oxidizes the cholesterol. This is a major contributor to hardening of the arteries. Chlorine is

also a known thyroid suppressant, which contributes to elevated cholesterol, as discussed previously in option #1.

21. **Adequate water is a simple solution that we can all afford.** Dr. F. Batmanghelidj, M.D., in his book *Your Body's Many Cries for Water* (1992/1998), pointed out that without making any dietary changes, a patient was able to drastically reduce his cholesterol level, just by drinking more water before meals. By doing so, he was able to reduce his cholesterol level from 279 to 203 (76 points) within two months! Adequate water intake has many additional benefits regarding our overall health. One benefit in relation to our cardiovascular health, which we are all currently focusing on, is regarding the viscosity (thickness) of our blood. When we are properly hydrated, the viscosity of our blood is lower (basically thinner). This allows better delivery of oxygen and nutrients to the cells, and more effective removal of toxins. The added bonus is the reduced risk of the formation of blood clots leading to heart attacks and strokes. Sometimes our best solutions turn out to be the cheapest. I tend to think that Our Creator might possibly of planned it that way.

22. **Mangosteen or Goji Juice.** From clinical experience, Dr. Templeman found that **mangosteen (XanGo™) <u>equals or outperforms</u>** the popular cholesterol-lowering medications Lipitor™, Zocor™, **and Pravachol**™. One of his patients claimed that she was able to lower her cholesterol 55 points in only 30 days with mangosteen. Although mangosteen has proven as effective as statin drugs in lowering elevated cholesterol, that is actually not as significant as some of its other abilities. And rather than depleting many important nutrients as the statin drugs do, mangosteen instead donates many, as well as providing 43 biologically active substances known as xanthones.

Dr. Victor Marcial-Vega, M.D. did extensive research regarding goji juice, and just one of his discoveries was that **high cholesterol levels decreased a minimum of 50 points in four weeks in 67 percent of the patients tested, while drinking goji juice.**

To read about the full benefits of mangosteen and goji juice, please see the chapter earlier in this book titled "A Few of Nature's Miracles".

Just be aware that in regards to this particular issue (cholesterol), as well as others covered in this book, I am just scratching the surface. I am basically attempting to provide enough facts, sufficient to convince you that in every single case, the benefits of natural supplements far outweigh any provided by drugs, and with all the potential dangers eliminated. For instance, if we looked closely at the many benefits provided by each one of the twelve nutrients depleted by statin drugs, you could better appreciate the risks to your health from their use. If we then contrasted the many proven benefits of the mangosteen or goji juice, you could better recognize the tremendous differences between the two. The very same principle applies, no matter what condition you are addressing. Every single nutrient has many different uses in both the body and brain. Therefore, we should be adding (not depleting) those nutrients. Any substance that is responsible for stealing nutrients (i.e. drugs) should be recognized as the enemy it is, and dealt with accordingly.

As we can easily see, we have a multitude of natural solutions for adequately maintaining healthy cholesterol levels. And, when it comes to cholesterol, lower is not necessarily better (in fact, at times it can actually be much be worse). And, especially that the statin (cholesterol lowering) drugs are not only totally unnecessary, but also potentially dangerous. So, the question is: Armed with this knowledge, could you possibly justify using statin (cholesterol lowering) drugs when so many natural, safe, and very effective options are easily available (and without a prescription)?

CHAPTER TWELVE
THE TRADITIONAL APPROACH TO TREAT DEPRESSION

When a patient indicates that a problem with depression exists, no matter what the underlying cause might be, the majority of doctors will immediately respond with a prescription for an antidepressant. Most doctors are not trained in mental disorders or depression, and are seldom aware of the many serious side effects associated with the use of the antidepressants they prescribe. When the patient begins experiencing major symptoms from the use of these antidepressants (especially problems from long-term use), the doctor is usually totally unaware of how to safely assist them with their withdrawal. There is a potential for both physical and mental reactions associated with immediate withdrawal. This is a concern that Dr. Ann Blake Tracy, author of the book *Prozac – Panacea or Pandora?* (1991/1994), and Dr. J. Glenmullen, author of *Prozac Backlash* (2000), both warn of.

This pertains to the most popular class of antidepressants known as Selective Serotonin Reuptake Inhibitors (SSRIs). The first developed, and most widely used, is Prozac™, but there are others such as Zoloft™, Paxil™, Celexa™, etc. which are potentially just as dangerous. The only safe and effective solution for withdrawal from antidepressants, is addressing the basic underlying causes of depression in the first place.

There are several potential contributors to depression, and many people can easily have more than one of the predispositions. Unless the underlying problem is accurately identified and resolved, the depression will likely persist. Just eating foods that we are allergic to or sensitive to, can easily affect our mood. The conditions hypoglycemia, hypothyroid, or adrenal fatigue, as well as the use of many prescription and over-the-counter medications, can easily contribute to depression. The good news is there are solutions for each one, and without the use of toxic drugs, which only treat symptoms, deplete many important nutrients, produce side effects, and create toxins in the process. The more drugs a person is using, (legal or illegal), the less healthy they are likely to be, and the greater the risk for depression.

Are Your Medications Making You Depressed?

Far too many are being prescribed drugs that are contra-indicated (combined with other drugs that are considered risky). They are also being prescribed major drugs known to be potentially dangerous, for relatively minor problems. Two prime examples are the statin drugs being prescribed for a disease that never really existed, and antidepressants often prescribed for pain or just about anything else you can think of. Unfortunately, most doctors have absolutely no idea just how potentially dangerous these drugs can be (they must be safe – Prozac™ is even approved for children!). Although the statin (cholesterol-lowering) drugs can easily be eliminated (just by stopping them), antidepressants are another matter.

Even though I believe I can safely withdraw antidepressants fairly rapidly, most doctors who prescribe them are not trained in nutrition, and basically have no idea how to assure their safe and effective withdrawal. I actually devoted eighteen months of extensive research regarding different causes of depression resulting from chemical imbalances in the brain, as well as the many problems associated with the use of antidepressants. Not only can the antidepressants create either a bipolar (manic depressive) disorder, or even a worsening of depression, but also when taken in combination with other medications or drinking alcohol, they can potentially create even more serious reactions.

The SSRI antidepressants such as Prozac™, Zoloft™, Paxil™, Celexa™, etc. are all highly protein-binding, making them extremely difficult for the liver to metabolize. If we then consider that any other drugs a person might be also taking are waiting their turn to be metabolized and eliminated by the liver, you can easily see the potential for serious problem associated with drug overdose. When prescribing drugs, one thing that doctors seldom consider is the more drugs a person might be taking, the higher the dosage they can expect to be getting (and the greater the potential for an overdose). More of each drug can potentially get around your liver (it knows drugs are toxins, and is attempting to eliminate them.) The more drugs that manage to get through, the greater the potential for interactions and side effects. Also, more vitamins and minerals will be depleted, which can then lead to a serious deficiency. In the case of minerals, an imbalance is a concern as well. The late Dr. Carl C. Pfeiffer, Ph.D., M.D., author of the book *Nutrition and Mental Illness* (1987), discovered that depression, as well as many mental and behavioral disturbances, often resulted from either vitamin or mineral deficiencies, or possibly mineral imbalances (something prescription medications are known to contribute to).

Your medications could quite easily be a major contributing factor to your depression in several ways. First, on a list of the top 200 most prescribed drugs, there were a total of 109 prescription medications (54.5%) that actually listed <u>depression</u> **as a potential side effect.**

Then, on that same list, we also encountered a total of 163 prescription medications that depleted vitamins that often result in depression when deficient. And, of the 37 medications that did not list the depletion of vitamins that can result in depression, 20 simply had not been evaluated to determine the specific nutrients depleted, (although that does not mean that none were depleted). That means that <u>more than 90.5% of the medications</u> **deplete nutrients that, when deficient, are responsible for contributing to** <u>depression</u>**!**

The depletion (or a deficiency) of the following nutrients can result in depression. In addition to the nutrients listed, are the drugs, class of drugs, substances, or conditions such as stress that can contribute to their depletion. Anyone suffering from depression will likely be able to identify multiple risk factors:

1. **Vitamin B$_3$ (niacin)** – depleted by sulfa drugs, **SSRI antidepressants,** steroids and corticosteroids, sleeping pills, **estrogen (and oral contraceptives),** caffeine, antibiotics, alcohol, sugar, and physical and mental stress.
2. **Vitamin B$_5$ (pantothenic acid)** – depleted by sulfa drugs, sleeping pills, **estrogen (and oral contraceptives),** caffeine, alcohol, sugar, cooking, and physical and mental stress.
3. **Vitamin B$_6$ (pyridoxine)** – depleted by vasodilators (i.e. nitroglycerin), sulfa drugs, steroids and corticosteroids, smoking, sleeping pills, **estrogen (and oral contraceptives),** diuretics, diabetic medication, caffeine, asthma medications, **antidepressants and MAO inhibitors**, antibiotics, alcohol, sugar, heat (canning & roasting), and physical and mental stresses.
4. **Vitamin B$_{12}$** – depleted by sulfa drugs, **SSRI antidepressants**, smoking, sleeping pills, proton pump inhibitors (i.e. Nexium™), muscle relaxants, mineral oil and laxatives, Histamine H$_2$ blockers (i.e. Tagamet™, Pepcid™, Zantac™), **estrogen (and oral contraceptives),** diuretics, diabetic medications, **all cholesterol-lowering drugs,** including statins and bile acid sequestrants (i.e. Questran™, Colestid™), calcium deficiency, caffeine, antiseizure medication (i.e. barbiturates), amphetamines and diet pills, antibiotics, and alcohol.
5. **Biotin** – depleted by sulfa drugs, **estrogen and oral contraceptives,** caffeine, antiseizure medication (i.e. barbiturates, phenytoin), antibiotics, alcohol, and saccharin.
6. **Folic Acid (folate)** – depleted by sulfa drugs, **SSRI antidepressants**, steroids and corticosteroids, smoking, NSAIDs (i.e. ibuprofen), mineral oil and laxatives, Histamine H$_2$ blockers (i.e. Tagamet™, Pepcid™, Zantac™), **estrogen (and oral contraceptives),** diabetic medication (especially Metformin), diuretics, decongestants (i.e. pseudoephedrine), caffeine, **all cholesterol-lowering drugs,** including statins and bile acid sequestrants (i.e. Questran™, Colestid™), aspirin, antiseizure medication (i.e. barbiturates), antibiotics, antacids, alcohol, food processing, heat and boiling, and physical and mental stress.
7. **Inositol** – depleted by sulfa drugs, lithium, food processing, **estrogen (and oral contraceptives),** caffeine, antiseizure medication, antibiotics, and alcohol.
8. **PABA (Para-Amino benzoic Acid)** – depleted by sulfa drugs, **estrogen (and oral contraceptives),** food processing, and alcohol.

9. **Calcium** – depleted by sulfa drugs, steroids and corticosteroids, **SSRI antidepressants,** NSAIDs (i.e. ibuprofen), mineral oil (laxatives), Histamine H_2 blockers (i.e. Tagamet™, Pepcid™, Zantac™), high fluoride intake (Prozac™), **estrogen (and oral contraceptives),** diuretics, caffeine, **all cholesterol-lowering drugs,** including statins and bile acid sequestrants (i.e. Questran™, Colestid™), aspirin, antiseizure medication (i.e. barbiturates), antifungals, antibiotics, antiarrhythmic agents (i.e. digoxin), antacids, alcohol, high protein diet, high sugar diet, high saturated fat diet, soft drinks, excess salt or white flour, excess sweating, smoking and emotional and physical stress.

10. **Copper** – depleted by Histamine H_2 blockers (i.e. Tagamet™, Pepcid™, Zantac™), penicillamine™ (chelating agent for copper removal), excess zinc, ethambutol™ (tuberculosis treatment), bile acid sequestrants (Questran™), antiviral HIV medication, and antacids.

11. **Iron** – depleted by NSAIDs (i.e. ibuprofen), mineral oil and laxatives, narcotics, histamine H_2 blockers (i.e. Tagamet™, Pepcid™, Zantac™), choline magnesium trisalicylate (an anti-inflammatory), **all cholesterol-lowering drugs**, including statins and bile acid sequestrants (i.e. Questran™, Colestid™), Carisoprodol™ (pain reliever), caffeine (especially the tannic acid in coffee and tea), aspirin, antibiotics, antacids, high phosphorus diet (bran), excess sweating, heavy bleeding (i.e. menstruating women, bleeding ulcers), candida yeast infection, phosphate food additives and EDTA (disodium ethylenediaminetetraacetate – a food preservative).

12. **Magnesium** – depleted by steroids and corticosteroids, **SSRI antidepressants,** NSAIDs (i.e. ibuprofen), Immunosuppressants, high levels of zinc, **estrogen and oral contraceptives,** diuretics, diabetic medication, all cholesterol-lowering drugs, including statins and bile acid sequestrants (i.e. Questran™, Colestid™), antiseizure medication (i.e. barbiturates, phenytoin), antifungal medication, antibiotics, antiarrhythmic agents (i.e. digoxin), antacids, alcohol, antihypertensive (blood pressure lowering) drugs (including ACE inhibitors, beta-blockers and calcium channel blockers), large amounts of fats, sugar, refined flour, fluoride, soft water consumption, and physical and emotional stress.

13. **Potassium** – depleted by steroids and corticosteroids, sodium bicarbonate (Alka Seltzer™), smoking, Parkinson's disease medication, NSAIDs (i.e. ibuprofen), muscle relaxants, laxatives, immunosuppressants, diuretics, caffeine, antiarrhythmic agents (i.e. digoxin), asthma medication, aspirin, antifungal medication, antibiotics, amphetamines and diet pills, alcohol, Acetazolamide™ (a carbonic anhydrase inhibitor), ACE inhibitors and other blood pressure lowering drugs (including beta-blockers), excess sugar and refined foods, large amounts of licorice, and physical and mental stress.

14. **Sodium** – depleted by narcotics, muscle relaxants, laxatives, diuretics, beta-blockers (blood pressure lowering drugs), aspirin, antigout medication, antifungal medication, **antidepressants (especially SSRI antidepressants),** Acetazolamide™ (a carbonic anhydrase inhibitor), ACE inhibitors and other blood pressure lowering drugs, dehydration (fever, heat, diarrhea, vomiting).

15. **Tyrosine – depleted by estrogen and oral contraceptives.**

16. **Essential Fatty Acids (EFAs)** – depleted by NSAIDs (i.e. ibuprofen), **estrogen (and oral contraceptives),** antiseizure medication (i.e. barbiturates, phenytoin), high saturated fat diet, bronchodilators, aspirin, and food processing.

Microwave Cooking and Nutrient Depletion

An adequate level of B vitamins is especially important for healthy brain function, and those most often depleted by drugs. Although avoiding food processing in general is important, the primary concern is in regard to **microwave cooking**. In Dr. Lita Lee's book, *Health Effects of Microwave Radiation – Microwave Ovens*, she stated that every microwave oven converts substances cooked in it to dangerous organ-toxic and carcinogenic products (http://www.vaccinetruth.org/microwave.htm), and goes on to quote portions of the Russian investigations published by the *Atlantis Raising Educational Center* in Portland, Oregon, as follows:

DECREASE IN NUTRITIVE VALUE OF MICROWAVED FOODS

*Russian researchers reported a marked acceleration of structural degradation leading to **a decreased food value of 60 to 90% in all foods tested.** Among the changes observed were:*

   a. **Decreased bio-availability of vitamin B complex, vitamin C, vitamin E, essential minerals and lipotropic factors in all food tested.**
   b. *Various kinds of damage to many plant substances, such as alkaloids, glucosides, galactosides and nitrilosides.*
   c. *The degradation of nucleo-proteins in meats.*

This is a very serious concern that very few are even aware of. This is especially a concern as microwave cooking destroys the majority of some of the most important nutrients we all need. Even heating water in a microwave is a concern, as the structure of water is also changed, and important to the body as well. I would guess that by far, the majority of people in the nation use their microwave on a regular basis for convenience. If they only knew, (now you know!)

Now let's take a moment and evaluate what we just learned, so we can better understand why depression, (due to nutrient depletion), is such a widespread problem in the nation today.

Of the sixteen nutrients important for preventing depression, we find that:

1. **Seven (nearly half) are actually <u>depleted by antidepressants</u>.** We also find that one of the potential side effects of antidepressants is depression.
2. Also, **seven (nearly half) are depleted by the cholesterol-lowering medications** (basically for a non-disease).
3. If we look closely, we can also see why **far more women than men suffer from depression. Estrogen and oral contraceptives actually top our list by far, at <u>twelve of sixteen</u> contributing to the problem!**
4. If we then consider that many are also taking NSAIDs for pain, or H_2 blockers for acid reflux, or possibly various medications for lowering blood pressure, we can better understand why anyone on prescription and over-the-counter medications is a prime candidate for depression.
5. Many eat fast food quite often, as well as frozen TV dinners heated in a microwave oven, which depletes nutrients (60% to 90%). It is quite easy to see how both depression and disease in general are not only possible, but also quite likely.

As you can see, there is always an underlying cause of poor health or depression, and as we just discovered, even prescription medications can be a major factor contributing to depression. Although a nutritional deficiency or a chemical imbalance in the brain is the most likely suspect, there are other possibilities, as you will soon learn.

Additional Contributors To Depression

✓ **Hypothyroidism (reduced metabolism).** Not only is depression one of the most common symptom of hypothyroidism, but the resultant reduced metabolism causes reduced enzyme action in the liver. Just one more way you can expect even more of an overdose of all your drugs.

✓ **Drinking alcohol** (which is incidentally detoxified by the very same P450 enzyme in the liver that most drugs are), results in the increased potential for serious physical and mental disorders and depression. That is especially true regarding the SSRI antidepressants, and becomes especially apparent when you consider that **alcohol depletes ELEVEN of the 16 nutrients previously mentioned as necessary for preventing depression.**

✓ **Stress,** which most of us experience all too often, creates an elevation of the hormone cortisol, known to suppress the thyroid, resulting in lowered metabolism. This then often leads to either one or both of the most common side effects associated with suppressed thyroid function, (depression and mood swings). And as you have just seen, **physical and mental stress contributes to the depletion of SEVEN of the 16 nutrients previously mentioned as necessary for preventing depression.**

✓ **Combining different prescription medications along with occasional over-the-counter medications** considerably increases the risk for depression.

✓ **Drinking grapefruit juice** can actually suppress the major detoxifier in the liver, the P450 enzyme, for up to 24 hours. That alone could easily complicate matters even further, and potentially lead to a serious overdose of both alcohol and drugs.

✓ **SSRI antidepressants such as Prozac™** cause your body to respond as though you were stressed, (even though you might not be). And as we just noted, stress is another contributor to depression. Dr. Ann Blake Tracy warns that only **one 30 mg dose of Prozac™ actually raises the stress hormone cortisol level by 200%,** which would automatically suppress the thyroid, and thus the metabolism, a common cause of depression. Cortisol also causes damage to brain neurons, and leads to elevated blood sugar. In fact, it was found that **SEVEN of the 16 nutrients listed as necessary for the prevention of depression, are actually depleted by antidepressants!**

✓ **Elevated estrogen**. One common side effect of elevated estrogen levels is depression. You may also have noticed that **estrogen and oral contraceptives (another form of estrogen) contributes to the depletion of ELEVEN of the 16 nutrients previously listed as being necessary for the prevention of depression!**

✓ **Fluoride** not only disrupts the binding of iodine in the thyroid (reducing the metabolism), but also is a known enzyme inhibitor (reducing the liver's enzyme action), as well as a contributor to elevated estrogen. Every single molecule of Prozac™ actually contains three molecules of fluoride. The end result will be the reduction of the liver's ability to detoxify drugs, through two different mechanisms. Remember, drugs (legal or illegal) are inorganic chemicals, thus the liver will attempt to eliminate them.

✓ **Suppressed dopamine** levels also contribute to depression. According to Dr. Glenmullen, SSRI antidepressants can actually promote depression, as they are known to suppress another important feel-good hormone, dopamine, by approximately 50%. It's quite amazing how many ways antidepressants can actually contribute to depression, (even one potential side effect), and we can easily see why.

✓ **Chronic back pain** may seem unrelated to depression, however **a chiropractic adjustment is just might be in order,** as we find that back pain may alter brain chemistry.

> *Back pain doesn't just affect patients' backs – it also influences their brains, say scientist. According to a recently published report in the journal* Pain, ***chronic back pain (CBP) alters patients' brain chemistry.***
>
> *Researchers at SUNY Upstate Medical University in Syracuse, New York used a magnetic resonance spectroscopy to measure the relative concentrations of several brain chemicals (N-acetyl aspartate, creatine, choline, glutamate, glutamine, gamma-aminobutyric acid, inositol, glucose and lactate) in 9 CBP sufferers and 11 pain-free volunteers. Measurements were conducted in six different brain regions. Patients with CBP also underwent evaluations for pain and anxiety.*
>
> *Findings revealed that, "in chronic back pain, the interrelationship between chemicals within and across brain regions was abnormal, and there was a specific relationship between regional chemicals and perceptual measures of pain and anxiety. These findings provide direct evidence of abnormal brain chemistry in chronic back pain"* (Pain – December 2000, 15;89:7-18) (http://hub.elsevier.com/pii/S0304395900003407).

CHAPTER THIRTEEN
EVALUATING ANTIDEPRESSANTS

The Many Serious Problems Associated with Prozac™

In the April 1997 issue of *Life Extension* magazine, the editor, Saul Kent, wrote an editorial titled "What's Wrong with Prozac?" regarding the book titled *Talking Back to Prozac* by Peter R. Breggin and Ginger Ross Breggin. In that editorial, Kent noted that: *"Peter R. Breggin is a psychiatrist – formerly a consultant with the National Institute of Mental Health – who is a long-time critic of drug-based psychiatry. Ginger Ross Breggin is a writer and Director of Research and Education at the Center for the Study of Psychiatry."* According to Kent:

> *One of the most startling accusations the Breggins level is that* **Prozac is a chemical cousin of amphetamine and cocaine-drugs which also inhibit serotonin reuptake.** *It is those properties, the Breggins believe***, that make Prozac dangerous. And dangerous it is.** *Ordinary people have done things such as getting out of bed in the middle of the night and hanging themselves after taking it.* **There are numerous reports of 'speed'-like behavior and aggression.** *People have reported having nightmares where people are coming at them with knives, or they are going to kill others or themselves.*
>
> **One woman, put on the drug for weight loss, ended up trying to shoot herself in front of her children.** *(Her husband got the gun away from her). According to the Breggins,* **this type of behavior is consistent with what people sometimes do on cocaine or "speed." Is Prozac legalized "speed"?**

Sounds rather like a nightmare, doesn't it? For someone like Andrea Yates, who was on three different antidepressants, and suddenly forced to stop her medications due to a lapse in her insurance, it turned out to be not only a nightmare for her, but also her children. Unfortunately, misperceptions can seem very real to someone with a severe chemical imbalance in the brain. I can't help but wonder if Andrea is the one who actually belongs in prison, or those who are knowingly promoting these potentially dangerous drugs just for the sake of profit. The manufacturers, and their representatives, attempt to downplay the serious concerns associated with these antidepressants.

Kent also mentions that *"A meticulous dissection of FDA documents reveals that there is no proof that Prozac works better than tricyclic antidepressants – or that it works at all."* Apparently, the Breggins discovered that *"***One of the main studies the FDA used in approving Prozac is based on data from only 11 patients! And it was conducted by a doctor who has been accused of fraud in other trials.***"*

In addition, *"***None of the studies lasted for more than 6 weeks, and patients frequently rated Prozac as no better than placebo.*** There are millions of people taking this drug, trusting that clinical trials proved its safety, its efficacy, and long-term benefit, yet there is apparently no such data."*

Another important issue that the Breggins pointed out is that:

> **None of the patients who participated in the Prozac studies were suffering from severe depression.** *While some of this type of thing might occur in a large study, what the Breggins show is that juggling the data, and* **"cookin' the books" was the norm for the Prozac studies. One can only conclude that the real clinical trials for Prozac are being done on the American public – without its knowledge.**

Finally, Kent stresses that *"One of the most chilling aspects of the book is the possibility that Prozac may cause a type of social withdrawal and emotional flatness reminiscent of the worst sex offenders/murderers."*

Dr. Ann Blake Tracy, in her book *Prozac – Panacea or Pandora?* (1991/1994), mentions that when a drug is used to stimulate the adrenals, there is an internal loss of glandular control. The **adrenals begin to rush at the slightest provocation. She also warns that this can cause** *"mania, depression, akathasia type reactions (inability to rest or relax, anger, irritability, violence, etc.), hallucinations, electrical surges throughout the body, etc."* (p. 86). The body normally controls excess steroid levels through the release of the hormone or neurotransmitter, acetylcholine. Once the liver becomes impaired through the use of toxic drugs, or as the brain and nervous system can no longer produce acetylcholine, the body loses its ability to control its steroid levels. Dr. Tracy poses the question:

> *Why raise serotonin when it in turn raises steroid levels and produces a wide variety of mental and physical disorders?* *Animal studies demonstrate that in the initial administration Prozac actually causes the brain to shut down its own production of serotonin, thereby causing a paradoxical effect or opposite effect on the level of serotonin* (p. 87).

Dr. Tracy then goes on to describe the basic problem with all mind-altering drugs such as Prozac™, noting that any disruption, whether it be a raising or lowering of any neurotransmitter, can cause drastic changes in brain function, behavior, mood, memory, sleep patterns, cognitive reasoning abilities, etc. The neurobalance of the brain is very delicate and sensitive, and repercussions from any disruption of that balance are often very extensive.

The *Physicians Desk Reference* (PDR) states that Prozac™ binds to *"human serum proteins, including albumin and glycoprotein."* **All the serotonergic drugs, including Prozac™, are highly protein binding, (94.5%),** in theory blocking the reuptake of excess serotonin in the brain for extended periods. However, they also bind to other proteins or toxins in the blood, **making them too large to be broken down and metabolized readily by the liver.** This binding to various proteins causes excess stress to be placed on the liver and kidneys, which are involved in the metabolizing and detoxification processes. These are concerns that need to be addressed when attempting to withdraw from Prozac™. Dr. Tracy also warns that:

> ***Those who are mixing Prozac with other drugs,*** *those with pancreatic, liver and kidney weaknesses, those in a weakened physical condition, or those with a past history of diseases affecting those organs, including a past history of excessive alcohol usage or drug abuse, or* ***years of constant prescription drug use,*** *especially psychoactive drugs or drugs which include psychiatric side effects* ***are the ones having immediate extreme adverse effects*** (p. 91).

One of the more frequent complaints of adverse reactions made to the FDA about Prozac™ is *impaired liver function*, and Dr. Tracy asks:

> *If a patient is taking a drug which impairs the organ essential in controlling the amount of medication the body retains in the blood, how safe is the drug? Once liver function is impaired, any chemical can rapidly accumulate within the body to toxic levels, producing adverse reactions and* <u>even death</u> (p. 92).

Research indicates that serotonin is normally reduced in those who experience depression, insomnia, or those who abuse alcohol, as the chemical structure of the serotonin, and many drugs of abuse are actually quite similar. According to Dr. Tracy, *"it has been shown that LSD, causing an increase in serotonin, acts much the same as an SSRI."* She then goes on to explain that:

> *Cocaine blocks serotonin reuptake leading to an initial increase in serotonin levels. Alcohol increases levels of serotonin. The levels then subsequently drop just as they do with LSD. Steroids (cortisone, prednisone, etc.) directly affect serotonin and are known to create psychotic behavior* (p. 114).

It appears that all drugs that cause this initial increase in serotonin levels in the brain, no matter what their mechanism might be, eventually produce an accompanying increase in serotonin resistance in the serotonin receptors. Thus, prolonged use of antidepressants tends to produce effects in opposite directions. Forcing an increase in the amount of any neurotransmitter results in decreased receptor sensitivity. Neuroscientists have learned that different neurotransmitters do not function independently of one another, and thus a dramatic change in one, like boosting serotonin, can trigger compensatory changes in the others. A drop in dopamine, to compensate for the artificially elevated serotonin levels, is basically how the brain reacts in an attempt to maintain a healthy balance. Dr. Glenmullen stresses that, ***"drugs producing a dopamine drop are well known to cause the dangerous side effects that are now appearing with Prozac and other drugs in its class."*** This is what he refers to as the *"Prozac Backlash"*. He goes on to say that *"a critical variable determining the degree of damage appears to be total cumulative exposure to the drugs"* (*Prozac Backlash*, Glenmullen, 2000, p. 20). Not only other neurotransmitters, such as dopamine in the brain, but the entire body, can be influenced by these dangerous serotonergic drugs. Caffeine or nicotine, along with medications, tends to increase the chances of drug interactions. **Prozac™ greatly multiplies the effects of many other drugs, and thus increases the possibility of adverse reactions.**

The diet is one important factor that could help explain the many varied symptoms that people experience when on Prozac™, as many foods can also influence a person's moods or behavior. For instance, any food that a person is allergic to, or has a sensitivity toward, can easily lead to depression, mood swings, or possibly hyperactivity. Like alcohol and drugs, these are often the very foods that people tend to crave. Simple sugar, for example, which people often crave the most, can result in many behavioral problems. As sugar does not contain the nutrients necessary for its own metabolism, it will actually deplete them from the body.

Similarly, Dr. Tracy noted that many people on Prozac™ do not properly metabolize milk, which then results in the formation of caso-morphine, an addictive substance in the brain. Dr. Peter D. D'Adamo, N.D. tells us, in his book *Eat Right For Your Type* (1996), only those with blood type "B" properly metabolize milk. That might possibly explain why, according to Dr. Tracy, many schizophrenics found they returned to normal after removing milk from their diet. Also, different alcoholic drinks are made from different grains, and some grains are also a problem for many people, but especially those containing gluten. It is thought that an allergy to the particular grain might be a more important factor regarding the addiction than the alcohol itself, and probably the reason a person often prefers one alcoholic beverage over another.

The problem apparently lies with the fact that Prozac™ is so hard on the pancreas that it can actually push a healthy pancreas into a diabetic or hypoglycemic state. This can cause the pancreas to malfunction, thereby upsetting the blood sugar balance in the body. This blood sugar imbalance or hypoglycemic condition would, in turn, cause the "craving" for alcohol which people often experience as the body attempts to increase the blood sugar level.

In her book *Prozac – Panacea or Pandora?* (1991/1994, pp. 157 – 270), Dr. Tracy shares some of her patients' experiences while on Prozac™, as follows:

> *The rage and violent feelings are often referred to by the patients as:* ***"indescribable", "an anger unlike I have ever felt before", "only two weeks on Paxil I cannot believe I did not kill myself or someone else."***
>
> *"My wife told me that while she was on Prozac she could have killed me once or twice. Yet she is the most gentle, kind and sympathetic person I've ever known in my life! Contrary to what Lily would have to say about it, it was not a pre-existing condition. Everybody has ups and downs and depression and so forth, but this is different. This is a thousand times worse than the original problem they took the Prozac for to begin with."*

"I would wake up each morning thinking, 'Oh God, I'm still alive! I have to live another day of this hell of wanting to die!' I thought of running into trees at a high rate of speed."

"During the month I spent on Prozac I could think of nothing but various ways of killing those closest to me – my family, my mom, my dad and my brothers and sisters." (A very sweet and sensitive 14-year-old girl who took herself off Prozac because of these thoughts it was causing her).

"I felt I had to kill myself but I could not leave my family alone. I planned how I would accomplish the deaths of my husband and children in detail. How could I ever have had such thoughts?!"

"Throughout my life I have always been known as 'Mr. Mellow,' but the rage I felt on Prozac helped me to understand how someone could murder another."

"I became obsessed with dying. I thought dying was the only way out, and I never contemplated suicide before that time."

"Nothing mattered to me, especially my life or anyone else's. I didn't care bout anyone or anything!"

"After being on Prozac for one week I had an argument with another motorist and attempted to run over him with my car!"

"I've been a reformed alcoholic for twelve years, but while on Prozac I started craving alcohol again!"

"I thought I had someone else's brain in my body!"

"After using LSD in my past, I can tell you that taking Prozac is like taking half a hit of LSD, except that it also made me angry and aggressive."

"Although it was completely out of character for me, the compulsion to drink was so strong after starting on Prozac that it became impossible for me to drive past a bar."

"I wanted to stop using Prozac, but I was addicted. How could I be addicted to a drug that my family practitioner gave me?"

"I felt as though I was on a combination of speed and cocaine."

"Wicked! That's exactly how you feel on Prozac, wicked, just plain wicked!"

As my father often said: *"If something seems too good to be true, it probably is!"* That certainly applies to Prozac™, which is obviously not a panacea as advertised, but instead, a Pandora, as Dr. Tracy discovered, and something that many learned the hard way, from their own personal experience.

What About the Elevated Cortisol Caused by Prozac?

As we learned, just one 30 mg dose of Prozac™ increases the level of the stress hormone cortisol by 200%, and stress depletes both vitamin B_6 and zinc (as does Prozac™). The body reacts to the elevated cortisol by breaking down muscle tissue. According to Dr. Carl C. Pfeiffer, Ph.D., M.D., the breakdown of muscle results in the abnormal production of pyroles, which depletes both vitamin B_6 and zinc. Incidentally, muscle wasting is one well-known side effect associated with Prozac™. In his book *Nutrition and Mental Illness* (1987), Dr. Pfeiffer helps identify the problem. He discovered that **"B_6 and zinc are the missing link,"** and he states that **"Perhaps the most significant discovery in the nutritional treatment of mental illness is that many <u>depressed</u> and mentally ill people are deficient in vitamin B_6 and zinc"** (p. 33).

Vitamin B_6 is necessary for removing the acid from the amino acid L-tryptophan, converting it to serotonin (the feel-good hormone). Thus, anything that contributes to the production of stress hormones, such as cortisol produced by Prozac™, would reduce the amount of L-tryptophan that would be converted to serotonin. This is one more way Prozac™ can actually contribute to depression, as well as a reducing the sensitivity of serotonin receptors in the brain. Another important function of serotonin is the storage of energy. As a result, any reduction in serotonin would contribute to fatigue, as well as depression.

Although many assume that the serotonergic drugs such as Prozac™ increase serotonin levels, that is not actually true. Their only function is overriding the body's regulation of "excess serotonin" in the brain, (a very bad idea). This not only upsets the normal hormonal balance in the brain, but its systemic influence is evidenced by Prozac's extensive list of potential side effects (some major). Many systems are influenced because there are serotonin receptors in not only the brain, but also throughout the entire body.

An article in the February 2003 issue of the *Life Extension magazine* (pp. 87-88) quotes brain specialist Dr. David Perlmutter, M.D., one of the speakers at the American College for the Advancement of Medicine (ACAM) on May 17-19, 2002 in Fort Lauderdale. At this conference, he presented a lecture on the effects of chronically elevated cortisol on the hippocampus, an area of the brain important in the formation of memory as well as in the regulation of the hypothalamic-pituitary-adrenal (HPA) axis. One slide demonstrated the **neuroprotective effects of cortisol <u>reduction.</u>**

Dr. Perlmutter pointed out that ***"Humans with pathologically elevated cortisol,*** *such as the victims of Cushing's syndrome, have overactive adrenals, and* ***show much more cognitive decline than individuals with lower cortisol levels"*** (*Life Extension Magazine*, February 2003, pp. 87-88).

Dr. Tracy stated that the Cushing syndrome is one of the more serious conditions that result from excessive levels of cortisol stimulated by Prozac™. This results in a wasting of muscle tissue, similar to a serious muscle wasting condition that many AIDS patients also experience.

In the *Life Extension* article, Dr. Perlmutter also notes that ***"Alzheimer's disease patients show elevated levels of cortisol in their cerebrospinal fluid;*** *in these patients, the degree of hippocampal atrophy accurately reflects cognitive decline."* He then poses the question:

> *How does cortisol damage the hippocampus? It increases levels of glutamate, an excitatory neurotransmitter. Excess glutamate causes neural mitochondria to produce defective ATP (ATP, **a**denosine **tri**phosphate, is our energy molecule). This defective ATP eliminates the "magnesium block" guarding the neuron against excess influx of calcium ions, followed by generation of free radicals and cell damage or cell death. **Elevated evening cortisol indicates damage to the HPA axis. Evening cortisol elevation is related to sleep fragmentation (frequent awakenings) and less REM sleep. Even modest elevation in cortisol has been found to correlate with memory deficit** (pp. 87-88).*

Dr. Perlmutter goes on to discuss the important issue that *"Stress in childhood may set the HPA axis at an over-reactive level, so that the individual reacts to even minor stressors with an exaggerated cortisol response"* (*Life Extension Magazine*, February 2003, pp. 87-88). Considering the serious issues just discussed, along with the 575 potential side effects listed by the FDA associated with Prozac™ use, the question remains: How could the FDA possibly approve, and so many doctors prescribe Prozac™ for anyone, and **especially for children**?

Then, Dr. Glenmullen, M.D., in his book *Prozac Backlash* (2000), says that in his experience:

> ***As many as 75% of patients are needlessly on these drugs for mild, even trivial, conditions...[such as] anxiety, obsessions, compulsions, eating disorders, headaches, back pain, impulsivity, drug and alcohol abuse, hair pulling, nail biting, upset stomach, irritability, sexual addictions, attention deficit disorder, and premenstrual syndrome*** (pp. 11, 14).

He then notes that some employee assistance programs have even used SSRIs to *"prop up exhausted factory workers putting in grueling overtime shifts as result of corporate downsizing"* (p. 14). It basically sounds like a stimulant to me, which in fact it is.

Dr. Glenmullen also states that Prozac™ was on the cover of *Newsweek* (March 1990), boasting that the *"medical breakthrough"* had already been prescribed for so many conditions in addition to depression that *"even healthy people have started asking for it."* And, *New York* magazine called Prozac™ a *"wonder drug"* and the *National Enquirer* described it as a miracle diet pill. Another cover of *Newsweek* announced, *"Beyond Prozac: How Science Will Let You Change Your Personality with a Pill"* – seemingly, the voice of the scientific establishment (p. 13).

While the pharmaceutical companies have marketed these drugs as "selective" for serotonin, these serotonergic drugs are anything but selective in regards to their widespread effects. In fact, there is no known depression center in the brain, but instead, serotonin has a vast influence throughout the body. Although only about 5% of serotonin is found in the brain, and is one of the chemicals by which brain cells communicate, the other 95% is distributed throughout the rest of the body. The majority is produced in the gastrointestinal tract, and just one function of serotonin is the storage of energy throughout the body.

The Politics of Prozac™

In light of the literature reviewed on the effects of Prozac™ and other SSRI antidepressants, the question remains: Why are these drugs continuing to be prescribed by many doctors throughout the United States, and even approved by the FDA for children's use?

To better understand the rationale behind this situation, it might be beneficial to evaluate the politics of Prozac™ to understand why it is still legal, especially in spite of the proven potential for serious physical and mental damage associated with its use.

A major problem is regarding the drug approval process. First, most studies done to determine the safety of a particular drug, are normally conducted by the company that created the drug. The results of the study would be expectedly biased in favor of the drug's approval. Secondly, the company is required to pay a huge sum to the FDA for the drugs' approval. The FDA often evaluates drugs similar to drugs already approved in the past. According to Dr. Glenmullen (*Prozac Backlash*, 2000, p. 21), although the FDA only reviews about 25 new drugs a year, a professional staff of 1,500 doctors, scientists, toxicologists, and statisticians are assigned to review the results of studies normally conducted by the manufacturer on approximately 25 new drugs. Yet they allot a staff of only five doctors and one epidemiologist to monitor the safety of more than 3,000 drugs already approved, and being prescribed for millions of patients! The commonly held belief is: The drug approval studies are far from adequate to effectively determine their safety, suggesting that the FDA would rather not know about the results of a flaw in the approval process. As Dr. Glenmullen suggests, it would make more sense to assign a larger portion of the staff to evaluating the complaints filed, and long-term side effects from the 3,000 drugs being prescribed daily to millions.

In her book, *Prozac - Panacea or Pandora?* (1991/1994), Dr. Ann Blake Tracy recalls the time when she first uncovered the research that demonstrated the similarity between Prozac™ and other SSRIs, and the psychedelic drugs. She approached a well-respected scientist with this information, which appears to be a very common problem with many doctors. Dr. Tracy explains the basic problem:

> *I knew of his interest because he had been approached two years before by two doctors who were looking for a leading expert in the field of psychoactive drugs to help their brother. Their brother was an attorney who had experienced terrible long-term reactions while on Prozac for only five months. Help had been impossible to find. Every new doctor wanted to try another drug to stop his reactions and the reactions continued to become*

more and more severe with each new drug. After working with this patient for over a year, this doctor could offer no hope either. He tried everything he could think of, but he was baffled. He remained convinced that the patient was suffering what drug experts would call post drug syndrome. The symptoms were electric surges throughout the body which would leave him breathless and wondering if after the attack he could begin breathing again or retain the ability of his heart to continue beating, constant ringing in the ears, plus a large majority of the other side effects we have discussed. The doctor felt sure that what the patient was suffering was the result of damage to the cholinergic nervous system, like he had seen in conjunction with illicit drug use. This is something that we are being told does not happen with Prozac use. He was still looking for answers when I shared with him my newfound research. Obviously shocked, he responded, **"That means that LSD has the same effect upon serotonin as the Serotonin Reuptake Inhibitors! No wonder!"** *He asked for a copy of the research material. I then requested that he go public with this very critical information. He sighed deeply and replied,* **"Lilly will crush whoever comes forward with this information."** *It was clear that he felt the action may put an end to his career and that I was on my own –* **thanks once again to the politics in medicine in America** *(pp. 370-371).*

In case you wondered, he was referring to the pharmaceutical company Eli Lilly, who produces Prozac™, (a very profitable drug).

Suppression of this kind of information helps explain why the general public is unaware of the dangerous side effects that can result from Prozac™ and other SSRI drugs. Even more serious is the concern that many doctors who write the prescriptions for Prozac™ or other SSRI antidepressants know little about how dangerous the drugs really are. Their information normally comes from the literature provided by the company attempting to promote their product, or their sales staff, both obviously biased. The drug companies also promote the antidepressants for many uses other than depression, although depression was the only condition the drug had been approved for by the FDA.

Now let's look at some other very serious concerns:

1. According to Dr. Ann Blake Tracy, regarding Prozac™: *"As of October, 1993, 28,623 complaints of adverse side effects had been filed with the FDA, including 1,885 suicide attempts and 1,349 deaths"* (*Prozac – Panacea or Pandora?*, 1991/1994, p. 55).

2. In the *Journal of the American Medical Association*, **the FDA commissioner, David Kessler indicated that** *"only about 1 percent of serious events are reported to the FDA"* (*Prozac – Panacea or Pandora?*, Tracy, 1991/1994, p. 55). Notice he said **"serious events"**. And that statement was made by the FDA commissioner himself. If Dr. Kessler's statement is true, that would translate to 2,862,300 adverse reactions, 188,500 suicide attempts, and 134,900 deaths associated with Prozac™! These figures are unheard of in the history of the FDA – never have they seen anything that compares.

3. We need to keep in mind that although these figures are unbelievably serious, they were actually taken from statistics that are more than 15 years old, and as the prescribing of Prozac™ by doctors is continuing to escalate at a rapid pace, they could easily have doubled, or even tripled since then.

4. According to Dr. Ann Blake Tracy, in her 1999 audiotape titled *Help! I Can't Get Off My Antidepressants!*, one person in seven in our nation was currently on antidepressants. Although she didn't state how many were on antidepressants six years prior, when the statistics were current as she quoted in her book *Prozac – Panacea or Pandora?* (1991/1994), I am sure the percentage she quoted would reflect a much larger percentage of the population.

5. Then on November 16, 2002, during a lecture by Dr. Tracy at the *Symposium for Health Freedom* in Anaheim, California that I attended, she stated that since the 9/11 incident, the figure had actually doubled from *"one in seven"* to *"one in 3½"*, showing the potential rate of acceleration. Especially if we consider that the rate of prescriptions actually doubled in approximately 3 years, and was obviously precipitated by just one incident.

6. Another concern Dr. Tracy stated in her Anaheim lecture was that in the four years from 1995 to 1999, regarding children under 6 years of age, Prozac™ usage increased by an astounding 580%! This was before Prozac™ was actually approved by the FDA for use by children.

7. And finally, the decision by the FDA in February 2003 to approve Prozac™ for use by children. That would certainly indicate an obviously disproportionate appropriation of staff by the FDA to evaluate the 3,000 drugs they approved, as Dr. Glenmullen noted.

Candice Pert, M.D. was one of two developers to discover the serotonin binding processes, which made all of the serotonergic medicines possible. In *TIME* magazine, October 20, 1997 issue (p. 8), she talks about the widespread use of these drugs, and declares: ***"I am alarmed at the monsters I have created."*** According to Dr. Tracy, never in the history of medicine has the developer of any medication come out with such a strong negative statement about the drug in question, especially while the medications are still on the market.

MAO Inhibitors –Another Class of Widely Used Antidepressants

MAO Inhibitors – one more problem anti-depressant. Frankly, I would rather not deal with any more anti-depressants, as just evaluating them is rather depressing. Unfortunately, my conscience would somehow not allow me any peace of mind if I chose not to address this one also. The major concern regarding the MAO Inhibitors is the very extensive list of contra-indications (things to avoid) associated with their use. These contra-indications include the majority of healthy foods most people normally eat on a daily basis. Also, included on the following "Avoid" list are many commonly used prescription medications, and even several natural supplements, including some of the most important amino acids necessary for avoiding depression.

As we go through this extensive list of foods that anyone on the MAO Inhibitor therapy should avoid, I believe that we could all easily identify many <u>Healthy Foods</u> that should normally be included in any healthy diet. We will now allow Dr. James Balch, and his wife Phyllis, to take us on a tour through this extensive list as follows:

> ***MAO Inhibitors also have a high potential for dangerous interactions with other substances, including drugs and foods.*** *Persons taking these drugs must adhere strictly to a diet that includes no foods containing the chemical tyramine, such as almonds, avocados, bananas, beef or chicken liver, beer, cheese (including cottage cheese), chocolate, coffee, fava beans, herring, meat tenderizer, peanuts, pickles, pineapples, pumpkin seeds, raisins, sausage, sesame seeds, sour cream, soy sauce, wine, yeast extracts (including brewer's yeast), yogurt, and other foods. In general, any high-protein food that has undergone aging, pickling, fermentation, or similar processes should be avoided. Over-the-counter cold and allergy remedies should also be avoided (*Prescription for Nutritional Healing, *3rd edition,* Balch & Balch, 2000, p. 318).

I believe we would all likely benefit from eliminating the beverages beer, wine, and coffee, and just replace them with water. I have yet to identify any contra-indication associated with drinking water. But what about the brewer's yeast we must avoid? Although not all brewer's yeast is the same, the one I use daily from Lewis Labs, contains all the essential amino acids, (or the co-factors necessary for their conversion). Brewer's yeast is also known to be beneficial and often recommended for both diabetics and hypoglycemics. The beef and chicken we are told to avoid are normally part of most people's diet, unless they just happen to be a vegetarian by choice. Now lo and behold, we also have to avoid both cheese and cottage cheese. This is already getting depressing (which we are attempting to avoid), and we are just getting started!

We can easily see how difficult it would be to adhere to such a restrictive diet that excludes so many healthy foods essential for maintaining not only mental health, but also our health in general.

Apparently many of the sugars and starches that the American Diabetic Association (ADA) recommends avoiding, in order to reduce diabetes and hypoglycemia, are considered perfectly acceptable foods. Unfortunately, most of the proteins and fats important for maintaining our health and stabilizing our blood sugar should be avoided when using MAO Inhibitors. Unstable blood sugar or insulin levels often result in an increased accumulation of arterial plaque, and a greater risk for stroke or heart attack, as well as the increased potential for developing diabetes, or hypoglycemia. So, in our attempt to resolve depression, we are increasing our risk of acquiring two major diseases instead.

Keep in mind that according to Dr. James F. Balch, M.D.:

> **Tyrosine is needed for brain function**. *This amino acid is directly involved in the production of norepinephrine and dopamine, two vital neurotransmitters that are synthesized in the brain and the adrenal medulla.* **A lack of tyrosine can result in** *a deficiency of norepinephrine in certain sites in the brain, resulting in* **mood disorders such as depression** (*Prescription for Nutritional Healing, 3rd edition,* Balch & Balch, 2000, p. 51).

As we can easily see, a deficiency of the amino acid tyrosine, (which we are attempting to avoid), can actually result in mood disorders such as depression, something the MAO Inhibitors are supposed to be eliminating! Now let's see what Dr. Balch's concern is, regarding the use of tyrosine supplements with MAO Inhibitors. He cautions that **"If you are taking an MAO Inhibitor drug for depression, <u>do not</u> take tyrosine supplements, and avoid foods containing tyrosine, as drug and dietary interactions can cause a sudden, dangerous rise in blood pressure"** (*Prescription for Nutritional Healing, 3rd edition,* Balch & Balch, 2000, p. 318). What a contradiction we seem to have, as we are required to avoid the very foods and supplements we should be consuming. These foods are necessary for producing some very important neurotransmitters for avoiding depression.

We will let Eva Edelman, author of *Natural Healing for Schizophrenia* (1996/1998), shed additional light on the subject. First, she adds some more items to our "Avoid" list, (as if Dr. Balch's wasn't enough). Although pork was not on Dr. Balch's list, it was on Eva's list, along with one of our best sources of protein, <u>EGGS</u>. But if we look a little further, we also find <u>FISH</u>! Eva also listed dairy! So we are basically down to a strict vegetarian (vegan) diet. Most nutritionists don't recommend a vegan diet, as it is very restrictive and makes it extremely difficult to get an adequate amount of complete proteins, as well as vitamin B_{12}. Both are necessary for producing the amino acids and enzymes important for maintaining mental stability. Protein is also important for helping stabilize the body's pH, and the production of collagen to help build strong bones and healthy blood vessels.

At this point, we have been forced to eliminate most sources of protein, and resort to a strict vegan diet. Unfortunately, I can see another problem emerging also, as we will be restricting that diet even further once we combine the two lists of contra-indicated foods. We should be aware that any food or beverage that contains either of the amino acids, tyrosine or tyramine, is considered contra-indicated with MAO inhibitors, and in that case, the amino acid phenylalanine would also be a contra-indication, as it is a precursor to tyrosine.

Now that we understand what we are basically attempting to avoid, let's take a look at two more basic food groups we must exclude according to Eva's list: the legumes and nuts. Apparently some nuts have tyrosine, and others contain tyramine. Anyone familiar with a vegetarian diet is aware that nuts, seeds, and legumes, are the major source of a vegetarian's protein, and essential fatty acids. For example, soybeans are legumes, and soy products such as tofu, are often used as a meat substitute for protein for vegetarians. Grains such as wheat, rye, and barley contain gluten (unless sprouted), and must be avoided by many who have a gluten sensitivity. Many nutritionists recommend supplementing with Brewer's yeast, when on a vegan diet, but as we discovered, it is also an "Avoid" on Dr. Balch's list, but so are wheat germ, and Spirulina, on Eva Edelman's list. Obviously, we are left with a very restrictive, and extremely unhealthy diet.

It might be helpful if we now evaluate what Eva Edelman has to say about the importance of the two neurotransmitters, dopamine and norepinephrine, produced from the amino acid tyrosine, which we are attempting to avoid, and just how important they both are, as follows:

> *Dopamine (DA) mediates emotional and hormonal response, and the integration of experience, emotion (limbic system), and thought (cerebrum). It also stimulates the pleasure center of the brain, and plays a role in sexual arousal. Dopamine exercises crucial control over movement. The muscle tremors and rigidity in Parkinson's patients result from insufficient dopamine.*

> *Norepinephrine traverses pathways related to intellectual performance, subtle complex motor tasks, pleasure, and anxiety. It mediates learning ability, mental acuity, attention span, alertness, arousal and mood, and plays a role in the association of reward with stimulus.* **Norepinephrine deficiency is often implicated in <u>depression</u>** (*Natural Healing for Schizophrenia,* Edelman, 1996/1998, p. 142):

Now that we are aware of the tremendous importance of tyrosine, we can't help but ask: Why are we going to so much trouble attempting to avoid tyrosine, especially when we are also required to exclude most of the healthy foods from our diet, in order to do so?

Another consideration we still haven't discussed is the influence on the thyroid. Tyrosine, along with iodine, just happens to be necessary for producing the thyroid hormones. Also, just as 5-HTP is a step closer to serotonin than tryptophan is, tyramine is also a step closer to several hormones, including the thyroid hormone, than tyrosine is. But, unfortunately we need to avoid tyramine. How can we possibly expect to have a normal thyroid function if we conform to the dietary restrictions imposed by the MAO inhibitors? Let's just take a closer look at how important the thyroid hormones really are, and what we can expect when they are not adequately supplied. Eva Edelman will help us understand the serious potential for a problem in that regard, when she states that:

> **Thyroid hormones regulate metabolism, and thus, energy and oxygen availability to the brain.** *They also influence nerve receptor accessibility to mood messages.* **Hypothyroidism causes a progressive slowing of mental and physical functioning,** *compromising memory, concentration, comprehension, and energy, and depressing reflexes.* **Other symptoms can include depression, suicidal ideas, emotional instability, delusions, fear, suspiciousness, and resentment.** *If untreated, symptoms, in some cases, progress into obsessions, terrifying dreams, auditory or visual hallucinations, paranoia and psychosis* (*Natural Healing for Schizophrenia,* Edelman, 1996/1998, p. 118).

From the above, we can easily see that anything that could compromise the function of the thyroid is a major concern, and deserves serious consideration.

Another important issue regarding the dietary restrictions associated with the MAO inhibitors is the amino acid tryptophan, which was often used for depression in the past, but thanks to the FDA, only available by prescription, (at least until recently). It is currently available without a prescription, although at a considerably higher price. Fortunately, we can find tryptophan in several foods, and the best sources of tryptophan are: poultry, cottage cheese, bananas, eggs, nuts, wheat germ, avocados, milk, cheese, and the legumes. Unfortunately, every single one of these foods is on the list of foods we must exclude from our diet while on MAO inhibitors. It appears that MAO inhibitors are much better at causing, than resolving depression, which incidentally is also true regarding the SSRI antidepressants.

Eva Edelman also mentions that one of the biochemical factors leading to depression is imbalances of MAO, an enzyme that normally breaks down the monoamine neurotransmitters, that the MAO inhibitors are attempting to suppress. Eva also notes that dopamine, norepinephrine, serotonin, and acetylcholine, are all considered monoamines. If we also consider the importance of those four critical neurotransmitters, we can easily see the potential for damage by the MAO Inhibitors, as they don't even pretend to be selective as the SSRI drugs do. If you noticed, I said they "pretend to". If you recall, SSRI antidepressants also suppress dopamine, although they are by definition supposed to be selective to serotonin only.

One more problem we are facing is, according to Eva, ***"Excess MAO has been linked to depression with attendant anxiety and agitations."*** But we also have another potential problem as, ***"Deficient MAO has been associated with social and psychiatric problems, alcoholism, and increased risk of suicide"*** (*Natural Healing for Schizophrenia,* Edelman, 1996/1998, p. 132). One common denominator between all anti-depressants is their inability to maintain proper balance. In their attempt to override the body's natural processes, by either stimulating or suppressing something, they actually disturb the critical chemical balance in the brain by doing so. We should normally expect to have either one or both of the problems associated with either excessive or deficient MAO levels. Only our body has the ability to effectively accomplish, and maintain that delicate balance, and we will soon discover that we have more than one natural resource that can assist our body in doing just that.

Now that we are more aware of the many dangers associated with drugs normally prescribed for depression, we should be concerned about resorting to their use. Although all drugs are rather scary by nature, that is especially true regarding any mind-altering medication, such as the SSRI antidepressants or MAO Inhibitors. As we learned, they can potentially contribute to depression in several ways, while dulling the senses and emotions. We should not accept being more like zombies void of any emotion. That is not a normal healthy condition that anyone should be willing to accept.

We should strive instead to be healthy vibrant individuals, with both feelings and emotions, alert and energetic and living life to its fullest. This is only possible when depression is properly dealt with in a natural (drug-free) manner. Not only can these antidepressants disrupt the delicate balance in the brain, but they can also create permanent brain damage (especially from long-term use). Our brain is one of our most valuable resources, and thus we must avoid anything that could in any way contribute to dementia and loss of critical function. By resolving depression the proper way, not only can we help prevent brain deterioration, but possibly even reverse the process. For example, at 75, both my retention and recall are far better than they were when I was much younger.

The first priority should be stopping the damage (all the drugs), and then concentrate on restoration, which I believe is entirely possible. So now we'll learn some drug-free solutions to depression.

CHAPTER FOURTEEN
HOW DEPRESSION CAN BE RESOLVED WITHOUT DRUGS

Although some people just seem to cope more effectively than others, there is normally a good explanation. The late Dr. Carl C. Pfeiffer, Ph.D., M.D., author of the book *Nutrition and Mental Illness* (1987), discovered that a chemical imbalance in the brain is often the major underlying factor that influences how we might possibly respond to various events in life. **Some of the most important neurotransmitters, critical for our brain's functioning, are dopamine, norepinephrine, and serotonin, and doctors have concluded that depression occurs when these levels become too low, or <u>out of balance</u>.**

It was once believed that the brain could somehow protect itself from nutritional deficiencies, but we now know that is not really true, and that the brain actually requires certain nutrients. A sufficient supply, as well as the proper balance, of vitamins, minerals, and amino acids, is important for healthy mental function. If this supply is not met, biochemistry changes take place, resulting in symptoms such as fatigue, depression, and irritability, just to name a few. One potential problem arises when people choose to rely solely on their doctors' advice for their healthcare. Most traditionally trained doctors are all too quick to prescribe medications for any symptom, while failing to consider the importance of nutritional deficiencies. At times, doctors even discourage taking vitamins, suggesting that they are just a waste of money. In some cases, doctors also warn of the potential for some supplements interacting with their medications. Interestingly, those at the greatest risk of taking the most medications are patients unfamiliar with nutrition (the majority of people), who are also the most concerned about their health. Unfortunately, although few doctors have any training in nutrition, they tend to discredit its value. The problem lies in many people's total confidence in their doctors' opinion, which they seldom, if ever question. We must all become better informed, and then take a more active part regarding our healthcare, which is our ultimate responsibility.

Earlier in this book we discovered some potential underlying causes of many people's depression, and why so many in the nation are currently on antidepressants; just one more drug that quite often leads to even worse depression or mood swings. Due to most doctors' restricted training in medical school, as well as the limited time normally allotted for each patient, another drug is often the most likely solution (just one more quick fix). It is rather difficult for a doctor to justify charging for an office visit unless he either writes, or renews a prescription, or recommends some surgery. Unfortunately, the only solutions available to most medical doctors are those approved by the American Medical Association (AMA).

Our Emotions Can Be Controlled

We all normally experience various episodes in our lifetime that can contribute to either stress or depression. These events are normally transient, and should soon resolve. It is how we deal with the adverse incidents, such as the death of a loved one, divorce, or possibly a financial reversal, in the interim that makes the difference.

If a loved one passes on, we must remember that death is beyond our control, and something no one can escape. Only God can make that decision, and although we obviously will miss them, life must go on until our time comes. Making the most of the remainder of our lives is the very best thing we can do for them, as well as ourselves. You might begin by making a list of your goals and blessings, and then review them the first thing every morning. You can continually expand your list, whenever new ones come to mind.

Learn to focus on positive uplifting thoughts only. Negative thoughts tend to lead to stress or depression, two conditions that far too many are unnecessarily taking medications for. Whenever a thought comes to mind that is not uplifting, remove it immediately, and replace it with another that is.

Remind yourself to review your list each morning, and it will soon become a habit. Abraham Lincoln summed it up pretty well when he said: ***"Most folks are about as happy as they make their minds up to be,"*** so make up your mind to be happy every single day. Happiness is basically a state of mind that seems to come naturally for some, although something others need to work at. Parents' attitudes and moods are often reflected in their children. If your parents tended to be pessimistic, rather than optimistic toward life, you might have to work a little harder at developing a positive attitude than others.

Actually, service to others can be very rewarding. It allows us to focus on others who are less fortunate, which not only brings a great deal of satisfaction, but also reminds us just how fortunate we really are. By focusing on the problems of others, we also tend to forget our own. Service to others was an important principle Jesus taught by example during His lifetime.

If your depression is possibly the result of an unwanted divorce, keep in mind that it was likely for our own good. No matter how much you might love someone, if that person does not share that love, whatever the reason, you can never be truly happy. You must give them their freedom, and avoid any hostile feelings, even though it may seem justifiable. Harboring negative feelings is basically self-destructive, and can negatively influence your personality. It will just make your chances of finding another spouse (or happiness) much more difficult. For example, if a man meets a divorced woman with a bad attitude toward men, due to a bad experience from her previous marriage, he will likely assume that she was the problem, although though that might not necessarily be true.

I just happen to be aware of a prime example. It is regarding a woman I knew since she was a teenager, (over 50 years ago). She was very pretty back then, and married a good man. Unfortunately, her good looks provided her opportunities outside her marriage. This resulted in an affair that led to a painful divorce. She became very hateful, even though she had brought the problem on herself. Every time I ran into her, she would immediately start in on her ex-husband, who appeared to be a very good person. Her hatred continued for years, and became a major part of her personality. Her good looks began to disappear, as her features began to reflect the years of harbored hatred. Although she was blessed with good looks that many women would have given anything for, due to her lack of self-discipline and negative spiteful attitude, in her case it turned out to be a curse.

A cheerful optimistic personality is a characteristic that both women and men are drawn to, not only in the opposite sex, but also as a choice of friends. In order to attract a mate, or just develop good friendships, we should begin developing those positive attributes that we admire the most in others. Nothing can be more depressing than being around someone with a negative attitude. On the other hand, a cheerful person with a positive attitude is rather like a ray of sunshine, or a breath of fresh air (something we all can use more of). So let's see if we can begin developing the characteristics that we so much admire in others.

It is not necessarily our experiences in life that dictates our happiness, but rather how we react to them. We can't always control the events we encounter throughout our lifetime, although how we respond to each is our choice. We must learn to adapt to our environment, and look for the good in every situation, no matter what our initial response might possibly be. We must remember that it is difficult to retract something inappropriately said in haste, and an apology might not always undo the damage. It is rather like the judge during a trial, instructing the jury to disregard a statement made by a witness (believe me - they won't forget!) We must learn to control our emotions when appropriate. It is much easier than damage control after the fact. Just by developing good social skills, we can often avoid the depression we might possibly experience from dwelling on foolish mistakes, by preventing them in the first place.

While conducting research on addictions, I discovered that many alcoholics tend to suffer from personality disorders, which often leads to depression, thus influencing their interactions with others. Depression then leads to excessive drinking, which then results in worse behavior. It is basically a vicious cycle that often repeats itself over and over. Our interaction with others (not only who we interact with, but also how we interact with them) can have a major influence on our quality of life in general. Serious introspection might be necessary, and remember to be objective. Recognizing that a problem exists is the very first step in the recovery process. Motivation is important, and input from others might be helpful, as we might tend to rationalize at times, in an attempt to justify our actions.

Let There Be Light – Lots of Light

Years ago, I took a course on Interior Decoration (one of my interests), taught by a prominent decorator with many years experience. She mentioned that psychiatrists would often have her consult with many of their patients who were depressed. She noticed that their homes were often very drab with dark colors and insufficient light, and that normally a few decorating changes would dramatically improve their overall mood. Sunlight stimulates the production of serotonin, so we want to let as much light in as we possibly can, and use light colors to reflect as much light as possible.

On the other hand, we should eliminate as much light from our bedrooms as we possibly can. Doing so would stimulate the production of melatonin necessary for the quality REM sleep to promote the restoration of our mind and body. Sleep deprivation is just one contributor to depression. Prozac™ and other SSRI antidepressants cause an elevation of the stress hormone cortisol, which also disrupts the REM sleep cycle.

Light therapy has proven to reverse the winter depressive symptoms of Seasonal Affective Disorder (SAD). In one study, 80 percent of 112 patients improved significantly with light therapy. Bright full-spectrum fluorescent lights (not ordinary light bulbs), are necessary. Even the average household or office lighting, which emits an intensity of 200-500 LUX, is not enough. The minimum dose necessary to be beneficial is 2500 LUX, although more is often required. The intensity of a bright summer day can be as much as 100,000 LUX! In the winter months, using a 10,000-LUX Full Spectrum Light Box for 30 minutes each morning is normally enough to help produce serotonin and reduce depression. This is especially beneficial in the winter months of the northern latitudes, when sufficient natural sunlight is not normally available. Keep in mind though, that using the light box in the evening can cause overstimulation, and thus insomnia, as serotonin is stimulating. Taking 3 mg of melatonin approximately ½ hour before bedtime is one way to promote deep sleep.

Light therapy consists of sitting two to three feet away from a specially designed light box, usually placed on a table, allowing the light to shine directly through the eyes. Tinted lenses, or any device that blocks the light to the retina of the eye, should not be worn. It is not necessary to stare at the light, although it has been proven safe. You can carry out your normal activities such as reading, working, or eating, while sitting in front of the box. After a week or two, either reducing or increasing the daily duration may be necessary. Improvement is normally noticed within three to four days, and should continue as long as necessary. There are several companies that sell light boxes in the 10,000-LUX range.

Regular fluorescent light is actually rather stressful, and tends to be depressing. I replaced all the fluorescent lights in our home and my office, with full spectrum bulbs. We actually have twelve in our kitchen, and it is the most cheerful room in our home. I also replaced all reading lamps with full spectrum incandescent bulbs. When purchased by the case, full spectrum fluorescent bulbs are fairly inexpensive, and are well worth the price.

Because Light Therapy (phototherapy) is no longer considered experimental, and is a mainstream type of psychiatric treatment for SAD or depressive/anxiety conditions, many insurance companies will cover the cost of a therapeutic light box. The discovery that several forms of depression respond to daily exposure to bright light has called attention to the popular notion that sunlight is one effective therapy for depression.

In her un-dated booklet titled *"The Miracle of Simple,"* Susan M. Lark, M.D. sheds some light (pun intended):

Take us out of the sunlight for any length of time and we become depressed. *A blue light will make your pulse rate slow, your breathing relax, and your adrenal glands and immune system respond magically.*

A red light *heightens your sense of smell and taste, and awakens your libido by* ***stimulating all the endocrine glands****. Energy levels soar, blood flow increases, and* ***metabolic rates pick up****.*

My dad, who was a medical doctor and research scientist himself, built ***a simple light box*** *for my mom, and fitted it* ***with a red light filter****. She loved it – and said* ***it was as effective as a cup of coffee, but without the jitters*** *(p. 30).*

Our body responds to different frequencies, and different colors have varying frequencies, and thus our body responds accordingly. Light therapy, using a whole spectrum of colors, is one method proven beneficial for various conditions.

Of all the stimulants the human brain responds to, one of the most powerful is light. **The body has hundreds of biochemical and hormonal rhythms, all of which are governed by light and dark**. In a study done by a Harvard medical team, volunteers were taken through a series of light-exposure tests, experimenting with intensities ranging from 7,000 LUX to 12,000 LUX. Scientists measured the change in brain-wave patterns immediately following this exposure and were able to establish the link between the retina and an area of the brain known as the suprachiasmatic nuclei. According to professors Richard Kronauer, Ph.D., and Charles Czeisler, M.D., the two scientists who headed the three-year Harvard study, this confirms that there is a direct connection between light exposure and the part of the brain that is thought to play a key role in attention focus and energy production (*Low Fat Living*, Cooper, 1996, p. 71). Therefore, **if you have a hard time getting going in the morning**, try turning on every light in the house and see if that helps get you moving! The most benefit can be achieved when using full-spectrum lighting.

Natural Resources for Resolving Depression

1. **Check your thyroid!** Although depression can eventually lead to other conditions, depression can only be effectively treated and resolved by addressing the underlying problem. One seemingly unrelated contributor to depression might be the thyroid, and if you have a hypothyroid condition, that should be your very first focus (explained in detail in the Hypothyroidism chapter of the book). Just remember to use the natural hormone Armour™ thyroid, (not Synthroid™).

2. **Goji and/or Mangosteen Juice.** For thousands of years, goji has been known in Asia as "the happy berry". One to two ounces, one to two times daily, has been historically used to "uplift and elevate" mood. With 19 amino acids (including the 8 essential amino acids) and 21 trace minerals (as well as other important nutrients), goji also enhances energy and eliminates fatigue.

Drinking two ounces of mangosteen juice, three times daily is also very effective, and often all that is necessary for resolving depression. Although we are each unique, and results may vary based on many different factors, mangosteen has in many cases elevated the mood and eliminated depression. It also seems to be very effective in relieving chronic (long-term) pain. As told in his book *Tame the Flame* (2004), Dr Sam Walters, N.MD. discovered that mangosteen had effectively resolved the long-term pain he had been taking medications for due to a serious parachute accident over twenty years ago. In his book, Dr. Walters states that ***"Often chronic pain will lead to psychological responses such as anxiety, fear, sleeplessness, and even <u>suicidal thoughts</u>."***

Although we have yet to discover exactly how the these fruits resolve so many different conditions, I can see a few ways it could possibly help eliminate depression. First, according to Dr. Sherry Rodgers, M.D., 95% of the feel-good hormone serotonin that antidepressants are attempting to increase, is actually produced in the intestinal tract. Both the mangosteen and goji have been proven effective in resolving all the common intestinal conditions. They are also effective in eliminating a condition in the small intestine known as leaky gut syndrome, as well as acid reflux disease. Both conditions make the digestion and assimilation of proteins less effective, (especially when antacids are used). These proteins are important for producing amino acids required for building both the important neurotransmitters such as serotonin and dopamine, and the enzymes critical for our sense of well being.

One other beneficial influence that the mangosteen appears to have is on the thyroid gland. Dr. Sam Walters discovered it is sometimes effective in eliminating the need for thyroid medication. That can be an important factor, as a low thyroid condition, referred to as hypothyroidism, is one common cause of depression. Insufficient metabolism is also often the underlying cause of inappropriate weight gain, and the inability to effectively lose weight on any diet, and just being overweight can be very depressing. So, a low thyroid condition (insufficient metabolism) is often a potential contributor to depression in more ways than one. This condition is covered in considerable detail in the chapter in this book on Hypothyroidism. It is an absolute must-read for anyone suffering with depression (especially for women, who are ten times as likely as men to become hypothyroid). This condition is, in my opinion, the greatest contributor to depression. If it is a problem, it must be resolved in order to truly eliminate your depression.

Mary Lou soon experienced both an elevated mood and increased energy from using mangosteen. And if you recall, Mary Lou was able to eliminate a 16-year dependency on Prozac™, and do so in only two months, by using the mangosteen juice, along with a good vitamin B-complex and essential fatty acids (flax seed oil). Following her withdrawal, she not only experienced an elevated mood, but also an increased level of energy. Although Mary Lou used XanGo™, similar results would likely occur with other mangosteen juice, or the goji juice as well.

For more detailed information on goji and mangosteen, and their many health benefits, see the chapter earlier in this book titled "A Few of Nature's Miracles".

3. **SAMe.** **S**-adenosyl**m**ethion**e** (SAMe) is a natural substance, normally produced by the liver when an adequate supply of nutrients is available. Due to their nutrient depletion, prescription medications can quite easily reduce the liver's ability to effectively produce SAMe. It is especially beneficial for anyone attempting to phase out any of the SSRI antidepressants such as Prozac™, Paxil™, or Zoloft™, as it does not influence the serotonin level, and is safe to take until the antidepressants are phased out. Incidentally, SAMe normally becomes effective in resolving depression in approximately one week, although most antidepressants take approximately 30 days before they do. SAMe has proven beneficial for repairing any damage to the liver, and resolving elevated homocysteine, as well as resolving depression in most people. In a double-blind study, SAMe was found to have even **less** side effects than a sugar pill, (as we know, sugar is not good for us!). Just contrast that with Prozac's extensive list of potential side effects.

4. **B-Vitamins.** I suggest taking a high-potency vitamin B-complex, such as B-100 (100 mg of each B vitamin), or if you might possibly have poor liver function, you might consider taking a coenzyme form of B-complex vitamins instead. The coenzyme formula actually contains the B-complex vitamins in the form used by the body, and the conversion by the liver is not necessary. The B vitamins are critical to normal brain function, and are unfortunately depleted by many prescription medications. B vitamins are also necessary in assisting the brain in creating neurotransmitters that enable brain cells to communicate with each other. For example, vitamin B_6 is necessary for the conversion of the amino acid tryptophan to serotonin. Most people suffering with dementia were found to be deficient in the B vitamins, folic acid and B_{12}. Unfortunately, most physicians seldom recommend B vitamins to treat depression, (or any vitamins, for that matter).

5. **Essential Fatty Acids.** The essential fatty acids (EFAs) in fish oil, or flax oil, are extremely important in resolving depression, as they are essential for creating and maintaining the receptors for important neurotransmitters such as serotonin and dopamine. Just taking flax oil, along with a good coenzyme B complex, was sufficient for eliminating my granddaughter's depression.

Dr. Bruce West, in *A Special Report from Health Alert* (2001), states that flax seed and flax oil are *"Probably the most remarkable source of nutrition in our entire food chain… flax oil is the supreme source of essential fatty acids"* (p. 1). He goes on to point out that our bodies cannot manufacture EFAs, which is why they are called essential fatty acids. They must be consumed in our daily diet. Not only do they help control cholesterol and prevent cardiovascular disease, but **in a matter of just a few hours, *"your mood can be improved and a feeling of calm can be experienced, along with initial relief from depression"*** (p. 2).

It is important to note that EFAs are most commonly depleted by a diet high in saturated fatty foods, aspirin, **estrogen (and oral contraceptives)**, NSAIDS (i.e. ibuprofen), and bronchodilators (commonly used to treat asthma or bronchitis).

6. **Minerals.** A good multi-mineral that includes calcium, magnesium, zinc, and copper is also beneficial, as they are often depleted by medications as well, and you could quite easily be deficient in minerals if you have been taking medications. According to the late well-known and respected psychiatrist Dr. Carl C. Pfeiffer, Ph.D., M.D., a vitamin or mineral deficiency can result in various brain disorders, including depression. We just need to provide the resources and allow our brain to take care of the details (something it can do very efficiently). It's when we attempt to use drugs to force it to do what we think it should, that we soon encounter problems.

7. **Amino acids.** Because some amino acids act as neurotransmitters or as precursors of neurotransmitters, the chemicals that carry information from one nerve cell to another, certain amino acids are thus critical for the brain to receive and send messages.

Even if vitamins and minerals are absorbed and assimilated by the body, they cannot be effective unless the necessary amino acids are present, no matter how well balanced your diet. Impaired absorption, infection, trauma, stress, drug use, age, and imbalances of other nutrients can all affect the availability of essential amino acids in the body.

While a good multi-amino acid complex containing all essential amino acids should be taken, it is also suggested to take the following additional individual supplements (but at a separate time). Each amino acid has its own unique benefit. Some are more calming, while others are more stimulating. If an individual amino acid, such as Taurine for example, was taken along with the complex containing all essential amino acids (those that the body can't produce), you might not realize the same benefit. The Taurine could possibly be combined with other amino acids and used for some other purpose. When combined, they have multiple uses in the body, such as producing enzymes, red blood cells, tissue repairs, etc. We can more effectively regulate how they will be used by taking some separately from others.

It is normally wise to take the more stimulating amino acids such as tyrosine in the morning for most people, or when experiencing depression for anyone suffering from a bipolar condition. In contrast, the more calming amino acid would ordinarily be best if taken in the evening, or when experiencing a manic episode by those with the bipolar or manic-depressive disorder.

Following are some of the more beneficial amino acids for depression:
- ✓ **Glutamine** – an energizer, memory booster, and stress reliever. It is an alternate source of fuel for the brain and helps build and balance the neurotransmitters. It improves mental energy and promotes relaxation, as well as stabilizing blood sugar, thus reducing cravings for sugar and alcohol.
- ✓ **Taurine** – helps reduce anxiety, irritability, insomnia, migraine, alcoholism, obsessions, and depression. It also enhances the activity of the calming neurotransmitter Gama-Aminobutric Acid (GABA).
- ✓ **Tyrosine** – acts as an energizer and mood enhancer, and is a precursor to the neurotransmitters dopamine, adrenaline, and noradrenaline, as well as the thyroid hormone.
- ✓ **Acetyl**-L-carnitine – enhances mood, restores energy, and improves mental fatigue. Doctors have compared acetyl-L-carnitine against the prescription mood-stabilizer "amisulpride" and found that *"acetyl-L-carnitine was just as effective as amisulpride in treating depression, without any of the side effects"* (*Life Extension* magazine, September 2006, p. 67).

✓ **L-theanine** – last but certainly not least, this is another fairly new amino acid, discussed in the January 2002 issue of the *Health Sciences Institute* newsletter. One article explains how research has revealed that L-theanine effectively crosses the blood-brain barrier and induces several distinct chemical changes in the brain that reduce feelings of stress:

> *Approximately 30 minutes after it is ingested, L-theanine stimulates the production of alpha waves. Such brain waves leave a person feeling alert but deeply relaxed. Theanine also stimulated production of gamma aminobutyric acid. GABA, our most widespread neurotransmitter, limits nerve cell activity in those areas of the brain associated with anxiety, and consequently induces a state of relaxation, calmness, and serenity in stressed or agitated individuals* (pp. 1-2).

The newsletter mentioned that L-Theanine also "significantly increased" tryptophan, an amino acid that is the basis of serotonin, a mood-altering brain chemical that is essential to the feeling of well-being and relaxation and may help alleviate symptoms of clinical depression. Apparently, in addition to providing the foundation for substances essential to good neuron function, L-theanine may also prevent brain cell death.

8. **Phase Out Your Medications.** Although this step is important, it is important to first build up your body with sufficient nutrition. Once you have been taking the goji and/or mangosteen, SAMe, vitamins, minerals, amino acids, and essential fatty acids, you can begin slowly reducing (in an attempt to phase out) the dosage of your medications while carefully monitoring your blood pressure and blood sugar levels (when appropriate). Although it is helpful to maintain healthy levels of both blood pressure and blood sugar (unless extremely elevated), on a temporary basis neither should be life threatening. If you are on several medications, or are at all concerned, you might ask your doctor if he or she can assist you in the drug withdrawal process. As I have always stressed, you better than anyone else, can more effectively evaluate your pain and depression level, if that is what you are taking medication for. Keep in mind that one side effect associated with many medications is depression, thus just eliminating some medications might be sufficient to resolve your depression.

9. **Phase out antidepressants.** If you are currently taking any antidepressant, this is the most important step in your recovery process. It is critical for restoring the natural balance of neurotransmitters in the brain (something only the body can accomplish). It is also important to phase out **all other** prescription medications, **BEFORE** attempting to phase out any antidepressant (especially the SSRI antidepressants). This will help strengthen your body for the withdrawal process. And, regarding the SSRI antidepressants, such as Prozac™, Paxil™, or Zoloft™, there are many different benefits from phasing them out of your life once and for all. One thing people soon discover after withdrawal, is a return of their emotions, and often claim that it feels as though a fog is lifting. Just avoiding the potential long-term side effects, such as diabetes and adrenal fatigue, along with any of the 575 potential side effects associated with the drug Prozac™, definitely makes it well worth the effort. Any drug such as Prozac™ that can increase your level of the stress hormone Cortisol by 200% is obviously a major concern, and just one major contributor to many of the side effects associated with Prozac™.

Dr. Ann Blake Tracy, in her book *Prozac – Panacea or Pandora?* (1991/1994), recommends improving the diet, and reducing the dosage of your antidepressant very slowly. She said that at times it might take as long as two years, and would require slowly shaving the pill in the process. Although reducing your dosage of antidepressants slowly is sometimes advisable, in my opinion that would be extremely difficult to accomplish over that long a period, especially as some are in capsule rather than pill form. However, at the time Dr. Tracy wrote her book, the mangosteen was not yet available in the U.S.

Although I have actually seen some people go off their antidepressants cold turkey and do so without any problem, there are multiple factors involved, and thus is not normally advisable. It typically depends upon how long you have been taking the antidepressant, your overall health, nutrient intake, and daily stress levels. It is usually best to begin by reducing the dosage by ¼ for two weeks, and then go on a half-dose for another two more weeks, and finally reduce the dosage by ¾, to ¼ for dose the last two weeks. Although, if you have only been on the antidepressant for a few months, that is normally not necessary.

People often tend to have difficulty dealing with stress following the use of SSRI antidepressants, especially for an extended period of time. The continuous stimulation of cortisol caused by Prozac™ (200% increase from one 30 mg dose) for example, in time can result in adrenal fatigue, as well as a hair-trigger response to any stress. One of Dr. Tracy's patients discovered that when attempting to stop her antidepressants, after an unusually stressful day at work (she didn't deal well with stress). She found that drinking a cup of chamomile tea along with several hours of rest helped her recover. In her case, the mangosteen and SAMe are two valuable resources she was not taking, although both would have been beneficial.

There are many helpful herbs for dealing with stress (even better than the chamomile tea), without causing drowsiness. One I find very effective is called Valerian root. It is fast acting, very effective, and yet quite inexpensive. If you try to avoid stressful situations, (especially during the withdrawal process), and take Valerian root when necessary, you will be much more successful, and experience less symptoms during the withdrawal process.

10. **Remove/Eliminate Fluoride.** Another major issue concerning Prozac™ is the three molecules of fluoride found in each molecule of Prozac™. Fluoride is known for suppressing both the thyroid function, and enzyme action throughout the body. This is just one more reason for finding a better solution for dealing with depression. Very few doctors that prescribe SSRI antidepressants such as Prozac™ are fully aware of these two major concerns associated with their use. One very important step to take is eliminating the accumulation of fluoride in the thyroid (especially after using Prozac™). This involves using a supplement called Iodoral™, which contains both iodine and potassium iodide. It will help kick start the thyroid gland by removing accumulated fluoride and replacing it with the proper form of iodine necessary for producing the thyroid hormone. In his book *Iodine: Why You Need It – Why You Can't Live Without It* (2004), Dr. David Brownstein notes that with many of his patients, he observed the detoxifying effect of iodine supplementation on heavy metals such as mercury, as well as bromine, chlorine, and fluoride, which are all known to inhibit iodine from binding to thyroid receptor cites. He also mentioned that **bromine** is used as a dough conditioner during the commercial baking process, and **can also be found in many prescription and over-the-counter medications.** Just one more concern regarding medications, and another reason to consider eliminating them from your life forever.

Dr. Brownstein also discovered that **91.7% of his patients he tested for a thyroid deficiency actually had low iodine levels.** He also stated that many different conditions such as thyroid disorders, chronic fatigue, fibromyalgia, and cancer of the breast and prostate are often the result of an iodine deficiency. I personally purchase Iodoral™ from the Women's International Pharmacy, as the owner Wally Simons, R.Ph. is a good friend whom I trust, although there are likely other sources.

11. **5-HTP.** An alternate solution that might work for you is 5-hydroxytryptophan (5-HTP), an amino acid derived from a West African herb, *Griffonia simplicifolia*. 5-HTP is easily absorbed and is highly effective at raising serotonin levels, with up to 300 mg per day often being effective. As a serotonin enhancer, 5-HTP has proven in studies to be a mood elevator for people who suffer from depression, anxiety, and stress. However, while attempting to withdraw from Prozac™, or any SSRI antidepressant for that matter, 5-HTP is not a good choice. It could help contribute to a condition called serotonin syndrome, which is caused from excessively elevated serotonin, and something to be aware of. Instead, SAMe would be a safe choice and better option, as it doesn't influence the serotonin level.

12. **Licorice Root.** High levels of the enzyme monoamine oxidase (MAO) can destroy dopamine, norepinephrine, and serotonin, leading to depression. Unfortunately, MAO is concentrated primarily in the brain, where it causes the most damage. While scientists believe that most forms of depression are caused either by neurotransmitter uptake, increased MAO levels, or both, they have just begun to realize that licorice root (*Glycyrrhiza glabra*) can be extremely beneficial when battling depression.

Studies in Japan suggest that **the most benefit comes from licorice's ability to inhibit MAO. Licorice has been shown to inhibit 44-64% of MAO, which is comparable to synthetic treatments,**

but without the side effects, thus making licorice nature's form of an MAO inhibitor. And you don't have to avoid all those healthy foods! If you read the section on MAO inhibitors in the Antidepressants chapter of this book, you will better understand the significance of this recent discovery. Keep in mind that licorice root can sometimes worsen hypertension.

The best form is deglycyrrhizinated licorice root (DGL), and should be available in your local health food store.

13. **Rhodiola Rosea** is another herbal supplement that proves to be highly beneficial. In the book *Arctic Root (Rhodiola Rosea) – The Powerful New Ginseng Alternative*, written by Carl Germano, R.D., C.N.S., L.D.N. and Zakir Ramazanov, Ph.D. (1999), it is stated that *"Rhodiola rosea not only decreases the levels of stress hormones in the body… but evidence also suggests that **Rhodiola rosea may help those people, buried by feelings of depression, climb out of their psychological hole"** (pp. 46, 139). Depression is normally a consequence of insufficient serotonin levels, and the book goes on to say that scientists have found that extract of **Rhodiola rosea definitely enhances the transport of the serotonin precursors into the brain, thus promoting serotonin production**.

An article in *Life Extension* magazine (2004/2005 winter special edition), explains: *"Rhodiola works primarily on the mitochondria in the central and parasympathetic nervous system. In small doses, **Rhodiola increases the bioelectric activity of the brain and stimulates norepinephrine, dopamine, and serotonin, all major neurotransmitters"** (p. 39). The article goes on to note that, although 17 varieties of Rhodiola rosea are available, positive effects were achieved using the **Russian Rhodiola**, standardized to 3% rosavins and 1% salidrosides.

14. **DHEA (dehydroepiandrosterone).** In a major study conducted in the UK, as many as 67% of men and 82% of women reported a noticeable decrease in their depressive symptoms while taking only 25 mg/day of DHEA. In the March 2003 issue of *Life Extension Magazine*, it was reported that researchers at the University of Newcastle upon Tyne, UK tested DHEA to see if it offered any protection against cortisol, a glucocorticoid known to be elevated in patients with depression. In their study, cortisol and DHEA were measured in saliva taken from 39 patients with unipolar depression who had been medication free for at least six weeks. These samples were then compared with those of 41 non-depressed subjects. The results showed that **the level of cortisol was significantly higher than that of DHEA in the depressed patients, when compared with healthy subjects** (pp. 27-28). The article concludes:

> *This indicates that reduced DHEA levels may be a marker for depressive illness and a contributing factor to the associated deficits in learning and memory. These results also suggest that the administration of DHEA or other anti-glucocorticoid treatments may reduce neurocognitive deficits in major depression (Am J Psychiatry 2002 Jul;159(7):1237-9).*

According to the book *DHEA – Unlocking the Secrets to the Fountain of Youth*, written by Beth M. Ley (1996): *"DHEA regulates **diabetes**, obesity, carcinogenesis, tumor growth, virus and bacterial infection, **stress**, pregnancy, **hypertension**, collagen and skin integrity, fatigue, **depression**, memory and immune responses"* (p. 32). Beth goes on to point out that:

> **Stressful events depress DHEA production. The Cortisol/DHEA ratio in individuals with panic disorder is depressed by about 50 percent**
>
> **A number of drugs, not only pharmaceuticals, but also alcohol and tobacco, lower levels of DHEA, probably due to the increased stress on the body. Birth control pills especially have a detrimental effect. Alcohol puts an added stress on the body.** *Alcohol has numerous and various effects on hormone production in the body* (p. 35).

It was also found that *"**people taking DHEA simply claim that they feel better; less stressed, less depressed, more energetic.** DHEA has shown to improve memory by increasing formation of brain cells. **DHEA has also shown to decrease aggressive behavior and <u>decrease depression</u>"*** (pp. 81-82).

As we can see, **both stress and the stress hormone Cortisol (increased 200% by <u>Prozac</u>™) <u>can reduce DHEA and thus contribute to depression!</u>**

15. **Relora™,** an extract from Philodendrons, is yet another safe and effective supplement, found to **increase DHEA levels, while also lowering cortisol**, both associated with depression. It is available at most health food stores and through mail order.

The cover story of the June 18, 2002 edition of *Woman's World* magazine, featured Dr. Jim LaValle explaining how Relora™ was tested in a human study and found to be a safe, effective, rapidly acting, non-sedating dietary supplement that helps control stress and its associated symptoms: irritability, emotional ups and downs, restlessness, tense muscles, poor sleep and concentration difficulties. The study was conducted in Dr. LaValle's clinic to measure cortisol and DHEA levels in patients with mild to moderate stress. **Elevated cortisol levels and depressed DHEA levels are associated with chronic stress.** A two-week regimen of **Relora™ caused a significant increase in salivary DHEA (227 percent) and a significant decrease in morning salivary cortisol levels (37 percent)**. These significant finds support **Relora's ability to relieve stress and its potential role in depression (a major issue).**

16. **NADH** is basically an **energizer that stimulates the production of the neurotransmitters serotonin, dopamine, and noradrenaline.** It is also an antioxidant, and improves mental clarity, memory, alertness, and concentration.

17. **Noni** has been used in the Hawaiian Islands for years, for all types of ailments. In her audiotape titled *Help! I Can't Get Off My Anti-Depressants!* (1999), Dr. Ann Blake Tracy suggests that, *"**Noni juice will help you to get rid of the disassociative state that comes from these drugs** [i.e. Prozac™]. That 'almost being in a dream state' that you feel in the withdrawal."* She goes on to say that *"**It will help prevent mania.** I have been amazed at what I have seen Noni do with those who have gone manic because of these drugs."*

In her book *Understanding the Nature and Cause of Addictions*, Dr. Mary L. Reed, CNHP, MH, ND also encourages the use of Noni, indicating that *"Tahitian Noni seems to be a lifesaver for many who have an addictive personality"* and goes on to say that, *"It has been used successfully by those with drug addictions, cigarettes, alcohol and sugar. **It is also helpful for <u>depression</u>** and vitality"* (p. 4).

18. **Pregnenolone** is a hormone that appears to be an excellent resource to assist in reducing stress and maintaining emotional health. Just be aware that pregnenolone is produced from cholesterol, (one of its many benefits). Because it is a precursor for all steroid hormones, pregnenolone helps regulate proper hormone balance. It is also involved in emotional health, proper sleep, and reduced stress, and is known for its ability to promote feelings of balance and harmony. Clinical studies have examined its role in relieving depression, improving memory, reducing stress, treating arthritis, and increasing longevity. Pregnenolone has been used for many years in high doses, and most importantly with no reported side effects.

19. **Protein-rich Diet.** Not only serotonin, but also another neurotransmitter, dopamine, is also suspected to decrease with reduced exposure to light. Dopamine is the brain activator, and it has been proven that people are more alert and think more clearly when dopamine levels are high. A dietary approach to low dopamine levels is a protein-rich diet. Foods such as cheese, extra-lean meat, chicken or turkey, fish and salmon, and eggs raise dopamine levels and help boost energy and mood. In addition, protein does not trigger a high insulin response, allowing the blood sugar to remain level.

20. **Vitamin D Supplementation.** Another vitamin level that drops during the winter months due to less sun exposure is vitamin D. Researchers at John Hopkins University showed in one study that people with SAD were more likely than others to have low levels of vitamin D in their blood. Additionally, moods improved when these people supplemented their diets with vitamin D. Another study, from the University

of Newcastle in Australia, reported that **forty-four healthy people agreed that their moods improved during the winter when they took vitamin D supplements.** Incidentally, fish oil is a good source of vitamin D.

21. **Light Therapy.** As noted earlier in this chapter, light therapy has proven to reverse the winter depressive symptoms of SAD (Seasonal Affective Disorder), in addition to assisting the body in naturally producing serotonin.

22. **Drink Sufficient Water.** An adequate supply of water (preferably 10 glasses a day) is essential for effective neuron transmission of critical hormones in the brain. The body basically responds to dehydration as a stressor, and any stress will suppress the thyroid function. Then, a typical symptom of suppressed thyroid is depression. When we are dehydrated, the viscosity (thickness) of our blood also increases. When the blood thickens, the amino acid L-tryptophan, (which is a relatively large molecule) finds it difficult to cross the blood-brain barrier. Tryptophan is the basic building block of serotonin, which is important for avoiding depression. Incidentally, vitamin B_6 (depleted by many medications) is necessary for the conversion process to take place.

No other drink can replace water, and some beverages such as coffee, caffeinated soft drinks, and alcohol are actually very dehydrating. Most fruit drinks are basically loaded with sugar, often in the form of high fructose corn syrup, which contributes to elevated insulin, and then hypoglycemia. One of the many symptoms associated with hypoglycemia is depression. The symptoms of hypothyroidism (low thyroid) and hypoglycemia (low blood sugar) are surprisingly similar, and depression is a common denominator. So as we can easily see, water is also helpful in avoiding depression, and basically something we can all afford. Just make sure there is no chlorine or fluoride in the water you drink, as both can suppress the thyroid function, which would just reduce the benefit of drinking water.

23. **Celtic sea salt.** Replace common table salt, which is acidic and missing the mineral potassium, as well as many important trace minerals, with Celtic sea salt. Celtic sea salt is instead alkaline, and contains both sodium and potassium, as well as 84 trace minerals in the ionic form, which is important for effective assimilation and utilization by the cells.

According to Dr. Balch (in regards to the mineral potassium), the secretion of stress hormones (caused by Prozac™) causes a decrease in the potassium-to-sodium ratio both inside and outside of the cells. This is just one more reason to get off Prozac™, which stimulates the stress hormone cortisol. Adding Celtic sea salt to your diet, during and after withdrawal, will help restore proper mineral ratios. This is an important issue, as the sodium-potassium pump is responsible for the transfer of nutrients into the cell, as well as the removal of toxins from the cell. Although common table salt contains only sodium, Celtic sea salt also contains the important mineral potassium.

24. **Exercise** is also beneficial, as it balances the nerve chemicals and hormones, increases endorphins, curbs hunger, relaxes the body, and improves the quality of sleep. Exercising outdoors whenever possible, is the best way to get more natural light exposure, which is something your body will definitely benefit from. When walking, get away from traffic as much as possible. The carbon monoxide fumes from vehicles can considerably reduce your oxygen level.

CHAPTER FIFTEEN
BIPOLAR DISORDER AND LITHIUM THERAPY

The Bipolar disorder is a condition that can easily result from the use of Prozac™ or any other SSRI antidepressants. The primary concern is the standard Lithium Therapy, normally prescribed for the bipolar disorder, which is a potentially dangerous drug! Although the bipolar disorder was not a condition I had initially planned to discuss, I soon discovered the wisdom in doing so, as it is such a common side effect associated with the SSRI antidepressants. I feel I would be remiss if I chose to exclude such an important part of the overall puzzle.

How Antidepressants Contribute to the Bipolar Disorder

Serotonin affects nearly every area of brain activity, with serotonin binding sites found throughout the brain. Although serotonin has a strong impact upon the function of the brain, 90% of the production of serotonin actually takes place in the intestinal tract. The body is normally very efficient at preserving and utilizing its resources. Given the fact that serotonin is used throughout the brain, and is important for storing energy, we can easily see that many potential problems could easily arise from Prozac™ use.

Prozac™ precipitates the bipolar condition by suppressing the reuptake of the excess serotonin in the synaptic space between the neurons. The normal function of the reuptake of serotonin that Prozac™ is attempting to inhibit is likely twofold: (1) the first priority of the normal serotonin reuptake process appears to be preventing the over-stimulation of neurons. This function is necessary in order to maintain the critical balance or stability of the various neurotransmitters in the brain. (2) The second function of the serotonin reuptake would be to save the excess serotonin in the synapses for use elsewhere in the brain where it is most needed. For example, the energy storage that serotonin plays a part in also.

As we have just learned, Prozac™ causes over-stimulation of serotonin receptors, by suppressing the reuptake of the excess serotonin. This is where the bipolar condition normally begins. An excessive stimulation of neurotransmitters naturally initiates a chain reaction that results in an unsteady environment in the brain. Most illegal drugs, as well as Prozac™ and other SSRI antidepressants, eventually contribute to similar problems.

Because one of the normal serotonin reuptake functions is preventing over-stimulation, as well as preserving any excess serotonin for use elsewhere in the brain, the serotonin receptors begin shutting down, (due to over-stimulation), and this is the basic source of at least one problem. That is the same basic concept that results in insulin resistance in Type II diabetes, although from excess insulin stimulation. But with a Bipolar disorder, instead of the insulin resistance in the body, the result is a toxic buildup of excessive serotonin in the brain, resulting in poor serotonin utilization, and then a resistance of serotonin in the brain. That is especially true with long-term usage, which can eventually become potentially life threatening, and can then lead to even worse depression.

Dangers Associated With the Common Lithium Carbonate Therapy

A local author Eva Edelman, in her book *Natural Healing for Schizophrenia* (1996/1998) discusses lithium carbonate, a highly reactive trace element commonly prescribed for bipolar disorders by many doctors. She mentions that, ***"Conventionally prescribed doses (starting at 900 mg Lithium Carbonate per day) <u>approach the lethal level.</u>*** *Since lithium accumulates in the body,* **this dosage range can be <u>particularly dangerous,</u>** *so blood levels are frequently checked"* and then goes on to warn:

> ***Lithium intake at the psychiatric dose range has been associated with reduced concentration, confusion, memory defects and <u>a blunting of emotions</u>, thought***

processes and personality. Some researchers warn that <u>lithium can cause progressive and irreversible intellectual deterioration,</u> and should be entirely contraindicated (p. 155).

The question is then posed: *"Is lithium an essential trace mineral?"* Eva Edelman states that *"No one knows how lithium works, but these actions might contribute to its effects"* and also that, *"Lithium influences* [the important neurotransmitters] <u>*acetylcholine, dopamine, serotonin* and *GABA* receptors in the limbic system and basal ganglia"</u> (p. 155).

Providing adequate resources necessary for producing sufficient amounts of the above neurotransmitters in particular, and in the proper ratios to each other, is critical. Our body is perfectly capable of maintaining that delicate balance as long as adequate resources are provided. There is no drug or inorganic mineral on the market with that capability. Only the body can effectively accomplish that goal, and is an important part if its design. Toxic amounts of any **in**organic mineral that has the potential to negatively influence several critical neurotransmitters could quite easily create numerous problems. As we will soon discover, extremely high doses of the **in**organic lithium carbonate normally prescribed for the bipolar disorder, can do just that. In contrast, it appears that trace amounts of the **trace mineral** lithium, in its organic form, could very well be beneficial to the brain. That is an issue we will discuss in more detail a little later.

In her book *Natural Healing for Schizophrenia* (1996/1998), Eva Edelman lists 36 potential side effects regarding lithium carbonate, in three different categories: mild, moderate, and severe.

A few of the "mild" symptoms, which appear to be the result of lithium therapy, are: *"fine tremor of the hands, slurred speech, and incoordination."*

Some of the "moderate" symptoms include: *"dizziness, sedation, rigidity, central nervous system effects."* We can easily identify the underlying cause of those particular side effects as typical symptoms associated with suppressed levels of both serotonin and dopamine, caused by lithium.

Other moderate side effects include *"<u>Depression</u>",* and *"Goiter or Hypothyroidism (in up to 10% of patients)."* The <u>suppression of the thyroid</u>, in this case, is more than likely at least one cause of depression. **Two well-known symptoms associated with hypothyroidism are depression and mood swings (another term for bipolar disorder), and yet these are actually the very symptoms that lithium is normally prescribed for in the first place.**

Eva Edelman states that *"Lithium is known to alter adrenal cortisol levels, deplete certain neurotransmitters, and depress the thyroid"* (*Natural Healing for Schizophrenia*, 1996/1998, p. 155). The altered cortisol levels she referred to is a problem normally associated with Prozac™ also, and one contributor to the thyroid suppression, just noted. Another concern is: Lithium bonds to, and removes iodine from the thyroid, and is sometimes even used to **reduce a hyperthyroid** (elevated thyroid) condition, meaning it would actually depress the thyroid, although that is obviously not our objective.

Then, under **"severe"** side effects (my interpretation: **rather scary**) we find: *"Impairment of consciousness, cardiac abnormalities (20%-30%), permanently increased kidney output, bedwetting, <u>irreversible kidney scarring</u>, other kidney damage, liver disorders, rise in blood sugar, increased white blood cell count, blood disorders, <u>coma</u>, <u>death</u>"* (*Natural Healing for Schizophrenia*, Edelman, 1996/1998, p. 155).

<u>The rise in blood sugar</u>, one of the severe side effects of lithium carbonate, again creates the same basic problems, just from a different route. One contributor to elevated blood sugar is surprisingly, a sodium deficiency, which is the problem lithium is best known for creating. An excessive rise in blood sugar normally stimulates insulin secretion, resulting in hypoglycemia, which, like hypothyroidism, also results in both depression, and mood swings – again, the symptoms we were originally taking the lithium for. The resultant combined side effects (of hypothyroidism and hypoglycemia) could be even more severe than either condition would be individually.

Considering the serious side effects of <u>increased kidney output, irreversible kidney scarring, and other kidney damage noted,</u> and that the two major functions of the kidneys are to

maintain proper levels of both the water and sodium in the body, a serious problem is evident. The kidneys control water levels by retaining an adequate level of salt, which attracts and helps maintain the appropriate water levels in the body. Sodium, (along with potassium), is involved in transferring nutrients into, and toxins out of all cells, as well as the transport of the various neurotransmitters (all extremely important functions). Eva Edelman explains that:

> *Lithium forcefully shifts sodium and potassium levels, which are critical to conveying nerve messages along the neural axon. Lithium may assist in sodium ion transport.* ***Rosenblatt believes lithium may act as a substitute for sodium. Snyder warns that lithium might disrupt critical sodium balances*** *(Natural Healing for Schizophrenia,* Edelman, 1996/1998, p. 155).*

The <u>damage to the kidneys</u> would obviously affect their ability to retain an adequate level of salt, and thus water, which would explain the increased kidney output. In time, this problem would likely worsen due to the <u>permanent kidney scarring</u>. Also, one problem associated with kidney scarring is elevated blood pressure. If the kidney scarring were irreversible, as indicated, hypertension would likely be also. Kidney dysfunction and the potential for dialysis is another serious concern. The potential for damage to the kidneys could be even greater for anyone also placed on cholesterol lowering medication, which can also damage the kidneys, and thus elevate the blood pressure even further.

I see another potential problem on the horizon. First, both Prozac™ and lithium often lead to elevated blood sugar, and eventually diabetes. Then, under the new established guidelines, the potentially dangerous statin (cholesterol lowering) medications are now approved and recommended for anyone with diabetes. What a tragic series of events, which is often perpetrated by the excessive, and unnecessary use of potentially serious medications. This is an occurrence that is all too common in medicine today.

<u>Edema</u> (fluid retention) is another problem associated with both lithium, and Prozac™ use, and is also one condition associated with hypothyroidism (low thyroid). According to Dr. Ann Blake Tracy, the brain might possibly swell also, and Cranial Massage has been reported by patients to be very beneficial, as it releases a lot of pressure if there is any swelling in the head. She also notes that Cranial Massage assists in getting rid of the panic or anxiety that comes from the adrenalin rushes in withdrawal, as some of these adrenalin rushes have been reported to go on for up to 4 hours straight. Another safe but little-known solution to the intracranial pressure mentioned (that could eventually result in blindness) is urine therapy. Excessive pressure in the brain from trauma for instance, can result in damage to the neurons (a potentially serious condition). Ingesting urine is very effective in reducing potentially dangerous pressure in the brain (and obviously free), as well as perfectly safe. Urine therapy has been practiced for thousands of years, and no one has ever had a reaction from their own urine. Preventing neuron damage in the brain is a critical issue that should be taken serious.

Additional, and possibly even more critical conditions associated with lithium use, include the following:

> **[These side effects]** *appear to be related to serum lithium levels, including levels within the therapeutic range: muscle hyperirritability (fasciculations, twitching, clonic movements of whole limbs), hypertonicity, ataxia, choreoathetotic movements, hyperactive deep tendon reflex, extrapyramidal symptoms including acute dystonia,* ***blackout spells, epileptiform seizures, vertigo,*** *downbeat nystagmus,* ***incontinence of urine or feces,*** *somnolence, psychomotor retardation,* ***restlessness, confusion, stupor,*** *tongue movements, tics, tinnitus,* ***hallucinations, poor memory, slowed intellectual functioning,*** *startled response,* ***worsening of organic brain syndromes,*** *cardiac*

arrhythmia, hypotension, **peripheral circulatory collapse***, bradycardia,* **decreased creatinine clearance and albuminuria** **[indicating kidney damage]***, blurred vision, and impotence/sexual dysfunction.*

A few reports have been received of the development of painful discoloration of fingers and toes **and coldness of the extremities** **[indicating suppressed thyroid] within one day of the starting of treatment with lithium.**

*Cases of pseudotumor cerebri (***increased intracranial pressure** *and papilledema)* **have been reported with lithium use. If undetected, this condition may result in enlargement of the blind spot, constriction of visual fields and** **blindness** **due to optic atrophy** (http://www.healthyplace.com).

And, although we discussed several "serious" conditions that result from traditional lithium therapy in the high doses normally prescribed, the two most serious of all still remain, which are namely **"coma and death."** According to the *Bantam Medical Dictionary, 3rd edition* (1981/2000), under "Lithium Carbonate" we find that *"Excessive doses can cause an encephalopathy and even death"* (p. 283). Encephalopathy is: *"Any of various diseases that affect the functioning of the brain."*

Now that you have learned many of the serious consequences associated with taking lithium carbonate and the nutrients it depletes, the challenge now is resolving the bipolar disorder while also protecting the brain from potential damage in the process. But first, we will attempt to identify some ways that lithium carbonate could contribute to such an extensive list of serious conditions.

How Does Lithium Create So Much Chaos in both the Body and Brain? (Answer: By Depleting Important Nutrients)

In the second edition of the *Drug-Induced Nutrient Depletion Handbook* (2001/2001), written by Ross Pelton, R.Ph.D., C.C.N., and three other registered pharmacists, we find one possible explanation. We learn that the vitamin **inositol is depleted by lithium,** and that *"although depletion has been noted, routine* **replacement of inositol is not recommended** *due to a possible relationship to lithium's therapeutic effect"* (p. 167). Apparently, "lithium's therapeutic effect" is something they chose not to discuss, so I'm not sure what the concern might be.

Dr. Balch observes that one important function for which inositol is known for, is assisting in the prevention of several cardiovascular problems, particularly helping remove fats from the liver. He also lists **irritability and** **mood swings** as two problems **related to inositol deficiency.** Once again, it appears that **lithium might be contributing to the very problem it is being prescribed for.** Interestingly, Dr. Balch also notes that *"Research has also shown that **high doses of inositol may help in the** **treatment of depression***, **obsessive-compulsive disorder, and anxiety disorders, without the side effects of prescription medications"** (*Prescription for Nutritional Healing, 3rd edition,* 2000, p. 19).

In the *Drug-Induced Nutrient Depletion Handbook* (2001/2001), although only inositol was listed under "Nutrients Depleted", in a study titled "Lithium and Sodium Depletion" in that very same handbook, it was discovered that the administration of lithium carbonate resulted in **"renal sodium wasting"** (a very important issue).

Also discussed was how lithium blocked the anti-diuretic hormone the kidneys use to retain both salt and water. So, although sodium was not listed under "Nutrients Depleted", we find that it actually is depleted. Just as we learned that sodium and potassium are necessary for both transporting nutrients into the cell and removing toxins from the cell, adequate sodium retention is also necessary for maintaining sufficient water levels in the body, an area in which lithium definitely falls short. This is because one important function of sodium (salt) is attracting water, and once sodium wasting begins, dehydration then follows, often resulting in elevated histamine or histadelia.

Histadelia is a term referring to a condition where the body has high levels of histamine, and in his book *Your Body's Many Cries for Water* (1997), Dr. F. Batmanghelidj, M.D. points out that when the body is dehydrated, histamine levels increase. Dr. Batmanghelidj also states that one of the most common causes of elevated histamine in the body is <u>dehydration</u>. And according to Dr. E. Denis Wilson, M.D., in his book *Wilson's Syndrome – The Miracle of Feeling Well* (1996), elevated histamine is also common when the thyroid function is reduced (another condition lithium is known to cause). Other conditions associated with elevated histamine are **depression**, compulsion, abnormal thinking and **the constant threat of suicide** (all potentially serious conditions). Elevated histamine is also a common contributor to asthma, which an adequate intake of Celtic sea salt and water will often resolve.

We must then consider that, although inositol was the only nutrient listed as depleted by lithium, Eva Edelman suggests otherwise, noting that ***"choline can be depleted in histadelia."*** Choline is the precursor of the neurotransmitter acetylcholine, a calming neurotransmitter, and one of the four that lithium affects. **Both choline and inositol have many important functions including efficient neurotransmitter function, <u>relieving</u> anxiety and <u>depression</u>, and also promoting sleep.** Edelman points out that **choline and inositol may also play a role in the absorption of calcium, magnesium, manganese, and zinc,** and goes on to explain that:

> ***Choline and inositol nourish and strengthen nerves and brain.*** *They have been used to help relieve anxiety and depression, and promote sleep.* ***Choline is the precursor of acetylcholine, a neurotransmitter essential to memory, nerve/muscle communication, and parasympathetic activity.*** *Choline also helps maintain the myelin sheath which surrounds certain nerve axons. DMAE* [**Dim**ethyl**a**mino**e**thanol]*, a potent form of choline, is reported to sometimes* ***benefit behavior disorders,*** *and frequently be effective in hyperactivity.*
>
> ***Choline can be depleted in histadelia,*** *and* ***supplementation may improve mood****. In certain cases, choline may be helpful (once biotype imbalances are reduced)* ***in moderating the racing thoughts and hypomania*** *which can occur in paranoid schizophrenia.* ***Inositol is reported to have a mild sedative action and be useful in promoting sleep and reducing anxiety*** *(Natural Healing for Schizophrenia,* 1996/1998, p. 31).

So as we can see, **anything such as lithium carbonate that can lead to <u>the depletion of choline, could actually contribute to hypomania</u> – again, <u>what lithium is normally prescribed to prevent.</u>**

Then, there is even the possibility of <u>calcium depletion</u> also. According to another fairly extensive report on lithium, obtained at <u>http://www.healthyplace.com/medications/lithium.htm</u>, not only was *"hypothyroidism"* and neurogenic *"Diabetes Insipidus"* mentioned, but in addition, *"hyperparathyroidism"* was also included as one of three conditions that **apparently can persist even after the discontinuation of the lithium therapy.** This raises the questions: Do these conditions eventually become resolved after lithium therapy is discontinued, or do they become permanent? And if not, what is the approximate time frame for resolution?

Hyperparathyroidism, which is the **over activity of the parathyroid glands** and normally treated by surgery, resulting in the removal of all, or part of the parathyroid glands. The next question is: If part is removed, then what part, (or how much), of the glands should be removed? **The "parathormone" hormone is produced by the parathyroid glands, and is responsible for the distribution of calcium and phosphate in the body.**

The *Bantam Medical Dictionary, 3rd* edition (1981/2000) states **that *"a high level of the hormone causes transfer of calcium from the bones to the blood"*** (p. 240). The first, and most obvious conclusion is: The onset of calcium depletion of the bones would lead to osteoporosis. Dr. Balch

(*Prescription for Nutritional Healing, 3rd edition*, 2000) stresses that *"a proper balance of magnesium, calcium, and phosphorus should be maintained at all times"* (p. 31). He then mentions that **"Excessive amounts of phosphorus interferes with calcium uptake."** This brings to light the importance of vitamin K supplementation, especially whenever an elevated level of calcium is present in the bloodstream, which can result from an overactive parathyroid hormone, potentially resulting from lithium therapy.

An adequate level of vitamin K is also important for maintaining the integrity, and permeability, of an important and delicate part of the vascular system (the critical blood-brain barrier). Its function, whether preventing unwanted toxins, or just the opposite, by allowing the many nutrients necessary for healthy brain function to penetrate, is extremely important.

Richard Wood, Ph.D., a researcher at Tufts University in Boston, in an article about the newly discovered importance of vitamin K in regulating calcium deposition (*Life Extension Magazine*, 2003, February, p. 86), states that vitamin K deficiency increases with age, and then goes on to point out that vitamin K helps prevent vascular calcification; and **"Poor vitamin K status has been found to triple the risk of severe vascular calcification"** (p. 86). **A deficiency of vitamin K, combined with an excessive level of calcium in the blood, could be a serious combination,** especially in light of vitamin K's ability to *"Reduce neuronal damage by protecting the vascular system, guarding against inflammation and blocking excess calcium into brain cells"* (p. 86). Dr. Wood mentions that *"Vitamin K is also involved in regulating important brain enzymes and growth factors."*

And statin drugs could compound the problem of vascular calcification even further (another strike against the statin drugs), as they deplete vitamin K (which was discussed earlier in this book), as well as many other critical nutrients. With excess calcium in the bloodstream, the problem could be much more severe than it normally would be.

Although vitamin K supplementation would be beneficial in reducing some of the elevated calcium in the blood, another factor might possibly be of even greater concern: The interaction of two very important minerals in the body, calcium and magnesium. As previously mentioned, according to Dr. Balch: *"The proper balance of magnesium, calcium, and phosphorus should be maintained at all times"* (*Prescription for Nutritional Healing, 3rd edition*, 2000, pp. 25-26), and he goes on to point out that excessive calcium levels would interfere with the absorption of the two critical minerals: magnesium and zinc. Many potential problems could easily result from a deficiency of either one or both of the two very important minerals.

First, according to Edelman (*Natural Healing for Schizophrenia*, 1996/1998), **magnesium is:**

> ***Calming to the nervous system.*** *In a study of 165 boys, those with schizophrenia, depression, autism or sleep disturbances had low levels of magnesium. In other studies,* ***psychiatric patients who tried to commit suicide were also found to have depressed levels.*** *Magnesium affects cell membrane permeability, helps maintain cellular electrical potential, and supports formation of tyrosine.* ***A deficiency may produce*** *apathy,* ***agitation, irritability, personality changes,*** *disorientation, bizarre movements,* ***sleep disturbances,*** *depression and, in some cases, hallucinations* (p. 35).

Also, according to Dr. Balch (*Prescription for Nutritional Healing, 3rd edition*, 2000), **magnesium aids in "maintaining the body's proper pH balance and normal body temperature,"** and he adds that *"some possible manifestations of magnesium deficiency include poor digestion, rapid heartbeat, chronic fatigue,* ***seizures,*** *and tantrums;* ***often a magnesium deficiency can be synonymous with diabetes. Magnesium deficiencies are at the root of many cardiovascular problems"*** (p. 30).

Dr. Balch also stresses that ***"a low magnesium level makes nearly every disease worse."*** Thus, as we can easily see, a magnesium deficiency definitely has widespread implications.

Then, Eva Edelman notes:

***Zinc** is abundant in the brain hippocampus and may function as a neurotransmitter.*

*It is needed in neuron development neurotransmitter synthesis, and **copper chelation.** Zinc also enhances resistance to stress; and helps maintain intellectual function, memory, and **level moods**. **Deficiency can lead to** headaches, lethargy, amnesia, other **memory impairment, irritability, behavior disorders,** and **paranoia.** Zinc is used in treating **histamine imbalances,** pyroluria, **and blood sugar disorders*** (*Natural Healing for Schizophrenia*, 1996/1998, p. 34).

Some other uses for zinc are blood pressure moderation, protein and **fatty acid synthesis, insulin storage, thyroid functioning**, and thiamin, phosphorus and **protein metabolism**.

Another important function of zinc is counter-acting some important excitotoxins. According to neurologists John Olney and Russell Blaylock, when certain chemicals exceed critical levels, they can overexcite brain neurons, causing nerve cell death (*Natural Healing for Schizophrenia,* Edelman, 1996/1998, p. 145).

It might be helpful if we now take a moment and evaluate some important issues that we just learned:

- **Lithium can contribute to elevated calcium in the bloodstream, which could potentially result in excessive calcification of arteries, the blood-brain barrier, and neurons in the brain.**
- **Excessive calcium levels can lead to a deficiency of the minerals magnesium and zinc.**
- **A magnesium deficiency can contribute to many different potentially serious conditions. Some associated with mental and behavioral problems are:**
    - o **Apathy**
    - o **Agitation**
    - o **Irritability,**
    - o **Personality changes**
    - o **Depression**
    So actually, the personality changes could just be another term for the bipolar disorder, which is obviously a personality change.
- **A low magnesium level makes nearly every disease worse.**
- **Although zinc has many important functions, it is necessary for neurotransmitter syntheses, and may also function as a neurotransmitter.**
- **Dopamine, serotonin, and acetylcholine are all important neurotransmitters that influence our mood.**
- **Another function of zinc is helping maintain level moods (basically preventing the highs and lows - normally referred to as bipolar disorder).**
- **A zinc deficiency can lead to irritability and behavior disorders, amongst many other conditions.**
- **Zinc also just happens to be used in treating two disorders – histamine imbalances and blood sugar disorders. They just happen to be conditions often caused by lithium therapy.**

Considering that according to Eva Edelman, ***"It is unknown whether lithium is needed or contraindicated for humans, much less, what daily intake should be,"*** and that ***"Rosenblatt believes lithium may act as a substitute for sodium,"*** and that ***"Snyder warns that lithium might disrupt critical sodium balances"*** (p. 155), one can't help but question the reasoning behind the conclusion that inorganic lithium therapy should even be considered, especially in light of the serious side effects associated with its use. As usual, there are much better options available.

CHAPTER SIXTEEN
LITHIUM WITHDRAWAL & SAFER OPTIONS

Toxicity and Withdrawal

Toxic levels of lithium are actually very similar to the excessive buildup of serotonin caused by Prozac™, which is referred to as serotonin syndrome. This brings us to the next important consideration: **Lithium withdrawal**. Eva Edelman quotes Dr. Carl C. Pfeiffer, Ph.D., M.D. and Dr. Richman, who both recommend increasing salt intake when withdrawing from lithium, as follows: *"For moderate excess, **Pfeiffer recommends withholding lithium and increasing dietary salt. Richman suggests salt water.** Stopping lithium may not initially reduce body storage enough to abort severe side affects. **In critical situations, dialysis might be indicated"** (Natural Healing for Schizophrenia,* Edelman, 1996/1998, p. 155). The question remains: How can we best eliminate the potentially toxic lithium carbonate, and replace it with safer alternatives?

The Therapeutic Benefits of Celtic Sea Salt

According to Dr. F. Batmanghelidj, M.D., **salt acts just like lithium in the body except it is excreted more rapidly.** But interestingly, one of the contra-indications (something to avoid) listed while on inorganic lithium carbonate therapy is "A Salt Free Diet" (*Natural Healing for Schizophrenia,* Edelman, 1996/1998, p. 155). So, apparently lithium is not effective without salt, although I believe Celtic sea salt might not only effective without any additional lithium, but could possibly eliminate the need for lithium carbonate therapy. And if salt will replace lithium during withdrawal from lithium, then why shouldn't salt be used in the first place?

One major difference between lithium carbonate and Celtic sea salt is the significant damage to the kidneys caused by the lithium. Even though the refined table salt most people consume is not nearly as damaging to the kidneys as inorganic lithium, any excess is not always adequately excreted. As a result, it could sometimes solidify, potentially resulting in some kidney problems. Quoting Dr. de Langre (*Seasalt's Hidden Powers,* 1992), *"Unrefined Celtic Salt has the opposite effect: its sodium drains out rapidly, keeping the kidneys at peak function, as well as promoting flexibility in the articulations"* (p. 87).

Celtic sea salt seems to have some qualities similar to lithium, and even contains the mineral lithium in trace amounts as nature intended. In nature, trace elements are found in trace (minute) amounts, and that is why they are referred to as trace minerals. Dr. de Langre stresses this important issue when he states that *"macro-nutrients as well as **trace elements should never be taken carelessly in any quantity.** Most of them have **a very narrow quantitive range between what is essential and what is toxic"** (Seasalt's Hidden Powers,* 1992, p. 21).

There is a major difference between **toxic doses of the inorganic lithium carbonate,** versus **trace amounts of organic lithium.** When doctors prescribe dosages of trace elements such as lithium, in an inorganic form and at a toxic dosage of 900 mg per day, many potential side effects are very likely. Just the severe irreversible damage to the kidneys alone, could easily result in kidney failure and the possibility of dialysis in the future. It is possible that many people with the bipolar disorder are just missing adequate sodium, potassium, magnesium, zinc, and organic iodine, all found in an easily assimilatable ionic form in Celtic sea salt. Even if just one important mineral is missing, some of the cellular reactions in the neurotransmitters might be influenced, as was mentioned with lithium usage. Some neurotransmitters are stimulating, while others are calming, and still others help modulate or balance emotions. If the lithium carbonate therapy were doing its job effectively, there would obviously not be so many serious side effects associated with its use.

Although lithium is just one trace mineral found in the Celtic sea salt, it is possible that organic lithium might also play an important synergistic role along with the sodium, chloride, potassium, and magnesium, in regards to the efficient function of the neurons in the brain. According to an article in the February 2003 issue of *Life Extension* magazine, Dr. David Perlmutter, M.D., a widely known author and lecturer on brain aging and regeneration, indicates that lithium is neuroprotective and neurotrophic. This basically refers to the protection of the brain neurons, and stimulating the growth of neural tissue in the brain. From the article, it is obvious that Dr. Perlmutter uses natural substances in his practice, and although he did not specify the form of lithium he was referring to, under the circumstances it would obviously be the organic form.

The trace element iron, also critical to our health, is found in Celtic sea salt. Although both copper and iron can be potentially toxic at elevated levels, fortunately trace minerals in the ionic form do not accumulate at toxic levels in the body, as other inorganic forms sometimes can.

Dr. Balch states that calcium (also found in Celtic Sea Salt) is important for both the maintenance of a regular heartbeat and the transmission of nerve impulses. He also mentions that *"Deficiencies of calcium are also associated with cognitive impairment, convulsions, **depression**, delusions, and hyperactivity"* (*Prescription for Nutritional Healing, 3rd edition*, 2000, p. 28).

Another important mineral found in Celtic Sea Salt is magnesium, and Dr. Balch notes:

*Magnesium is a vital catalyst in enzyme activity, especially the activity of those enzymes involved in energy production. It assists in calcium and potassium uptake. **A deficiency of magnesium interferes with the transmission of nerve and muscle impulses, causing irritability and nervousness.** Supplementing the diet with **magnesium can help prevent depression, and also aids in maintaining the body's proper pH balance*** (*Prescription for Nutritional Healing, 3rd edition*, 2000, p. 30).

One of the side effects associated with **in**organic lithium usage, is elevated blood sugar. Celtic Sea Salt contains chromium, which is an essential mineral for maintaining stable blood sugar levels through proper insulin utilization, and is especially helpful with diabetes or hypoglycemia. It has also been found that **some symptoms of a chromium deficiency are bipolar disease, depression,** obesity, **hypoglycemia**, and **diabetes**.

Vanadium is another trace mineral found in Celtic sea salt that is also beneficial for improving insulin utilization and improving glucose tolerance. It has been know for years that those with both diabetes and hypoglycemia do not properly metabolize sugar, causing them to be more prone to addictions. So, although lithium carbonate creates a problem by elevating blood sugar levels, Celtic Sea Salt contains minerals that will instead help stabilize blood-glucose levels.

The trace amounts of iodine, found in Celtic sea salt, is actually made up of two elements (lithium and tin), which benefit, rather than suppress the thyroid as lithium carbonate does. Thus, one potential problem might be resolved, rather than created. Dr. Jacques de Langre, Ph.D., explains in his book *Seasalt's Hidden Powers* (1992), that in the ocean the sea vegetation combine the two elements into organic iodine, which is then released into the ocean, and thus found in natural sea salt, along with the individual elements, tin and lithium.

In his book *Nutrition and Mental Illness* (1987), Dr. Carl C. Pfeiffer, Ph.D., M.D. mentions that trace elements are often the missing link in regards to mental illness, and that many schizophrenics and some manic-depressives not only have high copper levels, but low levels of zinc and manganese (both found in Celtic Sea Salt).

Dr. Balch explains how organic germanium (another trace mineral also found in Celtic Sea Salt) is effective in increasing tissue oxygenation, when he states that *"like hemoglobin, germanium acts as a carrier of oxygen to the cells"* (*Prescription for Nutritional Healing, 3rd edition*, 2000, p. 28). This is just one more way the Celtic sea salt can also increase the oxygen levels in the brain, which is another important issue.

Because of the diversity of the many important minerals and trace elements, and the ionic bioavailability of the organic ingredients, Celtic Sea Salt has the greatest potential for stabilizing the histamine imbalances in the brain, which are so very important, as well as preventing the dehydration that contributes to the histamine imbalances. In fact, according to Dr. Batmanghelidj, salt is the most effective antihistamine. It is also interesting that an organic form of lithium was once used as a salt substitute.

Additional Suggestions for Lithium Withdrawal

1. **Supplementing Vitamins and Minerals.** **The vitamins and minerals recommended for Prozac™ withdrawal should be included,** as they will benefit anyone who has been taking either Prozac™ or Lithium. They are also beneficial for anyone simply wishing to maintain their health.

2. **Essential Fatty Acids (EFAs)** are especially important. In addition to the information provided earlier in this book in the chapter on Depression, it is important to note that EFAs build our receptor sites and improve reception. In the book *Natural Highs* (2002), the authors Hyla Cass, M.D. and Patrick Holford discuss one study that proved that **when people with bipolar or manic depression were given 9.6 mg of omega-3 oils over a four-month period, they experienced "substantial" improvement** (pp. 148-149), although they recommend from 1,000 mg to 2,000 mg daily for anyone experiencing mental health problems.

3. **Withdraw from antidepressants and lithium at the same time.** If you are currently taking both Prozac™, (or some other SSRI antidepressant), in addition to lithium, it might be best to withdraw from **both** concurrently. Seldom are depression or mood swings nearly as dangerous as the antidepressants, or the inorganic lithium often prescribed for both conditions can potentially be. Also, as we learned earlier in the chapter on Depression, antidepressants are basically stimulants, and a major contributor to the bipolar disorder. As lithium is just the opposite (a suppressant), combining the two is obviously counter-productive.

4. **Lower serum lithium levels.** Two natural substances capable of lowering serum lithium concentration, by increasing the excretion of lithium in the urine, are urea and sodium bicarbonate. One-half teaspoon of Sodium Bicarbonate (baking soda) should be taken twice daily along with urea. This might be necessary during withdrawal, and only if elevated lithium is suspected. Urea is normally available in the powder form through the pharmacy without a prescription.

5. **The herb Golden Seal** is also very helpful in eliminating toxins, such as the inorganic form of Lithium carbonate.

6. **Re-hydration should begin** once the lithium carbonate is discontinued, with 10 glasses of water, along with 1 teaspoon of Celtic sea salt daily, as it contains organic iodine and lithium, as well as other important trace minerals, as we just discussed. These trace elements are much more easily absorbed and utilized by the body when in the natural organic ionized form found in the Celtic sea salt, and thus will not become toxic.

7. **Six tablets of kelp daily** might be helpful, in addition to Celtic sea salt. Kelp has many trace minerals, including organic iodine.

8. **Organic Lithium Orotate** is a **natural form of lithium,** which has been proven safe, and is normally sold in health food stores. It is important to remember that our body needs only trace amounts of the elements iodine and lithium, and trace amounts refers to micrograms, not hundreds of milligrams (basically thousands of times as much), which is usually the amount prescribed for the **in**organic lithium carbonate. Using the organic form of lithium might help reduce the manic phase in the beginning (which doctors are attempting to do with the inorganic lithium carbonate), or it might even be helpful to continue with the natural lithium orotate following withdrawal if it appears to be beneficial. Quite possibly, the organic form of lithium in the proper dosage might also prove to be a valuable resource to assist in repairing any brain damage that could have occurred from either lithium or Prozac™ use.

9. **"Serenity™",** a product developed by German physician, Hans A. Nieper, M.D., is another source of natural lithium. It is combined with organic orotate, which transports the natural lithium to the blood cells of our brain much more efficiently.

According to the Website http://www.healthyplace.com, *"Dr. Nieper is reported to have one of the highest cure rates for cancer in the medical world".* It was also claimed that his **success with depression**, migraines, **and bipolar disorder**, using the organic form of lithium orotate called "Serenity™" is unsurpassed.

10. **Inositol supplementation** might possibly be another safe and effective solution for replacing lithium, as lithium instead depletes the inositol and we learned of its importance. **One safe and inexpensive source is lecithin, which contains both inositol and choline, and is also known to be very important for healthy brain function.** I personally use lecithin granules, as they are the most reasonable source. If you substitute Celtic Sea Salt for lithium, along with the minerals necessary for healthy brain function, the synergism of both choline and inositol from lecithin could also assist in their efficient absorption. I personally use four tablespoons daily, as it has many other health benefits, including the homogenization of fats, and the brain contains a great deal of lecithin.

11. **Glycine** is an amino acid, necessary for central nervous system function. It functions as an inhibitory neurotransmitter, and has been **used in the treatment of bipolar depression,** as well as hyperactivity. While a good multi-amino acid complex containing all essential amino acids should be taken, it is also suggested to take additional glycine as an individual supplement (but at a separate time).

12. **Pregnenolone** is a hormone that modulates the neurotransmitters, and assists in stabilizing moods. It appears to be an excellent resource to assist in proper sleep, reducing stress and maintaining emotional health, and is known for its ability to promote feelings of balance and harmony. Clinical studies have examined its role in relieving depression, improving memory, reducing stress, treating arthritis, and increasing longevity. Pregnenolone has been used for many years in high doses, and most importantly with no reported side effects

13. **Goji and Mangosteen,** mentioned in the outline for withdrawal from the antidepressants (and in the "Nature's Miracles" chapter, earlier in this book), should both also be beneficial when eliminating lithium, especially as they doesn't interact with other medications. If you are on both an antidepressant, and lithium therapy, you might discover that once you have eliminated the antidepressant, your bipolar condition will likely lessen, or entirely disappear. Both goji and mangosteen also help reduce depression, as well as stress (mentioned next), without the stimulant effect of antidepressant medications.

14. **Avoid all forms of Stress.** The stress hormone cortisol is produced by emotional and mental stress (fear, confusion, worry, anger, rage, etc.), physical stress (exhaustion, physical discomfort, etc), illness, poor health (wrong diet, nutritional deficiencies), and toxins (pollution, any drugs legal, illegal or over-the-counter, especially SSRIs). According to a publication by the *Associated Press* (October 29, 2004), stressful situations trigger an enzyme in the brain called protein kinase C (PKC), which is also an active enzyme in bipolar disorder and schizophrenia. The active PKC enzyme not only impairs short-term memory, but it also affects the prefrontal cortex, the decision-making part of the brain as well, which researchers say *"could be a factor in the distractibility impulsiveness and impaired judgment that occurs in those illnesses."*

15. **Many natural supplements** are known to be either calming or stimulating. The objective will be to assist your body in maintaining that delicate balance that produces both calm and peace of mind. None of us can expect to experience an unnatural high without dealing with the depressing low that will ultimately follow. I am sure you are aware that we are describing the bipolar condition. Keep in mind that some of the supplements listed tend to produce more calming hormones, such as GABA or DHEA, while others are responsible for creating the more stimulating neurotransmitters, such as serotonin and dopamine.

You now have at your disposal, more than one safe yet effective way to balance your moods. If you sense a manic phase coming on, take advantage of the more calming ones. And of course, if you are feeling a little down, use the more stimulating ones. You can experiment and find which ones work the best for you. You are basically in charge, and you better than anyone, can evaluate what works best for you. The good news is: You have several options to choose from.

It is important to remember: Our bodies are each unique, and influenced not only by our diet, but also any nutrients or medications we might be taking. We will not all respond the same to a particular therapy or supplement, thus some supplements might be more beneficial for you, while others might possibly be more effective for someone else.

Another important issue: Although drugs can easily interact with each other, and can be potentially dangerous, that is seldom a concern with natural supplements. For example, I have taken many different vitamins, minerals, amino acids, and plant extracts for decades, and have yet to experience a reaction or interaction from doing so. Although it is very unlikely, it might be possible, as some people may have extremely compromised immune systems and are thus allergic to many different things, including many common foods. Some may also mistake a detoxification symptom for an allergic reaction.

Something else to consider: Although the traditional solution of high doses of the inorganic lithium carbonate is potentially dangerous, and possibly even life threatening, the bipolar condition it is prescribed for seldom is. Also, if you have been taking an antidepressant, and have a bipolar condition, it is more than likely a side effect from your medication.

As you probably noticed, under MARY LOU'S STORY, **she was able to safely and effectively eliminate a total of <u>nine medications</u> in only two months,** and is feeling so much better since her withdrawal. Most importantly, **one was a 16-year dependence on Prozac™, along with another antidepressant called Desyrel™, (as well as lithium).** She actually accomplished her amazing total withdrawal for the most part, by drinking two ounces of the mangosteen juice three times a day, along with such supplements as a high potency vitamin B-complex and flax seed oil. She had absolutely no problem with the withdrawal, and was totally amazed that something she considered impossible was surprisingly easy to accomplish.

CHAPTER SEVENTEEN
HYPOTHYROIDISM

Modern Medicine's Flawed Thyroid Evaluation and Treatment

Many of the symptoms associated with hypothyroidism are very similar to those associated with hypoglycemia, and both are often experienced by diabetics, with depression, mood swings, and behavioral disorders being the most common. The question is: Could these symptoms possibly be even more pronounced, when experiencing both conditions concurrently? If that holds true (which seems logical), depression would probably be even more serious, and a prescription for an antidepressant, (or possibly an additional antidepressant), would all too often be many doctors' solution.

There are also other symptoms associated with hypothyroidism, such as: brittle nails, dry skin and hair, low metabolism or inability to lose weight, fatigue or low motivation, headaches, fluid retention, heat or cold intolerance, as well as depression and mood swings to help identify the condition. Unfortunately, most medical doctors fail to take the time necessary to properly diagnose the underlying problem, thus a prescription for an antidepressant is all too often the typical response.

If you went to your doctor, who like most medical doctors studied traditional (allopathic) medicine, a hypothyroid condition could easily be misdiagnosed to begin with. Standard procedure practiced by most medical doctors (even endocrinologists, who specialize in hormonal disorders such as thyroid), would rely on the standard blood test evaluating your Thyroid Stimulating Hormone (TSH) and possibly T_4 thyroid levels. In many cases, the TSH and T_4 thyroid levels would be considered as normal, and you would thus be notified that your thyroid is not a concern (although it very well could be). Then, even if your doctor decided that thyroid supplementation might possibly be in order, he like most allopathic doctors, would likely prescribe Synthroid™, Levothroid™ or Levoxyl™, one of the artificial forms of T_4 thyroid. The problem is you are likely not experiencing a T_4 thyroid deficiency, and thus your medication will seldom work, and could at times make matters even worse, by shutting down even more of the active T_3 thyroid that would normally be produced by the thyroid.

Following The Money Trail -
(Why Thyroid Conditions Likely Remain Unresolved)

The basic problem is: A low thyroid condition can potentially lead to many different of symptoms (thirty or more), which are likely due to a reduction in the enzyme action of all 3,000 enzymes in the body. This then opens the door for a lot of prescriptions to deal with each of the potential symptoms. One of the most common symptoms associated with a hypothyroid condition is depression, and thus unnecessary prescriptions for antidepressants.

Unfortunately, the most common class, known as SSRI antidepressants such as Prozac™, Paxil™, Zoloft™, and Celexa™, etc., stimulate the adrenals to produce the stress hormone cortisol, which actually leads to elevated blood sugar. The SSRI antidepressants can thus not only worsen existing diabetes, but are also known to contribute to the development of diabetes in non-diabetics, from their long-term usage. That's not the only problem, as they also contribute to another serious condition known as adrenal fatigue, which is seldom properly diagnosed by most medical doctors. Only ample rest and natural supplements, (along with stopping the medication creating the adrenal fatigue), will heal the adrenals and finally restore their vital function, of creating several important hormones. **Although adrenal fatigue can be very debilitating, it was never classified as a disease! Interstingly, (three non-diseases) elevated cholesterol, acid reflux "disease," and obesity, are now classified as diseases, so your insurance will now cover the expensive medications, (and sometimes expensive surgery), for your non-diseases.** So, what's the basic problem?

The answer will soon become obvious, if we just follow the money trail for a moment. First, the majority of decisions most doctors make are influenced either directly or indirectly by the pharmaceutical industry (the most profitable enterprise in the entire world!). They have a strong impact on exactly what will, or will not be classified as a disease. The problem is, one of their most popular and profitable classes of antidepressants, the SSRIs (such as Prozac™), can easily lead to adrenal fatigue. And there is absolutely no drug that can possibly restore the health of the adrenals, or reproduce the many critical hormones the adrenals are responsible for.

Then, if you are required to stop taking a very profitable drug, and take natural supplements to resolve the condition instead, it creates an obvious dilemma (a conflict of interest). And what is their typical solution? Basically, just ignore its existence, and not classify it as a disease. Modern medicine can always come up with some profitable medication to treat the obvious symptoms that will result by ignoring the true problem. If you recall, **87% of the authorities that determine what is classified as a disease, and what is covered by your insurance, have financial ties to the drug industry.** There is a good explanation for why the major cardiovascular risk factor homocysteine, as well as adrenal fatigue are deliberately overlooked, and the hypothyroid condition is conveniently misdiagnosed. No drug can possibly resolve the associated symptoms, let alone the underlying problem, and natural therapies are never to be discussed, let alone be implemented.

Keep in mind that these are quite common scenarios, not just rare cases, but actually quite typical, normally due to superficial diagnosis (or lack thereof). This is what Dr. Bruce West often refers to as, resorting to *"Drugs for everything, and nothing but drugs for anything."* Basically a quick fix, although the problems you will experience as a result (normal side effects) can be long-term. The length of time you will be required to deal with the side effects depends upon how long you are allowed to remain on the medications you were prescribed, (all too often for a lifetime!).

Far too many are needlessly placed on two or three medications for treating the very same condition, and I found that even applies to antidepressants. Rather than replacing one antidepressant that is not working, they just add another (which was true in Mary Lou's case). Doctors often tend to ignore the warnings regarding combining some drugs that can be potentially dangerous when prescribed in combination. That is especially a concern regarding any mind-altering medication. And it's amazing how many women are constantly being placed on multiple contra-indicated antidepressants due to an undiagnosed hypothyroid condition. The thyroid condition continues to remain unresolved, and thus the depression normally does also. As a result, they are then left on antidepressants for years. Unfortunately, the low thyroid condition can also contribute to many other problems, including increasing the cardiovascular risk, as well as diabetes complications.

So what's the solution? Fix the underlying problem, and get off the medication! Those that chose to do so were totally amazed at how easily that could be accomplished. The bonus was, they were no longer required to deal with the many seemingly unexplainable side effects. And without exception, they began feeling better than they had in years, and no longer being tied to a lifetime of medications is an added benefit, and a tremendous feeling.

Effectively phasing out your medications is obviously much more difficult if your doctor is constantly warning you of the dangers of doing so. Some doctors are determined to be in charge, and can't accept the fact that their patient might possibly have the intelligence to somehow arrive at a more rational conclusion, in spite of the overwhelming evidence. There is absolutely no laboratory in the world that can more conclusively determine exactly what is the most beneficial for you, than your own body! We all know when we feel better, or worse.

Far too many doctors have an aversion toward anything derived from a natural source, rather than from some laboratory. If you happen to have such a doctor, I would suggest it might be time for a change. As I have always stressed, you and not your doctor, are in charge. All your health decisions should be yours alone, and your doctor's position should be in an advisory capacity only. If you are convinced that your conclusion is more valid than his, follow your instincts. Also, keep in mind that most of the conditions we are addressing can all be safely self-monitored, as well as utilizing natural supplements that don't pose the threat that drugs do. There are no supplements I recommend in this book, that I have not personally taken myself, at some time over the years. I have yet to experience a reaction from any of them, although I have never taken prescription medications.

Interestingly, those people that I have worked with so far, actually chose to eliminate their medications on their own, and then notified their doctor after the fact. Then, armed with absolute proof of their successful outcome, such as more stable blood sugar or blood pressure, more energy, or possibly less pain or depression, they now have conclusive proof that their decision to eliminate them was obviously a wise one. The most difficult problem some doctors have to deal with is admitting that all those medications they were prescribing were totally unnecessary. That is especially true when it is obvious their patient is doing much better without their medications. How can anyone argue with results? There is no better proof that most (if not all) medications were totally unnecessary. Eliminating the many side effects was just a bonus. Not only are those side effects troubling, and very uncomfortable, but the many symptoms normally experienced are also an indication there is likely some unseen damage taking place in the body as a result of their use.

Do The Self Test (Evaluating Your Own Thyroid Function)

You can either have your doctor do a test (for free T_3 thyroid), or you can do a temperature test yourself. This can be accomplished by placing a normal glass thermometer underarm, first thing in the morning before arising. Just lie still and leave it there for ten minutes and record your temperature. Repeat the process for five consecutive days, and then average your temperature. If your average temperature is 97.4° or less, natural thyroid supplementation will most likely help. The dosage might have to be titrated (adjusted) until you find the dosage that is right for you. Once it is, you should soon begin noticing a difference.

Considering the statistics, let's see what one of the foremost authorities on thyroid dysfunction, has to say on the subject. According to the late Dr. Broda Barnes, M.D., Ph.D., in his book *Hypothyroidism – the Unsuspected Illness* (1976), ***"Forty percent of the American people today are suffering needlessly and many dying for lack of an ingredient vital for health"*** (p. VII). The thyroid Dr. Barnes was referring to is a natural glandular extract, called Armour™ thyroid, which we will soon be discussing in detail. An important issue is: His book was published in 1976, so his statistical information is more than thirty years old. Today we should expect the statistics to reflect a considerably larger portion of the population experiencing hypothyroidism, as well as the associated problems, considering the many changes that have taken place the past thirty years (not for the better) that are known to contribute to reduced thyroid function.

Some Potential Causes of Thyroid Suppression

1. Diabetes / Hypoglycemia. I believe it's not just coincidental that approximately 80% of diabetics are also suffering from a hypothyroid condition, and it appears that the insulin resistance in the liver is likely the underlying problem. This insulin resistance in the liver reduces the efficiency of the conversion of the T_4 thyroid produced by the thyroid gland into the much more effective T_3 thyroid (approximately four times as effective). The metabolism is thus reduced due to the insulin resistance in the liver, which results in reduced body temperature. Enzymes are very sensitive to a body temperature change, and even a minor reduction in body temperature has been proven in lab tests to considerably reduce the enzyme action of all the 3,000 enzymes in the body. The enzyme in the liver responsible for the T_4 to T_3 conversion depends upon glucose (sugar). Not only is the availability of glucose to the liver reduced due to the insulin resistance, but the efficiency of the enzyme action is reduced also, due to the reduced metabolism, basically compounding the problem. In my opinion, this is the primary reason diabetics are much more prone to experience a hypothyroid (low thyroid) condition than non-diabetics.

2. **Iodine deficiency.** According to Dr. David Brownstein, M.D., in his book ***Iodine Why You Need – Why You Can't Live Without It*** (2004), after testing hundreds of patients, he discovered that **more than 90% exhibited laboratory signs of iodine deficiency.** Just one more reason so many people are hypothyroid and experiencing the many associated side effects, such as depression and increased cardiovascular problems.

3. **Excess Bromine.** Dr. Brownstein also discusses another problem that leads to insufficient iodine for effective thyroid function. Back in the 1960's, iodine was being used as a dough conditioner by the commercial baking industry, (a very good idea). Unfortunately, twenty years later due to an article published by the National Institute of Health (NIH), questioning the safety of using iodine in baking products, the iodine was replaced by Bromine, (a very bad idea). It wasn't as though iodine had created any problems after 20 years' use, (which it hadn't). It was just due to someone's concern, with no apparent valid basis. Dr. Brownstein identifies the basic problem when he states that: *"Bromine is halide (as is iodine, fluoride, and chloride)."* He then goes on to explain that ***"Bromine interferes with iodine utilization in the thyroid*** *as well as wherever else iodine would concentrate in the body"* (p. 38). In his opinion, ***"Iodine deficiency is a huge public health problem"*** (p. 41).

Bromine is actually made from fumigated grain products, and is often used as a clouding agent in many popular drinks. It has also been found that bromine *"Will replace chloride and accumulate, will also be taken up by thyroid gland instead of iodine,* **[causing]** *adverse effects on brain and thyroid function"* (http://www.hypoglycemia.asn.au/articles/rich_sources_nutrients.html).

4. **Dehydration.** According to Dr. F. Batmanghelidj, M.D., the enzyme action necessary for the T_4 to T_3 conversion is reduced by dehydration. One reason is because dehydration leads to insulin resistance in the liver, where the thyroid hormone conversion takes place. The enzyme responsible for that conversion requires glucose, which is reduced due to the resultant insulin resistance. Another problem is, the body recognizes dehydration as stress. This in turn results in the production of stress hormones, which are known to suppress thyroid function. Thus, your body obviously recognizes that dehydration is a serious issue, which we must never forget.

5. **Stress.** Stress hormones not only suppress the thyroid, but will also contribute to elevated blood sugar leading to diabetes. Stress (both physical and mental) also depletes the important mineral selenium, which is necessary for healthy thyroid function. Remember that according to Dr. Ann Blake Tracy, just one 30 mg dose of Prozac™ elevates the stress hormone cortisol by 200%. This becomes obvious if you consider that **SIX (over half!) of the 10 nutrients listed in the next section, which are necessary for healthy thyroid function, are depleted by stress!**

And as we just discussed, dehydration also is considered a stressor, although there are several. One discovery I made was, when a person is experiencing stress, their body temperature drops and their mood suddenly changes (and not for the better). They experience symptoms that are very typical of those normally associated with both hypothyroidism and hypoglycemia, as they are both very similar.

6. **Bad Fats (trans-fatty acids)** are found mostly in hydrogenated or partially hydrogenated oils. In his book *Overcoming Thyroid Disorders* (2002), David Brownstein, M.D. tells us that:

> *These foreign substances (trans-fatty acids) are actually incorporated into the cell membranes. This will **disrupt the normal functioning of the cells of the body, blocking the utilization of essential fatty acids. This can lead to the development of many chronic illnesses, including immune system dysfunction and hormonal imbalances, <u>particularly thyroid imbalances</u>** (p. 181).*

The nutrient depletion caused by bad fats, especially produces deficiencies of the fat-soluble vitamins A, D, E, and K, which is a major concern for anyone with a low thyroid. Insufficient vitamin A can cause a deterioration of the pituitary gland's basophil cells where the thyroid-stimulating hormone is synthesized, limiting the amount of iodine that the thyroid gland can absorb, and reducing the amount of thyroid hormone it produces. Vitamin D is required for healthy thyroid function, and vitamin E has been shown to protect against at least 80 diseases, including the ability to prevent heart attacks. And as we recently learned, vitamin K also serves many important functions.

7. **High Protein Diet**. This concern is explained best by Broda Barnes, M.D., taken from his book *Hypothyroidism: The Unsuspected Illness* (1976), as follows:

> *What was not realized was the effect of a diet high in protein on thyroid function – which explains why many patients have failed to lose weight on as few as 800 calories a day of such a diet and have been accused of cheating on their diet when, in fact, they did no cheating.*

> *…when the intake of carbohydrate and fat was kept low and I ate mostly veal and turkey, diarrhea soon developed and I had feelings of malaise and illness.*

> *…when the diet was changed so that it was low in fat but high in protein and with enough carbohydrate to prevent diarrhea, symptoms of hypothyroidism appeared. Cholesterol level in the blood became elevated and in order to keep it within normal range, four additional grains of thyroid daily were needed.*

> *Apparently, **a diet high in protein requires additional thyroid for its metabolism.** There were no symptoms of hyperthyroidism in spite of the extra thyroid until the diet was cut back to a normal amount of protein. Then typical hyperthyroidism appeared and the extra thyroid had to be discontinued.*

> ***It seems clear that a diet quite high in protein utilizes available thyroid hormone. Two studies in the medical literature indicate that excess protein lowers the basal metabolism*** (pp. 273-274).

8. **Iron deficiency.** An iron deficiency may impair the body's ability to manufacture thyroid hormone. Antibiotics, antacids, aspirin, all cholesterol-lowering drugs, and caffeine, as well as strenuous exercise, heavy perspiration, or heavy bleeding, often depletes this mineral.

9. **The Female Gender.** Approximately 90% of those who are hypothyroid are women. One reason is that the female liver is less efficient in producing the most active form thyroid (T_3 thyroid) than the male liver. Also, women have considerably more estrogen than men, and estrogen is a known thyroid suppressant.

10. **Elevated estrogen.** It appears that several of the symptoms associated with Estrogen Replacement Therapy (ERT) that many post menopausal women have received for years, are identical to typical hypothyroid symptoms. David Brownstein, M.D. (*Overcoming Thyroid Disorders*, 2002) explains that ***"Any orally prescribed estrogen will result in an increase in thyroxine binding globulin (TBG) which will decrease the amount of thyroid hormone that is available for the body to use."*** And he goes on to note that ***"I have seen many women with hypothyroid symptoms improve their condition when they stop taking their oral synthetic hormone replacement therapy"*** (p. 60).

Birth control pills contain estrogens also, and thus will effectively decrease the amount of thyroid hormone available to the body, just as ERT does, often leading to a hypothyroid condition. Dr. Brownstein comments regarding birth control pills: ***"I have successfully treated numerous women who have many of the signs of hypothyroidism by simply having them eliminate their use of birth control pills"*** (p. 60).

Although estrogen performs an important function during the childbearing years, its level should and does reduce following menopause. Even if a woman has had a total hysterectomy, and no longer has ovaries, her fat tissue, and even her adrenals are still capable of producing estrogen. This is one reason so many women find it difficult to lose weight, and why HRT just adds to the problem, and doesn't make a bit of sense. The more fat tissue a woman has, the more estrogen is likely to be produced, and thus the more thyroid suppression should be expected. This then reduces the metabolism, and the result is more fat storage. This is in my opinion, the basic reason so many obese women find it extremely difficult to lose weight. Another is, the more suppressed the thyroid is, the less energy you will experience, thus making exercise even more difficult. In my forthcoming book on weight loss, I will not only provide solutions to this particular problem, but also many others that could very well have been undermining the conscientious efforts of many to lose weight for years.

Estrogen and oral contraceptives also deplete **EIGHT of the 10 nutrients listed in the next section, which are necessary for healthy thyroid function!**

11. **Soy.** Unfermented soy products can mimic the effects of the female hormone, causing elevated estrogen levels, and resulting in thyroid suppression. In fact, one study found that *"daily soy consumption resulted in symptoms of hypothyroidism (i.e., malaise, constipation, sleepiness) and goiters in 50% of the subjects,"* and yet *"These hypothyroid symptoms resolved one month after stopping the soy ingestion"* (David Brownstein, M.D., *Overcoming Thyroid Disorders*, 2002, p. 63).

Another concern with soy is the phytic acid, which is present in processed soy powder and unfermented soy products, and binds with certain nutrients (calcium, magnesium, zinc, and other essential minerals). This inhibits their absorption, quickly leading to potential nutrient depletion and even more problems. According to Dr. Sherry Rogers, M.D. *"Soy foods can be toxic to the thyroid. Some components of soy foods inhibit thyroid peroxidase reactions that are necessary for making thyroid hormone"* (*Detoxify or Die*, 2002, p. 126).

12. **Simple sugars.** A diet consisting of too many simple sugars is just the beginning of a downhill spiral, beginning with insulin resistance. The metabolism is then suppressed by the insulin resistance, when then causes the body temperature to drop, thus reducing the enzyme action responsible for the conversion of the T_4 thyroid to the T_3 thyroid. This eventually results in Type II diabetes and hypothyroidism.

Sugar also contributes to the depletion of vitamins B_2, B_3 and B_6, all of which are necessary for healthy thyroid function.

13. **Overstimulation.** Thyroid and/or pituitary exhaustion can result from overstimulation with substances such as caffeine, sugar, or aspartame (NutraSweet™). The elevated stress hormone cortisol, also caused by SSRI antidepressants such as Prozac™, suppresses the thyroid as well. **Beta-blockers used for hypertension are known to suppress the thyroid,** as well (likely due to elevated adrenalin).

14. **Smoking cigarettes** increases the risk of developing hypothyroidism. One study from Japan showed **a 42% increase in hypothyroidism in smokers versus non-smokers,** while another study showed those who smoked had higher levels of TSH (thyroid stimulating hormone), indicating smoking worsens hypothyroidism (*Overcoming Thyroid Disorders*, 2002, p. 69). Elevated TSH is an indicator that the thyroid is not adequately responding to stimulation. This is normally due to a deficiency of nutrients necessary for producing thyroid hormones.

Also, both tobacco smoke and cigarette papers contain the toxic chemical cadmium, which actually replaces zinc in the receptors. And it has been found that a deficiency of zinc results in a decrease in the conversion of the T_4 thyroid hormone to the active form T_3 hormone. **Smoking also contributes to the depletion of vitamin B_6, B_{12}, and D, which are necessary for healthy thyroid function.**

15. **Alcohol. The presence of alcohol in the bloodstream inhibits thyroid function,** as well as overloading the liver's detoxification process. This is also one of the many contributors to a possible drug overdose, which can be a serious concern for some. Those taking the most medications would be at the greatest risk.

Alcohol has also been found to elevate estrogen levels in women (another contributor to suppressed thyroid), as well as **depleting EIGHT of the 10 nutrients listed in the next section as being necessary for healthy thyroid function!**

16. **Environmental Toxins.** There are many **thyroid "poisons"** in your environment, which greatly contribute to the suppression of the thyroid.

- ✓ Tobacco is a major contributor to <u>cadmium</u> toxicity.
- ✓ <u>Fluoride</u> can be found in drugs (every molecule of the popular SSRI antidepressant Prozac™ contains 3 molecules of <u>fluoride</u>!), juices, soft drinks, toothpastes, dental treatments, wheat flour processed with fluoride, and even the fluoridated water contained in processed foods. **Fluorides are cumulative,** and your body can only eliminate approximately half of your fluoride intake.
- ✓ <u>Lead</u> poisoning is another possible cause of thyroid imbalance, as is <u>nuclear pollution or exposure</u>. Lead may be in produce grown near highways with vehicles using petrol, or leached from metal cans.
- ✓ Occasionally, something as simple as <u>certain perfumes</u> can suppress the thyroid.
- ✓ Even some <u>fluorescent lighting</u> can cause thyroid imbalance. If you have fluorescent light fixtures in your home, make sure all the bulbs are replaced by the healthy full-spectrum bulbs. They are actually fairly inexpensive if purchased by the case, and they will definitely make a difference.

17. **Chloride (or Chlorine)** is another halide **known as a thyroid suppressant.** And according to Dr. Sherry A. Rogers, (*Detoxify or Die*, 2002), *"Chlorine drills holes in arterial walls."* She goes on to warn that chlorine is a *"Free radical initiator that elevates cholesterol and accelerates aging"* (p. 21), as well as promoting arteriosclerosis, and various types of cancers of the rectum and bladder.

Now that we are aware of the potential damage chlorine can cause, we need to evaluate where our greatest exposure might be, in order to avoid it as much as possible.

- ✓ The most likely source of chlorine is <u>city and community water systems</u>, so **if you have chlorine (and/or fluoride) in your household water, find a good filter system capable of removing them from your drinking water.**
- ✓ Unfortunately, you can also absorb chlorine through your skin, as well as inhaling the fumes, <u>when taking a shower</u>. There are now showerheads that will resolve that problem, by removing the chlorine.
- ✓ Also remember to <u>wear rubber gloves</u>, and <u>avoid breathing fumes</u> as much as possible if you use chlorine, or anything containing chlorine, such as a bleach, disinfectant, or tile cleaner, <u>when cleaning</u>.
- ✓ And last of all is the <u>exposure from swimming pools and hot tubs</u> that use chlorine. We use Baquasil™ in both our pool and hot tub in order to avoid chlorine, which is basically hydrogen peroxide and found in most pool supply stores. Most commercial pools and spas contain high levels of chlorine, which is normally evident from the obvious chlorine odor. Many women especially, tend to exercise in pools loaded with chlorine. They not only absorb it through their skin, but also by inhaling its vapors. Due to the higher water temperature of the water in the spa, you will inhale more chlorine, and due to the dilation of pores (from the higher water temperature), you will also absorb more chlorine through your skin.

Sucralose (Splenda™) – The Chlorine Connection

There is a fairly new artificial sweetener on the market called sucralose, sold under the name Splenda™. It is a white crystalline powder substitute for sugar, has zero calories, and is about 600 times sweeter than sucrose, resulting in intense sweetness. However, sucralose is produced by chlorinating sugar. This involves chemically changing the structure of the sugar molecules by substituting <u>three chlorine atoms</u> for three hydroxyl groups. Very few studies of safety for human consumption of this product have ever been published.

The FDA has admitted that sucralose, ***"increases in glycosolation in hemoglobin imply lessening of control of diabetes"*** (Federal Register, Vol. 63, No. 64, Rules and Regulations 16417-16433, Friday. April 3, 1998, age 16426, paragraph two).

And despite the manufacturer's claims to the contrary, **sucralose most definitely is significantly absorbed and metabolized by the body.** According to the FDA's *"Final Rule"* report, 11% to 27% of sucralose is absorbed in humans, and the rest is excreted **unchanged** in feces. **But according to the Japanese Food Sanitation Council, as much as 40% of ingested sucralose is absorbed**, (likely less biased and more accurate). Furthermore, **the absorbed sucralose has been found to concentrate in the liver, kidney, and gastrointestinal tract.**

Considering sucralose is most definitely absorbed and metabolized by the body, and each molecule of sucralose (or Splenda™) contains three atoms of chlorine, this would definitely interfere with iodine absorption in the thyroid, resulting in thyroid suppression.

Your Medications Could Be Suppressing Your Thyroid

On a list of the top 200 most prescribed drugs, out of the 180 prescription medications that were tested, **156 (nearly 87%!) were found to deplete nutrients necessary for healthy thyroid function.**

The depletion (or a deficiency) of the following nutrients can result in inefficient thyroid function. Also listed are the drugs, or class of drugs, substances, and conditions (i.e. stress) that can cause depletion:

1. **Vitamin A** – depleted by steroids and corticosteroids, NSAIDs (i.e. ibuprofen), laxatives (mineral oil), estrogen and oral contraceptives, caffeine, aspirin, all cholesterol-lowering drugs, including statins and bile acid sequestrants (i.e. Questran™, Colestid™), antiseizure medication (i.e. barbiturates, phenytoin), antibiotics, antacids, and alcohol.
    - **Insufficient vitamin A can cause a deterioration of the pituitary gland's basophil cells where the thyroid-stimulating hormone is synthesized, limiting the amount of iodine that the thyroid gland can absorb, and reducing the amount of thyroid hormone it produces.**
2. **Vitamin B$_2$ (riboflavin)** – depleted by sulfa drugs, steroids and corticosteroids, muscle relaxants, mineral oil and laxatives, estrogen and oral contraceptives, diuretics, diabetes medication, antidepressants (SSRI and tricyclics), antiseizure medication (i.e. barbiturates, phenytoin), antibiotics, alcohol, **antacids,** sugar, ultraviolet light, physical and mental stress.
    - **Vitamin B$_2$ strongly influences how well the thyroid gland synthesizes its hormones.**
3. **Vitamin B$_3$ (Niacin)** – depleted by sulfa drugs, SSRI antidepressants, steroids and corticosteroids, sleeping pills, estrogen (and oral contraceptives), caffeine, antibiotics, alcohol, sugar, and physical and mental stress.
    - **Vitamin B$_3$ is essential to healthy glands, especially the thyroid.**
4. **Vitamin B$_6$ (pyridoxine)** – depleted by vasodilators (i.e. nitroglycerin), sulfa drugs, steroids and corticosteroids, smoking, sleeping pills, estrogen (and oral contraceptives), diuretics, diabetic medication, caffeine, asthma medications, antidepressants and MAO inhibitors, antibiotics, alcohol, sugar, heat (canning & roasting), and physical and mental stress.
    - Diuretics and cortisone drugs also block the absorption of this vitamin.
    - **A thyroid gland deficient in vitamin B$_6$ has difficulty converting iodine into thyroid hormone.**
5. **Vitamin B$_{12}$** – depleted by sulfa drugs, SSRI antidepressants, smoking, sleeping pills, proton pump inhibitors (i.e. Nexium™), muscle relaxants, mineral oil and laxatives, Histamine H$_2$ blockers (i.e. Tagamet™, Pepcid™, Zantac™), estrogen (and oral contraceptives), diuretics, diabetic medications, all cholesterol-lowering drugs, including statins and bile acid sequestrants

(i.e. Questran™, Colestid™), calcium deficiency, caffeine, antiseizure medication (i.e. barbiturates), amphetamines and diet pills, antibiotics, and alcohol.

- Certain anti-gout medications, anticoagulant drugs, potassium supplements, medications for high blood pressure and Parkinson's disease, excess cholesterol, and a low thyroid interfere with the absorption of this vitamin.
- **Deficiency can result in a significant reduction in the conversion of T$_4$ to T$_3$ thyroid hormone.**

6. **Vitamin D (Calciferol)** – depleted by steroids and corticosteroids, smoking, muscle relaxants, mineral oil (laxatives), Histamine H$_2$ blockers (i.e. Tagamet™, Pepcid™, Zantac™), estrogen (and oral contraceptives), diuretics, diabetic medication, all cholesterol-lowering drugs, including statins and bile acid sequestrants (i.e. Questran™, Colestid™), asthma medications, aspirin, antiseizure medication (i.e. barbiturates, phenytoin), antibiotics, antidepressants, antiarrhythmics (i.e. digoxin), antacids, analgesics, alcohol, cooking (heat), light, high fever, physical and mental stress.
   - Some cholesterol-lowering drugs, antacids, and steroid hormones (cortisone) interfere with vitamin D absorption as well as depletion.
   - **Vitamin D is necessary for healthy thyroid function.**

7. **Iron** – a trace mineral depleted by NSAIDs (i.e. ibuprofen), mineral oil and laxatives, narcotics, histamine H$_2$ blockers (i.e. Tagamet™, Pepcid™, Zantac™), choline magnesium trisalicylate (an anti-inflammatory), all cholesterol-lowering drugs, including statins and bile acid sequestrants (i.e. Questran™, Colestid™), Carisoprodol™ (pain reliever), caffeine (especially the tannic acid in coffee and tea), aspirin, antibiotics, antacids, high phosphorus diet (bran), excess sweating, heavy bleeding (i.e. menstruating women, bleeding ulcers), candida yeast infection, phosphate food additives and EDTA (disodium ethylene diamine tetra acetate – a food preservative).
   - Excessive dairy products and eggs inhibit iron absorption.
   - **Iron deficiency has been reported to impair the body's ability to make its own thyroid hormones.**

8. **Selenium** – a trace mineral depleted by steroids and corticosteroids, SSRI antidepressants, excess zinc or copper, caffeine, alcohol, food processing, high fat foods, infection, injury, blood loss, aging, and physical and mental stress.
   - **Selenium deficiency is common in individuals eating a low protein diet.**
   - **Selenium is necessary for the conversion of the T$_4$ thyroid hormone to the active form T$_3$ hormone.**

9. **Zinc** – a trace mineral depleted by steroids and corticosteroids, SSRI antidepressants, HIV medication, Histamine H$_2$ blockers (i.e. Tagamet™, Pepcid™, Zantac™), estrogen (and oral contraceptives), diuretics, caffeine, all cholesterol-lowering drugs, including statins and bile acid sequestrants (i.e. Questran™, Colestid™), antibiotics, aspirin, antiseizure medication (i.e. barbiturates, phenytoin), antacids and ulcer medication, alcohol, ACE inhibitors and other blood pressure lowering drugs (including beta-blockers), diarrhea, perspiration, kidney disease, cirrhosis of the liver, food processing, physical and mental stress, a diet high in fiber, and the consumption of hard water. Zinc levels are lowered by diabetes.
   - **A deficiency of zinc results in a decrease in the conversion of the T$_4$ thyroid hormone to the active form T$_3$ hormone.**

10. **Tyrosine** – a nonessential amino acid depleted by estrogen and oral contraceptives.
    - **Tyrosine assists in the functions of the adrenal, thyroid and pituitary glands.**
    - **Tyrosine is necessary for the production of the thyroid hormones.**
    - **Deficiency of tyrosine can produce underactive thyroid and disrupted metabolism.**

How SSRI Antidepressants Can Contribute to Thyroid Suppression

One of the greatest contributors to thyroid suppression in my opinion, are the SSRI antidepressants, such as Prozac™, Paxil™, Zoloft™, Celexa™, etc. The first antidepressant in its class was Prozac™, which was announced in the U.S. in 1987 (more than 20 years ago). The others soon followed, as Eli Lilly experienced such success with Prozac™, the profit potential was obvious. This was especially apparent when, at a conference in Anaheim California that I attended several years ago, Dr. Ann Blake Tracy indicated that since the 9/11 incident, one in 3½ people in the nation were on antidepressants.

As Prozac™ was the first announced SSRI antidepressant, it is the best known. I don't want you, or the maker of Prozac™ (Eli Lilly), to think that I am picking on Prozac™, or that it is the only SSRI antidepressant involved in suppressing the thyroid. Although I may sometimes refer to Prozac™, the same would normally apply to the other SSRI antidepressants as well

Following are a few potential ways that SSRI antidepressants could contribute to thyroid suppression:

1. **Prozac™ / Fluoride.** According to Dr. Tracy, every molecule of Prozac™ just happens to contain three molecules of fluoride! The problem is, fluoride is a known thyroid suppressant.

2. **Prozac™ / Stress Hormones.** The stress hormone cortisol is another thyroid suppressant associated with Prozac™. Dr. Tracy states that just one 30 mg dose of Prozac™ increases cortisol by 200%! While on Prozac™, it's as though you are stressed every single day. This elevated stress hormone not only suppresses the thyroid, but also contributes to elevated blood sugar leading to diabetes (a major cardiovascular risk factor).

3. **SSRIs / Insulin resistance / Diabetes.** The increased level of blood sugar, stimulated by the elevated cortisol not only **contributes to insulin resistance** and thus type II diabetes, but is also contributing to damage to the arteries in the process. And of course once the insulin resistance is well established, we have another problem: **Insulin resistance in the liver.** The enzyme in the liver, necessary for the T_4 thyroid to T_3 conversion, becomes less efficient as it is dependent upon an adequate level of glucose. Less T_3 thyroid results in **reduced metabolism, and thus lowered temperature.** Then as we know, this also results in **less efficient enzyme action!** And unfortunately, there's more.

4. **SSRIs / Protein-binding.** The problem now is, the SSRI antidepressants are highly protein-binding, and thus very difficult for the liver to metabolize. Then, due to the reduced metabolism, you should begin getting a higher dosage of your antidepressant, as well as all your other medications, **greatly increasing the risk of thyroid suppression and possible drug overdose!**

5. **Prozac™ / Drug interactions.** An increase of side effects from all your medications can now be expected. And anyone who drinks alcohol is just adding to the risk. According to Dr. Tracy, the influence of alcohol is greatly potentiated by Prozac™ (basically 10 times!). The problem is the same P450 enzyme in the liver that is responsible for metabolizing toxins such as alcohol, is also attempting to metabolize your medications, including Prozac™.

6. **Paxil™ / Alcohol.** Although we have been focusing on Prozac™, as it was the first announced and most widely known, the same basic problem also applies to the other SSRI antidepressants. According to Dr. Tracy and Dr. Glenmullen, Paxil™ is likely the worst in its class. Dr. Tracy indicated that **although drinking one drink of alcohol while on Prozac™ is like drinking ten, with Paxil™ it is comparable to forty!** I could likely go on all day, but I will just take the problem of thyroid suppression by these antidepressants one step further and then quit.

7. **SSRIs / Bipolar Disorder and Lithium.** As Dr. Tracy noted, an antidepressant is basically a stimulant, such as cocaine, which also raises the level of serotonin. Any unnatural stimulation of any hormone leads to a rebound effect. The result is often an imbalance, such as the bipolar disorder. If you recall, Mary Lou was a prime example. She was first placed on Prozac™, after a stressful event suppressed her thyroid (a typical response).

141

One more problem associated with Prozac™ is a shutting down of serotonin receptors, or resistance to serotonin from the continual overstimulation caused by Prozac™. This then led to another potential side effect associated with SSRI antidepressants: Depression! So Mary Lou's doctor just left her on Prozac™, and added another antidepressant. And finally, the potentially dangerous lithium carbonate was prescribed for another side effect associated with Prozac™, (her bipolar disorder).

Along with the many potentially serious side effects associated with the lithium carbonate normally prescribed for bipolar disorder, such as permanent kidney scarring, is goiter (an enlarged thyroid gland). As we know, that is caused by a deficiency of iodine, necessary for producing the thyroid hormone. **One thing lithium is well-known for is its ability to bond to and remove iodine from the thyroid.** For that reason, high doses of lithium are often prescribed to treat hyperthyroidism (above-normal thyroid) to reduce the thyroid function. But the problem that by far the majority of people are suffering with is hypothyroidism (low thyroid), rather than elevated thyroid. Unfortunately, the majority of people are already iodine deficient.

What Do We Know About The Prescription Thyroid (Synthroid™)

1. Synthroid™ is a chemical form of T_4 thyroid.
2. In his book *Natural Hormone Replacement* (2001), Dr. Neal Rouzier, M.D. FACEP states that most of his new patients were experiencing typical thyroid symptoms, even though they had been taking the thyroid medication Synthroid™, (which was obviously ineffective).
3. The basic problem is, the majority of people have difficulty converting the T_4 thyroid, to the much more active T_3 form. Many different factors can easily undermine the efficient thyroid conversion process in the liver. One good example is Insulin resistance, associated with type II diabetes.
4. As with drugs in general, Synthroid™ not only has its share of associated side effects, but also some troubling potential risks, which should make any doctor think twice before prescribing it over a much safer, and proven effective alternative.
5. It has been reported in the *Journal of the American Medical Association*, that Synthroid™ depletes calcium (http://www.vitaminevi.com/Index/Drug_Index-F.htm).
6. Some **common side effects** associated with Synthroid™ include:
   * Diarrhea   * Irritability   * Headache   * Hand Tremors
   * Leg cramps   * Insomnia   * Vomiting   * Nervousness
   * Changes in menstrual periods
7. Then, some of the symptoms from possible overstimulation are:
   * Abdominal cramps   * Anxiety   * Chest pain
   * **Emotional instability**   * Hair loss   * Headache
   * **Heart attack or failure**   * Irregular heartbeat * Hyperactivity
   * Increased heart rate   * Irritability   * Tremors
   * Shortness of breath   * Nervousness   * Palpitation
   * Sleeplessness   * Muscle weakness
8. We are also warned that: Synthroid™ can interact with a wide variety of medications, which just happen to include some widely used medications, such as:
   * Oral Contraceptives   * Antidepressants   * Antacids
   * Blood pressure medications * Asthma medication   * Diuretics
   * Diabetes drugs   * Blood thinning drugs * Aspirin
9. A surprising number of women are placed on Synthroid™, (and **normally left on the drug**), yet we also find the warning that: ***"Postmenopausal women on long-term Synthroid™ therapy may <u>suffer a loss of bone density</u>, increasing the danger of osteoporosis [brittle bones]"*** (http://www.healthsquare.com/newrx/syn1421.htm).

10. Most importantly, the majority of diabetics are hypothyroid (requiring thyroid medication), and as we know the greatest common contributor to cardiovascular disease is diabetes. Thus, there is an obvious connection with all three conditions, yet from one source we find that:

If you have diabetes, or if your body makes insufficient adrenal corticosteroid hormone, Synthroid® will tend to make your symptoms worse. Synthroid® has profound effects on the body. Make sure your doctor is aware of all your medical problems, especially heart disease, clotting disorders, diabetes, and disorders of the adrenal or pituitary glands (http://www.healthsquare.com/newrx/syn1421.htm).

While another source additionally warns*:*

Tell your doctor if you have or have ever had diabetes; hardening of the arteries (atherosclerosis); kidney disease; hepatitis; cardiovascular disease such as high blood pressure, chest pain (angina), arrhythmias, or heart attack; or an underactive adrenal or pituitary gland (http://www.nlm.nih.gov/medlineplus/druginfo/medmaster/a682461.html).

As you can easily see, we have some obvious concerns regarding the use of the Synthroid™, which most doctors insist on prescribing for a thyroid disorder, as it is intimately connected with both diabetes, and cardiovascular disease.

Then there is the concern of possibly experiencing some of the more serious side effects associated with overstimulation (drug overdose), such as **emotional instability** or possibly even **heart attack or failure**, which is greatly increased when combined with any of the many commonly prescribed medications that Synthroid™ can interact with. I would assume that by far, the majority would be taking at least one of the medications on the list. For instance, women are already ten times as likely to experience a low thyroid condition as men, however many women are likely taking oral contraceptives, which is not only on the list of potentially interacting drugs, but is also a known thyroid suppressant.

Also, as mentioned earlier, depression is one of the most common symptoms associated with a hypothyroid condition, and even though Synthroid™ seldom resolves the condition, patients are normally left on Synthroid™, while another medication on our list of potentially interacting drugs (antidepressants) is often added, increasing potential risks.

Many in the nation are also taking at least one of the over-the-counter medications antacids or aspirin, which also increase the potential for drug interaction. The more potentially interacting medications you find on that list that you might be taking while on Synthroid™, the greater your risk will be. As usual, there is a much safer alternative, known as Armour™ Thyroid, which we will now examine.

Some of the Many Benefits of Armour™ Thyroid

1. Because Armour™ thyroid is a natural product, and not a chemical compound, your liver will not attempt to remove it, as it would with Synthroid™. Consequently, your effective dosage can be more easily controlled and maintained.

2. In Armour™ thyroid we find a combination of both T_4 and T_3, in the same proportion our body normally produces. Although T_3 is approximately four times as fast acting as T_4, both actually work well together, as the T_4 helps moderate the action of T_3. Sometimes the T_3 thyroid, (if not combined with T_4), can result in overstimulation unless slowly released, as only the body can efficiently do. Although a time-release form of T_3 is available, it can only be obtained through a compounding pharmacy, and there appears to be a concern. It is very difficult (if not impossible) to accurately achieve even distribution of the time-release agent with the T_3 thyroid hormone. Our thyroid normally produces an adequate level of T_4 thyroid, thus that is seldom the cause of the majority of hypothyroid conditions. It is instead an inefficient conversion process, and thus an insufficient level of free T_3 thyroid.

3. Companies such as Standard Process™, Inc., which produce quality supplements from natural sources only, include glandulars in their formulas that they refer to as protomorphogens. They contain extracts of organs such as heart, adrenals, kidneys, liver, thymus, or thyroid, etc. The extracts are normally from either bovine (beef) or pork organs. We find they are not species specific, but instead organ specific. This means, in our body they are not broken down as other proteins to individual amino acids, but instead go directly to the specific target organ, and are beneficial for maintaining or regenerating the specific organ intended.

As Armour™ thyroid is a glandular extract, it would likely strengthen the thyroid as well. Then, according to Dr. David Brownstein, M.D., it also contains T_1 and T_2 thyroid, as well as the beneficial cofactors calcitonin and selenium. Most importantly, **although Synthroid™ seldom works, Armour™ thyroid seldom fails.** The importance of proper metabolism cannot be over stressed, so getting the most effective form of thyroid hormone is essential.

4. We can only begin to appreciate the value of Armour™ thyroid, if we consider that many in the nation are needlessly placed on potentially dangerous antidepressants, when Armour™ thyroid would often resolve the condition (as well as many others). And by taking a thyroid hormone that truly works, the action of all 3,000 enzymes in the body will also begin working more efficiently. Then, many who were unable to lose weight, due to insufficient metabolism, would finally be much more successful.

5. And last but definitely not least, I believe we are all aware of the tremendous deterioration to the overall body, especially the cardiovascular system, the eyes, and kidneys, associated with diabetes. And then we have the **amazing discovery** of both Dr. C. D. Eaton and Dr. Broda Barnes, **that thyroid therapy (using Armour™ thyroid) prevented the normal complications normally associated with their patients' diabetes!** We also find that many of the conditions we normally attribute to diabetes, are actually influenced by a hypothyroid condition, which can only be truly resolved by Armour™ thyroid (not Synthroid™).

I rest my case.

The Natural Armour™ Thyroid Versus Synthroid™

A typical response by many doctors upon a patient's request for Armour™ thyroid seems to be that it is not as well regulated as Synthroid™. In reality, quite the opposite is actually true. The problem with Synthroid™ is, like other medications, it is a chemical compound, which is treated as a toxin by the liver. Then it also interacts with many other commonly prescribed medications, as we just learned. Especially when taking multiple medications, drinking alcohol, or even eating grapefruit (which suppresses the P450 enzyme in the liver responsible for detoxification), how can anyone accurately predict the effective dosage they might get on any particular day? So, even if the amount of T_4 thyroid in Synthroid™ was closely regulated, your effective dosage can still vary considerably.

Now, let's compare that with the Armour™ thyroid. First we'll evaluate the process for producing Armour™ thyroid, in order to assure that an accurate level, and ratio of both natural T_4 and T_3 are properly maintained. We find that:

Armour™ Thyroid is made from desiccated (dried) pork thyroid glands. The amount of thyroid hormone present in the thyroid gland may vary from animal to animal. To ensure that Armour™ Thyroid tablets are consistently potent from tablet to tablet and lot to lot, analytical tests are performed on the thyroid powder (raw material) and on the actual tablets (finished product) to measure actual T_4 and T_3 activity.

*Different lots of thyroid powder are mixed together and analyzed to achieve the desired ratio of T_4 to T_3 in each lot of tablets. **This method ensures that each strength of Armour™ Thyroid will be consistent with the United States Pharmacopoeia (USP) official standards and specifications for desiccated thyroid lot-to-lot consistency.***

The ratio of T_4 to T_3 equals 4.22:1 (4.22 parts of T_4 to one part of T_3) (http://www.armourthyroid.com/faq.html#q3).

We then find that Armour™ thyroid meets all the USP standards for accuracy and safety, as follows:

Armour™ Thyroid Tablets, USP contain the labeled amounts of levothyroxin and liothyronine, as established by the United States Pharmacopoeia (USP). To meet quality **standards it must also pass bacteriological testing and must meet other product quality tests.** *The ratio of Armour ™ Thyroid T_4 to T_3 is 4.22:1 (4.22 parts of T_4 to one part of T_3) (http://www.armourthyroid.com/faq.html#q7).*

If you want even more proof, which should convince any doctor with an open mind, we just happen to have another opinion from a very credible source: *The New England Journal of Medicine*!

NEJM STUDY PROVES ARMOUR THYROID BETTER THAN SYNTHROID

Patients with hypothyroidism show greater improvements in mood and brain function if they receive treatment Armour thyroid rather than Synthroid (thyroxine). Hypothyroidism, where the gland has ceased to function or been removed, is usually treated with daily doses of Synthroid. But the researchers found that substituting Armour thyroid led to improvements in mood and in neuropsychological functioning.

Not all tissues that need thyroid hormone are equally able to convert thyroxine to triiodothyronine, the active form of the hormone. But most patients with hypothyroidism (reduced thyroid function) are treated only with thyroxine. On 6 of 17 measures of mood and cognition -- a catchall term that refers to language, learning and memory -- the patients scored better after receiving Armour thyroid than after receiving Synthroid. No score was better after Synthroid than after combination treatment. The authors also detected biochemical evidence that thyroid hormone action was greater after treatment with Armour thyroid. The patients who were on Armour thyroid had significantly higher serum concentrations of sex hormone-binding globulin.
The New England Journal of Medicine 1999;340:424-429, 469-470
(http://internationalhealth.net/NewsArticles.htm#armour).

So the question is: Where did most doctors learn that Armour™ thyroid is not adequately regulated? Likely from the Abbott Laboratories representative who was promoting his company's product (Synthroid™). If he had done the research himself, he obviously would have known better.

Dr. Neal Rouzier discovered that many of his new patients were still suffering from typical thyroid symptoms, although they had been placed and often left on Synthroid™ (T_4) for years. The problem is, far too many don't efficiently convert the T_4 thyroid to the much more active T_3 form. However, Dr. Rouzier found that his new patients immediately noticed a major improvement when placed on Armour™ thyroid. Yet, in spite of the noted improvement, their own personal doctor normally insisted on placing them back on Synthroid™ (artificial T_4 thyroid), and absolutely refused to prescribe Armour™ thyroid. Is there something drastically wrong with this picture?

CHAPTER EIGHTEEN
THE NATURAL WAY TO ASSURE HEALTHY THYROID FUNCTION

What Is Normal Thyroid Function?

We find an interesting observation by Dr. Rouzier, in his book *Natural Hormone Replacement* (2001), (an area he specializes in). He noted that ***"In spite of 'normal' thyroid levels on standard blood tests, results are only seen with the restoration of the thyroid to <u>optimum levels</u>."*** He went on to cite an interesting study as follows:

> *One study in particular, reported in the Journal of the American Geriatric Society, attested to the above findings. In a five-year project, Dr. James C. Wren studies* **347 atherosclerotic patients** *– 174 women and 173 men – with only 31 considered clinically hypothyroid or with lab values below the normal range. With this in mind, all patients were given thyroid supplementation, and results were then calculated. Many of the patients experienced significant improvement and their mortality rate was cut in half of what is usual for this type of untreated patient.* **What is truly amazing about this study is that <u>only nine percent had diagnosed hypothyroidism,</u> yet a majority of participants reaped benefits from their thyroid supplementation** (p. 156).

I can easily see why the majority (91%) in the study, who appeared to have normal thyroid function, still experienced significant improvement from natural thyroid supplementation. For one thing, in my opinion the standard for thyroid evaluation is likely flawed. It appears the criterion was based on the <u>average</u> <u>population</u>, however, I would guess that approximately half the adults in the nation are either subclinical (borderline low), or actually hypothyroid (low). That percentage also runs considerably higher regarding both women and diabetics, (and many women are also diabetics). Thus, if "normal" was based on an average including those with low thyroid levels, wouldn't that result in "normal" actually being low?

The optimum level is obviously the one at which you perform the very best both physically and mentally. Your body is by far the best laboratory in that regard. For example, professor Dr. Lavene discovered that most of his brightest students were actually slightly hyperthyroid (high). The question remains: Are they really marginally high, or are they actually normal? Just the fact that people who are hypothyroid (low) are much more prone to experience many undesirable conditions, such as depression, heart disease, and diabetes, appears to be a good enough reason to maintain optimum, not marginal thyroid function.

The decision is up to you. Would you be satisfied being in the low-to-normal range, or would you prefer to maintain it in the optimal range? A good analogy is your I.Q. Although the range considered as normal is fairly broad, would you rather be at the bottom or the top of normal? The same would obviously apply to the thyroid, and its performance.

According to Dr. David Brownstein, M.D., author of the book *Overcoming Thyroid Disorders* (2002), some people simply require a higher dosage of thyroid to overcome the problem of cellular resistance. Once the problem of resistance is eliminated (if possible), the dosage may be reduced accordingly.

Another influencing factor, according to retired professor Dr. Ray Peat, Ph.D., is that people quite often require more thyroid hormone (sometimes up to four grains more) in the winter months than during the summer (http://www.thyroid-info.com/articles/ray-peat.htm). Additional thyroid hormone may also be necessary when consuming a high-protein diet (also up to 4 grains daily), according to Broda Barnes, M.D.

The **appropriate** dosage in my opinion, is the one which you feel your best. That amount often varies between individuals, and as you can see, there are actually many different factors involved. According to Broda Barnes, M.D. (*Hypothyroidism: The Unsuspected Illness*, 1976), quite simply ***"The proper dosage for any individual is the minimum needed to relieve symptoms"*** (p. 285).

Natural Solutions for Promoting Healthy Thyroid Function

Remember, resolving any health issue involves first eliminating as many contributors to the condition as possible, and then adding nutrients important for restoring good health.

Following are some do-it-yourself approaches you might try first that wouldn't require finding a doctor willing to prescribe Armour™ thyroid.

1. **Drug withdrawal (if necessary)** should be your first priority in order to restore your health to optimum levels. Unfortunately, taking supplements will have little value, as long as you also continue taking medications that are known to deplete them. Also, as drugs only suppress symptoms, and do so in an unnatural way, you have absolutely no way of determining if a condition has been truly resolved, as long as you continue taking the medication. Drugs would only suppress symptoms and undermine any effort you might be making to truly identify the underlying issue, or effectively evaluate your progress. If you recall, nearly 87% of the drugs evaluated for nutrient depletion, were found to deplete nutrients important for healthy thyroid function.

2. **Iodoral™** is critical to supporting healthy thyroid gland function. It is a natural iodine formula, consisting of both iodine and potassium iodide. Dr. David Brownstein, M.D. found in a study, that 91.7% of the patients that were tested for low iodine levels actually had an iodine deficiency. According to Dr. Brownstein, this appears to be a huge public health problem. He also confirmed, from clinical experience, that **the combination of iodine/iodide, called Iodoral™, was beyond a doubt, far more effective than a supplement that contained only iodine.** Dr. Brownstein also discovered that although the breasts in women, and the prostate gland in men, concentrate iodine, **the thyroid primarily concentrates <u>iodide</u> instead.** In his book *Iodine: Why You Need It, Why You Can't Live Without It* (2004), Dr. Brownstein also noted that *"Other tissues, including the kidneys, spleen, liver, blood, salivary glands, and intestines can concentrate either form"* (p. 50). So, we can easily see the thyroid gland must also share iodine with other glands and systems in the body. That would obviously increase the potential for an iodine deficiency, which according to Dr. Brownstein, is quite prevalent. He also stated that ***"All individuals with a thyroid disorder should be screened for an iodine deficiency"*** (p. 99).

Dr. David G. Williams suggests a simple self-test to determine if you are iodine-deficient, as outlined in the June 2004 issue of his *Alternatives* newsletter. Although he admits it is not 100% accurate, it is easy to do, inexpensive, and works very well as a screening tool. Simply dip a cotton swab or ball into USP tincture of iodine (available at most any drugstore), and paint a 2-inch circle of iodine on a soft area of skin such as your stomach or the inner part of your thigh or arm. If the yellowish stain disappears in less than one hour, your body is lacking in iodine. If the stain remains for more than four hours, it is an indication your iodine levels may be adequate.

3. **Celtic sea salt** is an excellent source of iodine, as well as many other minerals important for supporting thyroid function, and in their natural most efficient ionic form.

4. **Water.** Adequate water greatly influences every part of the body, and is necessary in all areas of health. It is especially important regarding the thyroid, as dehydration is considered a stressor, contributing to thyroid suppression. Dehydration also causes cells to become insulin resistant, which reduces the liver's ability to efficiently convert the thyroid hormones. I recommend ten 8-ounce glasses daily, along with 1 teaspoon of the Celtic sea salt.

5. **Thyromin™** is one natural option that doesn't require a prescription. It is a fairly new product used to nourish the thyroid, balance metabolism, and reduce fatigue. It was developed by Dr. N. Gary Young, N.D., and sold only through his company Young Living™ Essential Oils. Thyromin™ contains a combination of specially selected glandular nutrients, herbs, amino acids, minerals, and essential oils. All

the oils are therapeutic-grade and perfectly balanced to bring about the most beneficial and nutritional support to the thyroid. Thyromin™ contains vitamin E, Iodine, Potassium, CoQ_{10}, L-cysteine, and adrenal/pituitary extracts from bovine sources. It also contains the essential oils peppermint, spearmint, myrtle, and myrrh.

It is best taken at bedtime, starting with 2 capsules immediately before going to sleep. You then check your temperature first thing in the following morning, and if your basal temperature indicates no improvement, add 1 additional capsule that morning. If there is still no significant improvement by the next morning, then increase the dosage to 2 capsules in the morning and 2 at night, as Dr. Young notes it is best to take half of the total amount at night and half in the morning. Continue using this stepped approach until your temperature reaches the correct range (97.8˚ - 98.6˚). According to Dr. Young, another product called VitaGreen™ (also sold only through Young Living™ Essential Oils) will also enhance the effect of the Thyromin™.

6. **Selenium.** An additional consideration might also be a selenium deficiency. It has been found that **selenium-deficient individuals are almost always hypothyroid**. In fact, according to David Brownstein, M.D. (*Overcoming Thyroid Disorders*, 2002), he states that *"I have found significant numbers of patients in my practice who have selenium deficiencies, with resultant hypothyroid symptoms. When these deficiencies are improved, their hypothyroid symptoms often improve"* (pp. 65-66).

Selenium has also been shown to elevate mood and decrease anxiety, with the recommended daily dosage being 200 mcg of selenium yeast (the most absorbable form). The enzyme 5'deiodenaise responsible for converting the T_4 thyroid to the active T_3 form in the liver requires the mineral selenium, and that is likely the selenium connection.

Selenium is a trace mineral that can easily be depleted by SSRI antidepressants, caffeine, infection, and stress, as well as a high fat diet and many other factors. The level of selenium in food greatly depends on the levels of selenium in the soil where the food was grown, thus the vegetables grown in California's soil are likely to have a different concentration of selenium than the vegetables grown in New Jersey.

7. **Vitamin A.** Insufficient vitamin A can cause a deterioration of the pituitary gland's basophil cells where the thyroid-stimulating hormone is synthesized, limiting the amount of iodine that the thyroid gland can absorb, and reducing the amount of thyroid hormone it produces. Vitamin A can be depleted by all cholesterol-lowering drugs, antibiotics, caffeine, alcohol, and bad fats, as well as many other things.

8. **Vitamin B-complex.** Vitamin B_2 (riboflavin) strongly influences how well the thyroid gland synthesizes its hormones. Sufficient vitamin B_3 (niacin) is essential to the good health of all glands, especially the thyroid, by assisting in the respiration of cells and the efficient metabolism of carbohydrates, fats and protein. A thyroid gland deficient in vitamin B_6 (pyridoxine) has difficulty converting iodine into thyroid hormone. And in one study, when cattle were fed a diet deficient in vitamin B_{12}, there was a significant reduction in the conversion of T_4 to T_3. At the same time, low thyroid function decreases our ability to absorb vitamin B_{12}. Thus, the best solution is to take a good 100 mg B-complex vitamin daily, which includes all the B-vitamins. Keep in mind that microwave cooking can destroy the majority of B vitamins in your food.

9. **Vitamin D** is necessary for healthy thyroid function. Vitamin D is commonly depleted by such things as alcohol, antidepressants, antibiotics, aspirin, smoking, stress, and all cholesterol-lowering drugs, just to name a few.

10. **Tyrosine.** For thyroid hormone to form, a biochemical union of the amino acid tyrosine and iodine must occur. **Tyrosine is commonly depleted by estrogen and oral contraceptives.** Although meat, fish, and eggs contain tyrosine, some may benefit from 1,000 mg of supplemental tyrosine daily.

11. **Zinc** levels appear to be directly correlated with the levels of the active thyroid hormone T_3. According to David Brownstein, M.D. (*Overcoming Thyroid Disorders*, 2002), he states ***"My experience has clearly shown a decrease in the conversion of T_4 into T_3 in zinc deficient individuals"*** (p. 67).

12. **DHEA** (**dehydroepiandrosterone**) increases sensitivity to thyroid production, or conversion in the liver. It is also known to increase the insulin sensitivity of cells, (an important factor in diabetes). I would recommend 50 mg daily.

13. **Relora™** is an herbal formula containing magnolia and philodendron, and available at most health food stores. It has two important functions: Reducing the stress hormone cortisol, while increasing the level of DHEA. The recommended dosage is 150 mg, three times daily.

14. **Iron** deficiency has been reported to impair the body's ability to make its own thyroid hormones. Low iron can result from antacids, aspirin and antibiotics, among other things. In my opinion, the best form of organic iron is blackstrap molasses. Take one to two tablespoons daily.

15. **Some foods** that enhance your body's production of thyroid hormones are: Sea vegetables (kelp, dulse), garlic, radishes, egg yolk, wheat germ and brewer's yeast.

16. **Valerian root.** As we have learned, stress hormones are a major contributor to thyroid suppression, and Valerian is a very effective herb for relieving stress. It is fact acting, perfectly safe, and doesn't cause drowsiness. I would recommend taking two capsules, (450 mg each), anytime you experience stress. Valerian is inexpensive and should be available in your local health food store.

17. **TG100™** (available through Women's International Pharmacy) is a non-prescription item that contains 40 mg of thyroid tissue, along with 5 mg each of adrenal, pancreas, thymus, and spleen tissue, plus 120 mg of vitamin C (ascorbic acid). The other glandulars are important for supporting the thyroid function.

I found that the combination of Iodoral™ and TG100™ was effective in maintaining my wife's metabolism, without the necessity of using thyroid hormones. I have her take 1 capsule of TG100™, twice daily (in the morning and evening), along with 1 tablet of Iodoral™. The best dosage might vary, which is true with all supplements. It will obviously be more effective if you can also avoid as many thyroid suppressants as possible.

18. **Armour™ Thyroid.** One last thought: If all else fails, you can always attempt to find a doctor who would be willing to prescribe Armour™ thyroid. One solution to that problem is to call a pharmacy such as the Women's International Pharmacy at (800) 699-8143, which handles Armour™ thyroid, as well as other bio-identical (natural to the body) hormones, and ask for a list of doctors who prescribe Armour™ thyroid in your area. You can also find a complete list of doctors in your zip code area that prescribe Armour™ thyroid for their patients, by visiting their Website http://www.armourthyroid.com.

A Word Of Caution – And An Observation

Just don't ever allow yourself to get caught in the web (of the madness in medicine), as Mary Lou and many others unknowingly did. It all began with an undiagnosed and untreated hypothyroid condition that eventually led to nine unnecessary medications. So, sixteen years after Mary Lou received the original prescription for the new wonder-drug Prozac™, which was eventually followed by the other eight, I discovered that she was still dealing with a hypothyroid condition, because she had been taking the wrong form of thyroid (Synthroid™) that seldom works, although it is the thyroid most doctors insist on prescribing.

It is beyond belief that after decades of research and trillions of dollars invested, the obvious continues to be overlooked. The basic problem is: The true natural solutions, (as well as prevention), are not profitable. Unless we change our priorities in medicine, and place our health before profit, we will continue to experience an increase in our rate of disease, along with the constant escalation of our healthcare cost. We must finally take a stand and say: I will now take more responsibility for my own health, and my very first step will be to no longer be held hostage by my medications, and begin phasing them out of my life forever. And as I mentioned, those who chose to do so found it was perfectly safe, and surprisingly easy, as they normally never needed them all those years to begin with. Remember, just play it safe, monitor your levels, listen to your body and use caution during your withdrawal. It will definitely be worth your effort.

CHAPTER NINETEEN
TYPE II DIABETES – CAUSES AND POTENTIAL RISK FACTORS

The majority of diabetics (approximately 95%) have type II (non-insulin dependant) diabetes. It is predicted that by the year 2010, fifty percent of our children will have type II diabetes before they reach 20! (*Dr. Donsbach's Let's Talk Health*, http://www.letstalkhealth.com). This is especially a concern if you consider that the typical problems associated with diabetes likely contribute to more deterioration in the body (including aging), than any other disease. If those projections prove to be accurate, we could be in serious trouble in just a few years. Those statistics are likely based on the current trend (something we can and must change).

Diabetes begins when the insulin receptors in the cells become insufficiently responsive and insulin resistant, due to overstimulation. This then requires more insulin than normal in order to effectively utilize the glucose. And any time an organ, such as the adrenals or the pancreas, is required to produce an excessive amount of hormone such as insulin over an extended period of time, a couple of things normally take place. First, the organs tend to overreact to a normal stimulus, sometimes producing an inappropriate amount of hormone. And second, they eventually become fatigued, and thus less able to produce an adequate supply or quality of hormone. And without sufficient insulin, glucose cannot enter into cell, thus an excessive amount accumulates in the blood (increased sugar levels).

Insulin quality can also be compromised due to a vitamin or mineral deficiency, which can be caused by medications (even those prescribed for diabetes!).

Contributing Factors

According to Dr. Walter Willett, chairman of the Harvard School of Public Health's department of nutrition, based on his own long-term Nurses Health Study, along with dozens of other studies that have examined lifestyle habits and their effects on heart disease and diabetes, type II diabetes is at least 90 percent preventable. Following are many contributing factors:

✓ **Obesity / Abdominal fat.** Over the last decade, the number of Americans diagnosed with diabetes has increased by 50 percent. Coincidentally, over the same time period there was a 57 percent rise in obesity rates also (*Health Sciences Institute*, November 2002, p. 1). Apparently, excess weight increases the body's insulin requirement, thus pushing the beta cells (beyond their ability) for increased production, until the supply can't meet the demand any longer. Eventually this causes the body to simply become insensitive to insulin. This is especially a concern when you consider how much of the national population is considered obese.

It has been proven that excess abdominal fat, those with a waist circumference of 40 inches or greater, actually have **12 times** the risk of developing diabetes than someone of normal weight. Although obesity in general is the number-one risk factor for developing type II diabetes, apparently <u>abdominal</u> fat is a major contributing issue. So it might be helpful if we can at least identify some likely contributors to the problem.

According to *The Life Extension Foundation's Disease Prevention and Treatment, Expanded Fourth Edition* (1997/2003): ***"For the majority of Type II diabetics, the most important therapy to <u>prevent or reverse the disease is to reduce excess body fat"</u>*** (p. 682).

✓ **Hypothyroidism** (a low thyroid) and diabetes are very closely related, and I believe it is not just a coincidence that 80% of diabetics also suffer from a low thyroid condition. In fact, according to Dr. Broda Barnes, even when many of his diabetic patients were able to stabilize their blood sugar, most of the other symptoms of diabetes wouldn't go away until they were given (Armour™) thyroid therapy. He also notes: ***"Thyroid therapy prevented complications in Dr. Eaton's diabetic patients twenty years ago*** *and has been preventing the same complications in my patients, diabetic and nondiabetic, for twenty-four years"* (*Hypothyroidism – The Unsuspected Illness*, 1976, p. 227). That was in my opinion, quite an amazing discovery, with tremendous potential for diabetics.

When the thyroid is suppressed, the metabolism is reduced, requiring less sugar to be used for energy. Less glucose would obviously be required to maintain a lower-than-normal body temperature, than if the body temperature was maintained at the appropriate 98.6 degrees. If a person were still consuming the same foods, as well as the same amount, the result would be an excess of unused sugar in the bloodstream. This would then result in increased insulin production, leading to insulin resistance, increased fat storage, and eventually type II diabetes.

Possibly the worst combination that could contribute to obesity would be an excess of insulin (which is very efficient in storing fat), plus a deficiency of the thyroid hormone (which is responsible for fat removal), combined with an excess of unused sugar. The elevated blood sugar can be potentially dangerous, so it must be converted and stored as abdominal fat (another contributor to insulin resistance).

✓ **Diet**. Type II diabetes is largely a nutritional disease that can be easily caused by an unhealthy diet, and thus can also be controlled by a healthy diet. It may surprise you to learn that if an expectant mother eats a diet loaded with high sugar carbohydrates while deficient in good fats, she can actually pass on metabolic problems to her children that increase their risk for developing diabetes. Animal studies have shown that *"Insulin resistance, a precursor of type 2 diabetes, can be passed from an expectant mother to her child, and even worse, can alter the insulin sensitivity of the baby's eggs, thus possibly affecting the developing baby, and could affect that baby's children as well"* (Ron Rosedale, *The Rosedale Diet*, 2004, p. 35). This could be one reason why it is quite common for obese parents to have chubby children. They appear to have more fat cells than other children, at a very young age, which appears to contribute to insulin resistance.

✓ **The over-consumption of simple carbohydrates,** which seems to be the biggest offender, became much more prominent years ago, with the erroneous conclusion and announcement by the **"experts"** that it was the fats that made us fat. About that time, food manufacturers responded by producing processed foods that were either low fat or non-fat. They then compensated with an increase in carbohydrate content in order to maintain the taste that many seem to insist on, and which sells products. The general public was totally unaware that sugar and simple carbohydrates could easily be converted to a type of fat, and rapidly stored.

According to Dr. Rosedale, as presented at Designs for Health Institute's BoulderFest August 1999 Seminar, a study was done showing that heart attacks are two to three times more likely to happen after a high-carbohydrate meal. Apparently, **the immediate effects of elevated blood sugar brought on by a high-carbohydrate meal, means a raise in insulin.** This then immediately triggers the sympathetic nervous system, which causes arterial spasm (constriction of the arteries), thus increasing the potential for heart attack.

✓ **Simple sugars** also stimulate an immediate release of insulin. According to an article in *USA Today* (June 8, 2004), *"A study showed that women who drank the minimum of **one soda each day could increase their likelihood of developing type 2 diabetes by 85 percent** over the women who drank less than one can a day."*

With enough repeated stimulation and excess insulin release, insulin resistance in the liver results, eventually followed by resistance in the muscles. The very last to become insulin resistant is the fat tissue, and insulin just happens to be very efficient at storing fat in the interim. **Unfortunately, the body can very efficiently convert sugar into fat, and the more insulin resistant the liver and muscles become, the more efficient the fat storage will be.**

✓ **Lack of fiber in the diet.** Although a diet high in carbohydrates may be bad, a diet that is concurrently low in fiber is worse. Paul Zimmet, from the Lions-International Diabetes Institute in Melbourne, Australia, was involved in one group of studies in 1990, regarding fiber in the diet of several ethnic groups, who historically had a high-fiber, high-carbohydrate diet. The study revealed the following:

*Populations who are genetically inclined to develop insulin resistance and diabetes will do so at an alarming rate **when their diet is reduced in fiber and increased in refined carbohydrates even though the carbohydrate intake is relatively unchanged.** In all cases, high levels of insulin always occur before diabetes develops. Many of these people also have a dramatic increase in hypertension and heart disease* (Cheryle R Hart, M.D., *The Insulin-Resistance Diet*, 2001, pp. 69-70).

W. C. Knowler has been involved in several similar studies that support Zimmet's results about fiber, and came to the following conclusions regarding the Pima Indians of the Southwest United States:

*With their adoption of the typical American diet, one out of every two Pima Indians now develops diabetes. This is among the highest rates of diabetes in the world. Again, it is interesting that the traditional Pima Indian diet has always been high in carbohydrate content; only the fiber intake has decreased. Therefore, it is reasonable to conclude that **we should not be so concerned with a high-carbohydrate diet but rather with how much of the carbohydrates are refined and without fiber*** (Cheryle R Hart, M.D., *The Insulin-Resistance Diet*, 2001, p. 70).

✓ **The ADA recommended diet.** After completing nine years of medical training, specializing in endocrinology and metabolism at the University of California, Dr. Diana Schwarzbein, M.D., author of *the Schwarzbein Principle* (1999) and *the Schwarzbein Principle II* (2002), accepted a position at a medical clinic that was considered a premier diabetes center. The newly diagnosed diabetic patients were immediately placed on **the American Diabetes Association (ADA) diet.** The diet guidelines consisted of a low-calorie, high-carbohydrate, low-fat and low-protein program. The diet stressed fruit, milk, bread, and very little fat, which are common dietary recommendations of the ADA. Their primary function should be to find a cure for diabetes, although if anything would cause type II diabetes, it would obviously be following their recommendations.

In her book *The Schwarzbein Principle* (1999), Dr. Schwarzbein tells about the patients who "*ate a **perfect ADA breakfast** – a bowl of shredded wheat with non-fat milk, a banana and a glass of orange juice – and **watched their blood sugar rise one hundred to two hundred points. (A normal blood-sugar response to any meal is no more than ten to twenty points.)**" (p. xvii).

It's as though they were feeding their diabetic patients a diet of sugar! I would guess they could easily have done better by just eating as they normally would, without following any dietary recommendations. Diabetics usually test their blood sugar on a regular basis, as should any clinic treating diabetes. Any diet that can cause a rise in blood sugar ten times what is considered as normal, is obviously inappropriate, and that should soon become apparent. It's like so many things in medicine today that make absolutely no sense whatsoever. All I can say is, **if a therapy is not logical, it is likely inappropriate, and thus must be profitable.**

Currently, **the ADA places a priority on the amount rather than the source of the carbohydrate,** and notes that "*all carbs, from starches to just plain table sugar, share a basic biological property: They can be digested and converted into glucose*" (http://www.diabetic-lifestyle.com/articles/jul03_whats_1_.htm). I personally don't agree with the ADA in that regard, and neither do the results of studies. The source (or type of carbohydrate) should be in my opinion, the primary issue. **The ADA even <u>stopped</u> recommending that people with diabetes avoid sugar!** They now stress that we should instead focus on the total amount of carbohydrates in our diet. If you recall, we just discovered (under Fiber), that from studies conducted, the conclusion arrived at is that *"**We should not be so concerned with a high carbohydrate diet but rather with how much of the carbohydrates are refined and without fiber**"* (Cheryle R Hart, M.D., *The Insulin-Resistance Diet*, 2001, p. 70). This is not only a proven fact, but makes considerably more sense than the ADA's diametrically opposed conclusion. They are somehow ignoring the fact that there is a tremendous difference in carbohydrates. For example, the amount of both fiber and nutrients carbohydrates contain should be their primary concern.

All those years that the public was totally unaware of the many problems associated with simple carbohydrates, and just following both the food pyramid and the ADA recommendations, is when the dramatic increase in both diabetes and obesity took place. We also can't ignore the fact that a deficiency of several nutrients can contribute to diabetes, and they won't be found at all in sugar or in any quantity in simple carbohydrates. Also, due to their high glycemic index, they can rapidly spike an increase in both blood sugar and insulin, (both contributors to type II diabetes).

It's rather alarming that an organization established, and supposedly dedicated to finding a cure for diabetes, would instead be contributing to the problem. I can't help but wonder if they are just attempting to create an epidemic of diabetes, possibly in order to justify their existence. Have you ever wondered why it would be necessary to create large organizations, with extensive facilities and substantial annual budgets, just to find a cure for a particular disease? Where is the motivation to ever find a cure, as it would no longer require continued funding, and a lot of people would be looking for another job? Although type II diabetes is diagnosed and labeled as a disease, it is normally just a condition that is totally preventable by making simple dietary changes, and possibly minor supplementation.

Unfortunately, our entire medical system is entirely backwards. The less healthy patients are, the more potential for profit. The fact is, prevention is not profitable (and thus not part of your doctor's training). It's just that simple. Drugs just contribute to nutrient depletion and poor health, as does recommending a diet to control a disease that actually contributes to that very disease. Many doctors still suggest that taking vitamins are unnecessary and just a waste of money, while continuing to prescribe medications notorious for their depletion. Only by changing our priorities (and applying simple logic) can we possibly begin experiencing a reversal of the unnecessary deterioration of health in the nation.

✓ **Bad fats** are human-made fats, normally found in vegetable shortenings, margarines, "partially hydrogenated" oils, cookies, crackers, chips, and other ready-to-eat or processed foods. Hydrogenated oils and partially hydrogenated oils are made by heating vegetable oils in the presence of metal catalysts and hydrogen, which produces trans-fatty acids that are actually incorporated into the cell membranes, making them extremely hard and rigid. This disrupts normal cell functioning, as well as communication with the insulin receptors (and other hormone receptors as well), resulting in insulin resistance. Just remember: Bad fats equal bad receptors, which contributes to their resistance.

Approximately 95% of trans fatty acids come from partially hydrogenated vegetable oil, and according to a study published in an article in the June 2001 issue of *The American Journal of Clinical Nutrition*, **the worst offenders are trans fatty acids** (http://www.mendosa.com/newsletter_july.htm).

In the same study, it was noted that *"Polyunsaturated fatty acid intake was associated with a substantial reduction in risk."* Polyunsaturated fats and monounsaturated fats are found in nuts and seeds in their natural state, however, **most polyunsaturated oils are not good for you because they are processed using very high temperatures** (such as when corn oil is removed from the corn). And as heating and processing any fat renders them harmful, it is even worse to cook with this type of damaged fat. **The best oils are those that are liquid and cold-pressed (not heated in processing).** Any oil can be cold-pressed, and would be indicated on the label.

Bad fats not only poison the cells of the body and contribute to insulin resistance, but they also cause nutrient deficiencies, especially **depletion of the fat-soluble vitamins A, D, E, and K**, which are extremely important for anyone attempting to control or maintain healthy blood sugar levels. Insufficient vitamin A can cause a deterioration of the pituitary gland's basophil cells where the thyroid-stimulating hormone is synthesized, limiting the amount of iodine that the thyroid gland can absorb, and reducing the amount of thyroid hormone it produces. **A deficiency of vitamin D can cause insulin resistance, while a deficiency in vitamin K interferes with insulin release and glucose regulation.**

And vitamin E not only improves insulin sensitivity, but also reduces blood glucose levels, often lessening insulin requirements.

✓ **Blood type diet**. An important factor, regarding which foods you should eat or avoid, is based on your basic blood type (such as "A", "B", "AB", or "O"). According to Dr. Peter D. D'Adamo, N.D., **eating the wrong food for your particular blood type will result in reduced metabolism, insulin irregularity, fluid retention and fatigue.** Each blood type has a specific lectin. Foods also contain lectins that will influence how your body reacts to a particular food. It can upset the thyroid function as well as the production of insulin, which are both very important factors for a diabetic or hypoglycemic. You can find out more specific information, including which foods are the most beneficial and which foods you should avoid, in the book *Eat Right 4 Your Type* (1996), by Dr. Peter D. D'Adamo, N.D.

✓ **Stress** can be physical, emotional, or mental. It can be caused by substances such as caffeine, stimulants, nicotine, alcohol, sugar, steroids, and even most **over-the-counter, prescription, or illegal drugs.** When the body is stressed for any reason, it stimulates the secretion of insulin, as well as stress hormones, which results in a surge of glucose into a system that is often already burdened with excess sugar. **This can contribute to the destruction of the beta cells in the pancreas, as well as the suppression of insulin receptors, leading to insulin resistance.**

And then, stress also causes weight gain. This happens once the blood sugar is increased, due to the extra glucose that pours into your bloodstream. When unused, an excessive amount of insulin is then produced to control it. And because there is no metabolic need for energy production, the glucose is thus converted and stored as fat.

When the stress hormone cortisol is released, it does additional damage by depleting serotonin, sometimes creating overwhelming cravings for carbohydrates, often resulting in binging. As you can see, we have multiple contributors to **abdominal fat**, which greatly increases the possibility of developing **type II diabetes**. I can't help but wonder if the obesity leads to diabetes, or if the insulin resistance associated with type II diabetes is a major contributor to obesity, and which really came first (the chicken or the egg theory).

There is also strong evidence that stress can actually worsen the symptoms in preexisting diabetes, (as well as suppressing the thyroid). This becomes obvious if you consider that **SEVEN (half!) of the 14 nutrients listed in the next section, which are necessary for blood sugar regulation, are depleted by stress!**

✓ **Dehydration** is another possible factor we have to consider. In this regard, at least two problems will come into play. One is that **dehydration is considered a stress to the body,** thus we have one more contributor to elevated glucose from the resultant stress hormone produced. And another problem is, dehydration causes insulin receptors to become resistant, which allows the brain to receive more glucose for energy when there is insufficient water. According to Dr. F. Batmanghelidj, M.D., when the body once again receives adequate amounts of water following dehydration, many of the receptors do become active again. An additional benefit of water is, it flushes out the accumulation of acidic wastes and alkalinizes the body (see next).

✓ **An acidic pH** is often an underestimated precursor to diabetes, as well as a potential cause of weight gain. Acidosis (low pH) is considered extremely dangerous regarding the beta cells that produce insulin, as they are especially sensitive to pH, and thus find it very difficult to function efficiently, or even survive under very acidic conditions. This is likely the reason diabetes was historically treated with alkaline causing powders (baking soda), before insulin was introduced into medicine in the 1920s.

A low pH **(acidosis)** may go unnoticed for years, and according to *The McAlvany Health Alert* (June 2002), it *"leads to the progression of most, if not all, degenerative diseases including cardiovascular disease (the #1 killer in the U.S.), and diabetes,* as well as the never-ending frustration of excessive systemic weight gain"* (p. 2).

Once again, we find it is the **diet** that is the major influence in maintaining the body's proper pH balance. Certain foods naturally produce more acid, while others instead form more alkali. For example, while blood must maintain a pH of 7.35 to 7.45, other body fluids range between 4.5 and 7.5. Soft drinks such as cola have a pH of about 2.5 (extremely acidic). Incidentally, it takes 32 glasses of water (which is alkaline) to neutralize the acid from one 12-ounce cola. **Most all drugs are acidic, and their residues can accumulate in the fat tissue.** Also, be aware that vitamin C supplements listed as ascorbic acid are very acidic. The better choice is Ester-C, which is instead alkaline.

Other examples of highly acidic foods are: meat, sugar, pastas, rice, cheese, beans (pinto, navy, garbanzo, etc), grains and breads, high protein foods, sweetened yogurt, mustard, and ketchup, as well as caffeine and alcohol.

Some examples of alkalinizing foods are: Most vegetables, flax, unsalted butter, plain yogurt, eggs, all vegetable juices, cayenne pepper, gelatin, brewer's yeast, garlic, most herbs, almonds, fresh coconut, and most unprocessed, cold pressed oils, as well as good old-fashioned, non-chlorinated, non-fluoridated water.

Alfalfa is also an excellent alkalinizing agent that is easy to find, and very inexpensive. Sometimes referred to as the king of herbs, the roots of an alfalfa plant can extend as far as 130 feet into the earth. For that very reason, it is one of the most mineral-rich foods. I personally take four 1,000 mg tablets daily.

As done "historically", baking soda is still successful in maintaining a sufficient alkaline balance in your body, (as acidity is normally common in most people), by taking just ½ teaspoon with water each day. There is also a supplement available at most health food stores called "Alka-Aid™." It is a combination of sodium-bicarbonate (baking soda) and potassium. Just taking 100 mg of potassium along with the baking soda to balance the sodium would likely accomplish the same thing. You might also try drinking a glass of warm water with a teaspoon each of raw honey and organic apple cider vinegar each morning, to re-establish a slight alkalinity.

✓ **Hydrochloric acid (HCL) or stomach acid deficiency has been linked to diabetes.** One explanation might be that the inability to digest proteins is significantly compromised when there is insufficient HCL. This would then lead to a highly acidic condition, especially if you consider: *"When protein is inadequately broken down, it putrefies in the intestinal tract and tends to form nitrosamines and ammonia, highly toxic compounds and known carcinogens"* (Rita Elkins, M.H., *Digestive Enzymes*, 1998, p. 18). That would result in a more acidic condition in the body.

As we age, our HCL level tends to decline, and those with type "A" blood, normally have low levels also. Taking one teaspoon of Celtic sea salt with water daily will help the body produce HCL. If that is not sufficient, you can purchase hydrochloric acid (with pepsin) capsules, which you can take with any meal containing meat.

Also, keep in mind that starches such as potatoes or pasta can considerably slow the digestion of protein. The amylase produced to digest starch is actually alkaline, which thus counteracts the HCL necessary for digesting proteins. Organic unfiltered apple cider vinegar (2 tablespoons) with a meal works similar to HCL, and helps reduce the blood sugar in the process.

✓ **Caffeine** increases insulin levels, as well as stimulating the liver to release stored glycogen, which causes a short burst of high glucose followed by the sudden onset of hypoglycemia. Caffeine is also highly acidic, causes stress, and is dehydrating. And, caffeine is also responsible for **depleting SEVEN (half!) of the 14 nutrients listed in the next section as being necessary for blood sugar regulation!**

✓ **Alcohol** is a carbohydrate, derived from grain or fruit or both, which are forms of sugar. This means that it can dramatically raise your blood sugar response, as well as insulin levels. And the more you drink, the higher your levels of insulin can rise. After the initial sugar rush, alcohol creates even more trouble by causing extremely low blood sugar levels, potentially resulting in hypoglycemia, and contributing to insulin resistance and diabetes.

Chronic drinking also causes excessive amounts of fat to accumulate around the liver, resulting in an inability to digest fats properly and a slowing of all digestion, as well contributing to inflammation of the pancreas, which can all lead to diabetes (Balch & Balch, *Prescription for Nutritional Healing*, 3*rd* edition, 2000, pp. 147-149).

As well as being dehydrating, acidic, full of sugar, and a stress to the body, alcohol also depletes many important nutrients necessary for maintaining blood sugar levels and insulin. **Of the 14 nutrients listed in the next section as being necessary for blood sugar regulation, alcohol depletes TEN!**

✓ **Smoking.** Not only is smoking dehydrating, as well as contributing to acidosis, but also **the nicotine in tobacco causes insulin resistance.** Medical studies have confirmed that smokers have an increased risk of developing type II diabetes, as well as lung cancer and heart disease. Smoking also constricts the blood vessels and inhibits circulation. Lack of oxygen (due to poor circulation) and peripheral nerve damage are major factors in the development of diabetic foot ulcers, thus it is important to take measures to improve the circulation in the feet and legs. Smoking also severely depletes the body of vitamin C, which is important for circulation and a healthy immune system, essential to diabetics. Conversely, vitamin C destroys free radicals produced in smoke and lessens other negative effects of smoking.

✓ **Inadequate sleep** is another factor that triggers insulin resistance, according to researchers reporting at a meeting of the American Diabetes Association in June of 2001. In the reported study, **after eight days sleepers who averaged less than five hours of sleep per night were 40% less sensitive to insulin than those who averaged eight hours of sleep per night** (*Alternatives*, April 2002, Vol. 9, No. 10, p. 75).

✓ **Depression.** You may have noticed that many of the previously mentioned contributors to hypoglycemia, similarly also contribute to depression (as noted in detail in an earlier chapter of this book), such as hypothyroidism, bad diet (sugar, bad fats, etc.), stress, dehydration, and alcohol. However, it has been found that depression itself increases the risk of developing diabetes.

As reported in the British Medical Journal:

Depression may be the culprit behind both mental and physical health conditions.

According to studies, more than normal rates of depression can be found in patients with clinically manifest type 2 diabetes.

Researchers discovered a positive connection between higher levels of insulin resistance and severity of depressive symptoms in patients with impaired glucose tolerance, before the occurrence of diabetes (*British Medical Journal,* January 1, 2005; 330:17-18).

And, as reported in *Diabetes Care* (May 2005, Vol. 28, Number 5: 1063-1067):

Several factors may contribute to the depression-diabetes connection. For instance, fluctuations in weight spurred on by poor health habits (i.e. little to no exercise) and taking antidepressants that prompt weight gain are both prime candidates.

✓ **Statin drug use.** According to the *Annals of Internal Medicine* (April 20, 2004;140: 644-649), The American College of Physicians released a report stating new proposed guidelines, recommending that diabetics take cholesterol-lowering drugs, regardless of if they have good cholesterol levels or not. And undoubtedly, the doctors will follow these guidelines. However, as usual, these medications can actually be contributing to the problem by the nutrients they deplete. **Of the 14 nutrients listed in the next section, which contribute to blood sugar regulation, the statin drugs deplete SIX:** Vitamin D, vitamin E, vitamin K, magnesium, zinc, and CoQ_{10}. How are statin drugs supposed to help? I have yet to hear a good explanation.

✓ **SSRI antidepressants**, such as Prozac™, Zoloft™, etc., are also stimulants, and according to Dr. Ann Blake Tracy, just one 30 mg dose of Prozac™ elevates cortisol (stress hormone) levels by 200%! This type of constant stress then causes elevated blood sugar, an increase in insulin production, and eventually diabetes, (one common side effect). The constant stimulation caused by the SSRI antidepressants also suppress the thyroid, which is another risk factor contributing to insulin resistance and diabetes.

✓ **Lithium Carbonate therapy**, commonly used to treat the bipolar disorder, contributes to diabetes in much the same way as the SSRI antidepressants, as it elevates blood sugar levels, can result in diabetes, and suppresses the thyroid. In fact, according to a fairly extensive report on lithium (http://www.healthyplace.com), not only was **"hypothyroidism"** and neurogenic **"Diabetes Insipidus"** mentioned, but in addition, these conditions apparently persist even after the discontinuation of the lithium therapy.

Your Medications Could Be A Major Contributing Factor To Your Diabetes or Hypoglycemia

It is nearly impossible to maintain perfectly balanced blood sugar with drugs. Either your blood sugar drops dangerously low, resulting in hypoglycemia, or it spikes up, damaging your liver, kidneys, blood vessels, and even your heart. Not to mention what the drugs are actually doing (or not doing).

According to a list of the top 200 most prescribed drugs, a total of 102 prescription medications (51%) either listed diabetes, hypoglycemia or blood sugar fluctuations as a potential side effect, or noted that taking that drug would worsen the condition or interfere with its treatment.

On that same list, out of the 180 prescription medications that were tested, a total of **164 prescription medications were found to deplete nutrients that either assist in treating diabetes, controlling blood sugar, or potentially result in diabetes or hypoglycemia when deficient. Thus, more than 91% of the top 200 prescription medications that *are* known to deplete nutrients, are either causing deficiencies responsible for contributing to diabetes or hypoglycemia, or involved in blood sugar regulation.**

Following are nutrients important for preventing or regulating diabetes and blood sugar, along with the drugs, class of drugs, substances, or conditions such as stress, that can contribute to depletion, as follows:

1. **Vitamin B$_3$ (niacin)** – depleted by sulfa drugs, SSRI antidepressants, steroids and corticosteroids, sleeping pills, estrogen (and oral contraceptives), caffeine, antibiotics, alcohol, sugar, and physical and mental stress.
    * **Deficiency of vitamin B$_3$ can produce low blood sugar.**
2. **Vitamin B$_5$ (pantothenic acid)** – depleted by sulfa drugs, sleeping pills, estrogen (and oral contraceptives), caffeine, alcohol, sugar, cooking, and physical and mental stress.
    * **Deficiency of vitamin B$_5$ can produce hypoglycemia.**
3. **Biotin** – a member of the B vitamin family, depleted by sulfa drugs, estrogen and oral contraceptives, caffeine, antiseizure medication (i.e. barbiturates, phenytoin), antibiotics, alcohol, and saccharin.
    * **A deficiency of biotin can produce high blood sugar.**
4. **Vitamin C** – depleted by steroids and corticosteroids, smoking, NSAIDs (i.e. ibuprofen), muscle relaxants, estrogen and oral contraceptives, diuretics, **diabetic medication**, antihistamines, asthma medications, aspirin, anticoagulants, antidepressants (most), antiseizure medication (i.e. barbiturates, phenytoin), antibiotics, analgesics, amphetamines and diet pills, alcohol, caffeine, cooking (heat), high fever, physical and mental stress.
    * **There is an increased need for vitamin C in smokers, diabetics, the elderly, people under stress, and allergy sufferers.**
    * **May slow or prevent complications from diabetes.**

5. **Vitamin D** – depleted by steroids and corticosteroids, smoking, muscle relaxants, mineral oil (laxatives), Histamine H_2 blockers (i.e. Tagamet™, Pepcid™, Zantac™), estrogen (and oral contraceptives), diuretics, **diabetic medication**, all cholesterol-lowering drugs, including statins and bile acid sequestrants (i.e. Questran™, Colestid™), asthma medications, aspirin, antiseizure medication (i.e. barbiturates, phenytoin), antibiotics, antidepressants, antiarrhythmics (i.e. digoxin), antacids, analgesics, alcohol, cooking (heat), light, high fever, physical and mental stress.
   - **A deficiency of vitamin D increases insulin resistance.**
6. **Vitamin E** – depleted by NSAIDs (i.e. ibuprofen), all cholesterol-lowering drugs, including statins and bile acid sequestrants (i.e. Questran™, Colestid™), Orlistat™ (fat-blocking weight loss agent), mineral oil (laxatives), estrogen and oral contraceptives, aspirin, antibiotics, alcohol, heat, frying, oxygen, freezing temperatures, air pollution, inorganic iron, and chlorine.
   - **Improves insulin sensitivity.**
   - **Reduces blood glucose levels, often lessening insulin requirements.**
7. **Vitamin K** – depleted by sulfa drugs, antibiotics, aspirin, alcohol, antiseizure medication (i.e. barbiturates, phenytoin), anticoagulants (blood thinners), all cholesterol-lowering drugs, including statins and bile acid sequestrants (i.e. Questran™, Colestid™), blood thinners (i.e. Coumadin™), mineral oil (laxatives), rancid fat, x-ray therapy.
   - **All anticoagulants and antibiotics not only deplete vitamin K, but they also block the absorption of vitamin K.**
   - **Assists in converting glucose to glycogen for storage in the liver.**
   - **A deficiency interferes with insulin release and glucose regulation in ways similar to diabetes.**
8. **Coenzyme Q_{10} (CoQ$_{10}$)** – depleted by vasodilators (i.e. nitroglycerin), diuretics, **diabetic medications,** all cholesterol-lowering drugs, including statins and bile acid sequestrants (i.e. Questran™, Colestid™), phenothiazines (class of antipsychotic drugs), antihypertensive (blood pressure lowering) drugs (including ACE inhibitors, beta-blockers and calcium channel blockers), antihistamines, antidepressants (especially tricyclics), antiarrhythmics (i.e. digoxin).
   - **CoQ$_{10}$ is beneficial in treating diabetes.**
   - **A deficiency of CoQ$_{10}$ has been linked to diabetes.**
9. **Chromium** – a trace mineral depleted by **diabetic medication**, excess iron, processed foods, refined carbohydrates, and sugar.
   - **Chromium is necessary for maintaining stable blood sugar levels through proper insulin utilization.**
   - **Chromium assists in the treatment of diabetes and hypoglycemia.**
   - **A deficiency can produce glucose intolerance (especially in diabetics).**
   - **Deficiency symptoms parallel those of diabetes.**
   - **Diabetes and coronary heart disease have been linked to low chromium concentrations in human tissue.**
10. **Magnesium** – an essential mineral depleted by steroids and corticosteroids, SSRI antidepressants, NSAIDs (i.e. ibuprofen), Immunosuppressants, high levels of zinc, estrogen and oral contraceptives, diuretics, **diabetic medication,** all cholesterol-lowering drugs, including statins and bile acid sequestrants (i.e. Questran™, Colestid™), antiseizure medication (i.e. barbiturates, phenytoin), antifungal medication, antibiotics, antiarrhythmic agents (i.e. digoxin), antacids, alcohol, antihypertensive (blood pressure lowering) drugs (including ACE inhibitors, beta-blockers and calcium channel blockers), large amounts of fats, sugar, refined flour, fluoride, soft water consumption, and physical and emotional stress.
    - **Magnesium assists in the metabolism of sugar.**
    - **Assists with maintaining body's pH balance.**

- **A magnesium deficiency is often synonymous with diabetes.**
11. **Manganese** – a trace mineral depleted by steroids and corticosteroids, SSRI antidepressants, diuretics, caffeine, alcohol, excess sugar, and heavy consumption of meat or dairy products.
    - **Manganese assists with blood sugar regulation.**
    - **A deficiency can produce abnormalities in insulin secretion, impaired glucose metabolism, and pancreatic damage.**
    - **Low levels of manganese are often found in people with hypoglycemia.**
12. **Potassium** – an essential mineral depleted by steroids and corticosteroids, sodium bicarbonate (Alka Seltzer™), smoking, Parkinson's disease medication, NSAIDs (i.e. ibuprofen), muscle relaxants, laxatives, immunosuppressants, diuretics, caffeine, antiarrhythmic agents (i.e. digoxin), asthma medication, aspirin, antifungal medication, antibiotics, amphetamines and diet pills, alcohol, Acetazolamide™ (a carbonic anhydrase inhibitor), ACE inhibitors and other blood pressure lowering drugs (including beta-blockers), excess sugar and refined foods, large amounts of licorice, and physical and mental stress. Kidney disorders and **low blood sugar levels can cause potassium loss.**
    - **Potassium depletion can produce glucose intolerance.**
    - **Assists with maintaining body's pH balance.**
13. **Zinc** – a trace mineral depleted by steroids and corticosteroids, SSRI antidepressants, HIV medication, Histamine H_2 blockers (i.e. Tagamet™, Pepcid™, Zantac™), estrogen (and oral contraceptives), diuretics, caffeine, all cholesterol-lowering drugs, including statins and bile acid sequestrants (i.e. Questran™, Colestid™), antibiotics, aspirin, antiseizure medication (i.e. barbiturates, phenytoin), antacids and ulcer medication, alcohol, ACE inhibitors and other blood pressure lowering drugs (including beta-blockers), diarrhea, perspiration, kidney disease, cirrhosis of the liver, **diabetes,** food processing, physical and mental stress, a diet high in fiber, and the consumption of hard water. **Zinc levels are lowered by diabetes.**
    - **Food (especially dairy products, protein and fiber) interferes with the absorption of zinc.**
    - **Zinc is a constituent of insulin.**
    - **A deficiency can produce a propensity to diabetes.**
14. **Carnitine** – a non-essential amino acid, related to the B vitamins, depleted by antiseizure medication (i.e. barbiturates), HIV medication, and valproic acid and derivatives.
    - **Carnitine reduces the health risks associated with diabetes.**
    - **Stabilizes blood glucose levels.**
    - **A deficiency can produce impaired glucose control.**

As usual, your medications could either be the underlying cause, or at lease a contributor to your condition (in this case, it's diabetes).

Microwave Cooking Adds To Nutrient Depletion

It has been found that cooking foods in a microwave can entirely alter the biological structure of a food. The end result is: The majority of vitamins and minerals are destroyed, and many foods are converted to carcinogens (cancer causing). In *The Townsend Letter for Doctors and Patients* (June 2001), it states, *"Russian researchers also reported a marked acceleration of **structural degradation leading to a decreased food value of 60 to 90% in all foods tested.** Among the changes observed were: Decreased bio-availability of **vitamin B complex, vitamin C, vitamin E, essential minerals** and lipotropic factors in all food tested."*

This is a major concern if you consider that **vitamin B_3, vitamin B_5, vitamin C, vitamin E and several essential minerals are all included on the list of nutrients listed as important for**

preventing or regulating diabetes and blood sugar, yet they are all decreased by up to 90% by microwave cooking.

Something else to consider, as microwave cooking dramatically depletes many of the same vitamins that sugar does (necessary for its own metabolism), it could easily mean that healthy complex carbohydrates are actually being converted into simple sugars void of nutrients. Microwave cooking also dramatically changes the structure of foods, and could thus reduce the benefit of fiber in foods, which could have a considerable influence on the blood sugar levels.

Understanding Hypoglycemia

Although ninety-five percent of hypoglycemia is considered to be self-caused (by irregular eating habits, excessive amounts of carbohydrates, sugar, caffeine, or alcohol), unfortunately, diabetes medications, (especially when prescribed in combination, which is extremely common), tend to drive the blood sugar too low, leading to hypoglycemia. This is just one more example of complications associated with prescription medications that often create, rather than resolve a condition. Hypoglycemia can then lead to disorders such as: adrenal fatigue, thyroid disorders, pituitary disorders, kidney disease, pancreatitis, or liver disease.

Hypoglycemic symptoms are many and varied, and in his book *How to Eat Your Way Out of Fatigue* (1969), Dr. Clement G. Martin, M.D. does an excellent job of describing the symptoms of hypoglycemia as:

> *Recurrent seizures and coma; mental aberrations and optical troubles, such as double vision, occur.* **Market obesity is apt to be the eventual result** *of this disease if it is allowed to persist.* **Profound brain damage** *is, unfortunately,* **an anticipated result** *when the disease had progressed long enough* (p. 21).

> **The outstanding symptom is fatigue. Most commonly both mental and physical, though it can be only one or the other.** *Sudden sweating, varying from mild to an absolute drench, is a not too infrequent sign. These may be accompanied by chills, and usually the feeling of weakness grows greatest because the blood sugar is dropping rapidly in these sessions. This is the point where* **there is a real craving for food – some high energy food most likely. It might be candy, coffee and a sweet roll or some other pastry** (p. 31).

A person suffering from hypoglycemia might experience such symptoms as: fatigue, irritability, depression, anxiety, cravings for sweets, constant hunger, mental disturbances, and insomnia.

People with hypoglycemia can at times become very aggressive and lose their tempers easily. The onset and severity of symptoms are directly related to the length of time since the last meal was eaten and the type of foods that meal contained, most commonly occurring a few hours after eating sweets or fats.

According to Dr. S. Harris, M.D., the person who first discovered hypoglycemia:

> *Our brain is extremely vulnerable to changes in its fuel supply and can't work well when the fuel isn't furnished in a regular fashion.* **I have never met a patient with a sugar problem, either diabetes mellitus or hypoglycemia, who did not notice personality changes.** *Frequently, their complaint on coming in for the first visit would be, "I don't feel myself, something in me has changed." On questioning, you would get a great deal of material about personality changes and upsets* (Martin, *How to Eat Your Way Out of Fatigue*, 1969, p. 57).

Dr. Harris noted that in almost every case, the patient's first real feeling of satisfaction came once his diet changed and he felt his old and stronger thought processes and emotions coming back again.

The Effects of Alcohol on Hypoglycemia

In his book *How to Eat Your Way Out of Fatigue* (1969), Dr. Martin points out that ***"Alcohol is the quickest energy source known to man. Who needs energy this instantly? Hypoglycemics!"*** (p. 123). Although alcohol masks the symptoms, and provides a temporary increase in energy, it also lowers the body's supply of sugar even further, thus resulting in even worse low blood sugar problems. **Alcohol has a much more intense effect on a person with hypoglycemia than with others.** When a person runs out of sugar and uses alcohol as substitute fuel, the body may be overwhelmed, possibly to the point of death. **Deaths have been reported from hypoglycemia in alcoholics.**

How Hypoglycemia Influences the Thyroid

Anyone with hypoglycemia would likely experience an even worse low thyroid condition, as hypoglycemia means you also have less sugar (glucose) available to assist in the enzyme action in the liver responsible for the conversion of the T_4 thyroid to the much more active T_3 form. This can only be identified and resolved with the proper diagnosis, and treatment of the problem early on. Rather than the typical solution of medications for diabetics, in an attempt to reduce the blood sugar (often causing hypoglycemia), as usual there is a much better solution.

According to Dr. Broda Barnes, M.D., *"Treatment usually recommended for hypoglycemia is usually a diet high in protein and low in carbohydrate, with frequent feedings. **I have seen many patients with hypoglycemia who have responded to thyroid therapy.** Their symptoms have been ended and they have been able to eat normal diets"* (*Hypothyroidism – The Unsuspected Illness*, 1976, p. 238).

Dietary Suggestions For The Hypoglycemic

Just as the **cause** of this disease is often due to eating the wrong diet, the **solution** is often in eating the correct diet. In addition to the Dietary Recommendations for resolving diabetes, listed later in this chapter, following are a few dietary suggestions that should prove helpful in controlling or avoiding hypoglycemia:

- It is important to **eat a diet high in complex carbohydrates, fiber, vegetable protein, and plenty of fresh vegetables and good fats.** It may be helpful to also refer to the GLYCEMIC INDEX section in the DIETARY RECOMMENDATIONS FOR CONTROLLING BLOOD SUGAR.
- **Limit your intake of starchy foods (simple carbohydrates),** such as corn, noodles, pasta, white rice, white bread, and potatoes.
- **Avoid the following:**
  o **Simple sugars,** which include: sugar, fructose, glucose, corn sweeteners, corn syrup, fruit sugar, table sugar, and brown sugar.
  o **Fatty foods,** such as bacon, cold cuts, fried foods, gravies, ham, sausage, or dairy products.
  o **Artificial sweeteners**, such as aspartame and saccharin.
  o **Foods that contain artificial colors or preservatives.**
  o **Alcohol.**
  o **Caffeine, nicotine, stress, and other stimulants.**

CHAPTER TWENTY
THE DANGERS ASSOCIATED WITH SUGAR AND ARTIFICIAL SWEETENERS

What is one of the most widely consumed addictive substances on the planet? Would you believe: Sugar. Although sugar is both legal and acceptable by society, **there is very little difference between drug abuse and carbohydrate abuse.** In an article in his *Alternatives* newsletter (December 2000), Dr. David G. Williams, M.D. states his feeling **regarding sugar abuse and drug abuse:** *"Only when we begin to treat the former as seriously as the latter will be begin to see dramatic changes in our society"* (pp. 142-143).

Sugars cause significant increases in liver enzymes and an elevation of blood triglycerides, and these findings suggest that **the consumption of sugars can actually alter liver functions, perhaps even permanently.** Considering the high sugar intake of the average American, it is no wonder how profoundly it is implicated in chronic liver damage, with **high fructose corn syrup being perhaps the worst offender.**

High-fructose corn syrup is considerably different than *pure* fructose, but is usually labeled as just **fructose** in order to sound more acceptable to the unsuspecting public. According to a diabetes report in *Life Science* (2001), *"Look on the label of almost any fruit drink and you will discover **high fructose corn syrup which has single-handedly contributed to the rise of diabetes more than any other ingredient"*** (p. 4).

Pure fructose does not easily convert to glucose, thus it is lower on the glycemic index. However, studies have found that although the body absorbs and utilizes pure fructose much slower than it does glucose (table sugar), it actually causes much more damage inside the body than the glucose found in table sugar. In fact, **researchers have routinely fed fructose to laboratory mice to induce insulin resistant diabetes for antidiabetic drug testing** (Dr. Ron Rosedale, *The Rosedale Diet*, 2004).

The Dangers of Sugar

The following is part of a list (25 of 78), printed in the July 2002 issue of *The McAlvany Health Alert*, with some of the greatest concerns regarding how sugar can ruin your health:

1. Sugar can suppress the immune system.
2. Sugar can upset the body's mineral balance.
3. Sugar can produce a significant rise in triglycerides.
4. Sugar can cause kidney damage.
5. Sugar can cause hypoglycemia.
6. Sugar can contribute to weight gain and obesity.
7. Sugar can cause candidiasis (yeast infection).
8. Sugar can cause a decrease in insulin sensitivity.
9. Sugar can decrease growth hormone.
10. Sugar can change the structure of protein, interfering with protein absorption.
11. Sugar causes food allergies.
12. Sugar can contribute to diabetes.
13. Sugar can cause cardiovascular disease.
14. Sugar lowers the enzymes' ability to function.
15. Sugar can cause liver cells to divide, increasing size of liver.
16. Sugar can increase the amount of fat in the liver.
17. Sugar can increase kidney size and produce pathological changes in the kidney.
18. Sugar can overstress the pancreas, causing damage.

19. Sugar can increase the body's fluid retention.
20. Sugar can compromise the lining of the capillaries.
21. Sugar can cause hypertension.
22. Sugar can cause depression.
23. Sugar can cause hormonal imbalance.
24. Sugar increases the risk of Alzheimer's disease.
25. Sugar can increase blood platelet adhesiveness, (increasing the risk of blood clots.)

Studies show that just **one teaspoon** of sugar impairs the immune system by **50 percent,** for several hours after consumption, thus contributing to infections caused by its interference with the white blood cells' ability to kill germs. It has been found that **if you continually consume just a small amount of sugar at a time throughout the entire day, your immune system will be impaired by 50 percent ALL DAY LONG!** Is it any wonder that it has also been found in a study with rats, that when sugar is cut from their diet, they live almost twice as long as when their diet contains sugar?

Is There A Diabetes / Cancer Connection Related To Sugar?

Following is an extract from an article titled, *"People with high blood sugar levels more likely to develop disease,"* taken from *the McAlvany Health Alert Update* (March 25, 2005), as quoted from *The Associated Press*:

> *CHICAGO – A study of more than 1 million South Koreans suggests diabetes can raise the risk of developing and dying from several types of cancer, including digestive-tract tumors.*
> *This is not the first study to suggest such a link, but it sheds more light on exactly how diabetes might contribute to cancer.*
> *The highest risks for developing cancer and dying from it were found in people with the highest blood sugar levels,* *the South Korean researchers found.*
> *The study appears in Wednesday's Journal of the American Medical Association.*
> *Participants with diabetes were roughly 30 percent more likely than those without to develop and die from cancer.* *The highest risks were for cancer of the pancreas, the organ that produces blood sugar-regulating insulin. Diabetes involves inadequate production or use of insulin.*
> *Increased risks also were seen for cancers of the liver, esophagus and colon.*
> *[Elevated insulin might also play a part, as one function of insulin is the stimulation of cell growth, and] cancer is characterized by runaway cell growth.*

I believe there is an explanation as to why elevated blood sugar would increase the risk of cancer. **Sugar is cancer's primary source of energy,** and once a cell mutates, it would have an adequate source of energy. Also, our best defense against cancer is our immune system, which just happens to be suppressed approximately 50% by sugar. And a third influence would be the fact that sugar is very acidic. This creates an environment where oxygen will be depleted (and cancer hates oxygen).

We have thus created a perfect environment where cancer can both survive and flourish, (and we call it diabetes). There is always a logical explanation for any disease, or unhealthy condition we might possibly experience. It is also obvious that all diseases are somehow interrelated, and just the result of an unhealthy environment that we are unknowingly, and unnecessarily creating.

Sugar's Damaging Effects On Insulin

Repeatedly overloading the bloodstream with sugar every day causes **chronic over-stimulation of the pituitary and pancreas glands, which control insulin release.** Studies have shown that sugars and other simple carbohydrates in the presence of fats also cause an impaired insulin response. This allows large amounts of sugar to enter the blood without being controlled, which results in the body's release of even larger amounts of insulin. An excess of glucose in the blood is toxic, therefore as more glucose enters the blood, the body's first response is to turn this sugar into triglycerides (which make the blood thicker and "stickier") and subsequently, because there are now excessive amounts of insulin, the triglycerides must be stored in fat cells. The use of fat for energy is hampered with the presence of excess glucose in the blood.

According to Bryant Stamford, Ph.D., exercise scientist and director of the Health Promotion and Wellness Program at the University of Louisville in Kentucky, eating fats and sugars (simple carbohydrates) <u>together</u> is where the real problems begin. It is a common American practice to combine items like peanut butter and jelly on bread. Take a hamburger, French fries and a cola, for example. When your body gets the blast of simple sugars from soda (**a 12-ounce serving has an average of ten teaspoons of sugar**), **it releases a surge of insulin in response, causing the fat cells to open up and store fat.** Caffeinated beverages (i.e. soda) also contribute to dehydration, which leads to a host of problems and conditions.

And sweet sodas are not the only food that can produce this effect. **Any high-glycemic foods can produce an insulin response that results in rapid fat storage.** This is why the high intake of refined sugar has been linked to a variety of health problems, including elevated levels of cholesterol and other blood fats, as well as a chromium deficiency. Chromium, an important component of insulin, is unfortunately depleted by sugar. The majority of people in the nation are chromium deficient, often due to the high intake of sugar.

Simple carbohydrates currently make up 40% of the American diet. This explains why a very large proportion of those who are overweight show signs of insulin resistance, and also explains why 90% of diabetic adults are overweight. Highly elevated levels of insulin **damage** the body's ability to respond to this hormone, resulting in insulin resistance and obesity, and often eventually diabetes.

The Nutrient Depletion Caused By Sugar

It appears that sugar shares something in common with your prescription medications, (the extensive depletion of nutrients). What is sugar's excuse? It is totally devoid of nutrients (other carbohydrates normally have) necessary for its metabolism. Thus, it is forced to rob them from your resources. And if you are also taking nutrient-depleting drugs, they will likely be in short supply already.

Something to be aware of is, **of the 14 nutrients <u>previously listed as being important for preventing or regulating diabetes and blood sugar</u>, 7 (half!) can be depleted by sugar or sugar-substitutes!**

Although important nutrients are normally depleted by many sources, such as prescription drugs, stress, and food processing methods, just to name a few, **following are common nutrients depleted just by <u>sugar consumption</u>, along with some of their more important benefits.**

1. **Vitamin B$_1$ (Thiamine)** – Assists in blood formation, enhances circulation, prevents edema (swelling), reduces stress and anxiety, and enhances energy. Vitamin B$_1$ is also an antioxidant, which helps to protect cells against cancer, and the degenerative effects of aging, alcohol consumption, and smoking.
2. **Vitamin B$_2$ (Riboflavin)** – Necessary for red blood cell formation, assists in converting protein to energy, and promotes healthy skin, nails, and hair. A deficiency can produce hypertension (high blood pressure).

3. **Vitamin B$_3$ (Niacin)** – Necessary for proper circulation and healthy skin, enhances memory and prevents senility, reduces blood pressure and lowers cholesterol, assists in normal functioning of the nervous system. **A deficiency can produce low blood sugar,** fatigue, and depression.

4. **Vitamin B$_5$ (Pantothenic Acid)** – Required by all cells in the body, assists in the formation of antibodies and vitamin utilization, necessary for proper functioning of the adrenal glands, prevents certain forms of anemia, assists in the production of neurotransmitters, thus reducing stress, anxiety, and depression. **A deficiency can produce hypoglycemia.**

5. **Vitamin B$_6$ (Pyridoxine)** – Involved in more bodily functions than almost any other single nutrient, affects both physical and mental health, maintains sodium and potassium balance (pH), promotes red blood cell formation, enhances the immune system and antibody production, inhibits the formation of homocysteine (thus reducing cholesterol deposition surrounding the heart), maintains teeth and bones, and acts as an antihistamine.

6. **Choline** (A cofactor of the B vitamin family) – necessary for proper transmission of nerve impulses from the brain through the central nervous system, assists in gallbladder regulation, kidney and liver function, and hormone production. Prevents and treats arteriosclerosis, and important for cardiovascular health. A deficiency can produce hypertension (high blood pressure) and cardiac symptoms.

7. **Calcium** – Necessary for the transmission of nerve impulses, a regular heartbeat, and the entire nervous system, necessary for strong bones, teeth and healthy gums, lowers cholesterol and prevents cardiovascular disease, necessary for muscular growth and prevents muscle cramps, lowers blood pressure and assists with blood clotting. A deficiency can produce hypertension (high blood pressure), high cholesterol, and depression, and has been linked to colorectal cancer.

8. **Chromium – necessary for maintaining stable blood sugar levels and for proper insulin utilization,** lowers cholesterol, enhances energy, **assists in the treatment of diabetes and hypoglycemia**, and prevents osteoporosis. **A deficiency can produce glucose intolerance, and deficiency symptoms parallel those of diabetes.**

9. **Copper** – Although sugar is not specifically said to deplete the mineral copper, it has been discovered that **a copper deficiency is significantly worsened by high amounts of fructose.** Copper is necessary for healthy nerves and joints, reduces the degeneration of the nervous system, assists in the formation of red blood cells, hemoglobin, and energy production.

10. **Magnesium – More than 300 enzymes are activated by magnesium, and a low magnesium levels make nearly every disease worse.** Magnesium enhances energy, and is necessary for normal heart rhythm, muscular contraction, nerve transmission, and healthy nervous and muscular tissues. Reduces cholesterol and blood pressure, and increases the rate of survival following a heart attack. Assists in the prevention of cardiovascular disease, osteoporosis, and certain forms of cancer. Reduces stress, prevents depression, and relieves indigestion. **A deficiency can produce high blood pressure, cardiac arrhythmia (fatal), sudden cardiac arrest, and is often synonymous with diabetes.**

11. **Manganese** – Assists in reproduction, blood clotting, energy, and **blood sugar regulation.** Promotes a healthy nervous system and immune system. Necessary in the syntheses of thyroxine (the principal hormone of the thyroid gland), and for normal bone growth. **A deficiency can produce** heart disorders, high cholesterol levels and high blood pressure, **abnormalities in insulin secretion, and impaired glucose metabolism and pancreatic damage, and low levels of manganese are often found in people with hypoglycemia.**

12. **Potassium** – Necessary for a healthy nervous system, the transmission of nerve impulse, and assists in regular heart rhythm and proper muscle contraction. Prevents stroke, maintains blood pressure, and neutralizes the body's water balance (pH). **In addition to sugar, low blood sugar levels (hypoglycemia) can actually cause potassium loss.** Depletion can cause hypertension (high blood pressure), salt retention and edema (swelling), **glucose intolerance,** high cholesterol levels, fluctuations in heartbeat and respiratory distress.

The Dangers Of Artificial Sweeteners

It has also been found that **Biotin (a member of the B vitamin family) is depleted by saccharin, a common artificial sweetener.** Biotin assists in cell growth, maintains healthy skin, enhances energy, relieves muscle pain, and promotes healthy sweat glands, nerve tissue, and bone marrow. **A deficiency of biotin can produce high blood sugar.**

The artificial sweetener Aspartame is made up of three different substances. Two are the stimulatory amino acids phenylalanine and aspartic acid, and the third is **methanol (wood alcohol), a poisonous substance added during manufacturing.** Toxic levels of the methanol found in aspartame can cause disorders that include blindness, brain swelling, and inflammation of the pancreas and heart muscle. It has been proven that when these components are ingested, it not only affects both the nervous system and the blood pressure, **but it produces high insulin levels as well.**

Anytime there is something sweet in our mouth, our body assumes there is sugar coming. Our bodies weren't designed for artificial sweeteners that taste sweet, but have no carbohydrate content. So, insulin is produced in response to the anticipation of the arrival of sugar (which never came). And although there is no sugar, insulin has a job to do (transport sugar), thus it takes it from any place possible, which soon results in low blood sugar (hypoglycemia). The body then responds by craving sugar.

Dr. H. J. Roberts, an authority on aspartame, states that millions of people use NutraSweet™ or Equal™ instead of sugar in an attempt to avoid gaining weight, however it was proven years ago that **aspartame actually increases the appetite for sugar and carbohydrates** (*Second Opinion*, March 1996, p. 2). Diet sodas and other products containing the artificial sweetener aspartame, **can also block the formation of serotonin, worsening carbohydrate cravings, insomnia,** and **depression** in individuals who are already serotonin-deprived. **The carbon dioxide in these drinks may compete with oxygen, and possibly even enhance the effects of caffeine and NutraSweet™.** This could explain why many overweight people drink sugar-free beverages and do not lose weight, as they just eat more carbohydrates.

An article in the March 1996 issue of Dr. William Campbell Douglass' *Second Opinion* newsletter, lists the amazing number of complaints from aspartame use reported to the FDA. Just a few of those listed are as follows:

* Aggression	* Anxiety	* Blood pressure elevation
* Chronic Fatigue	* Death	* Depression
* Edema (fluid retention)	* Irritability	* Heart palpitations
* Irritability	* Phobias	* Shortness of breath

The artificial sweeteners saccharin, Equal™, and NutraSweet™, (as well as the prescription and over-the-counter drugs that too many tend to depend upon), were all developed in a laboratory, and because they are all unnatural to the body, they are treated by the body as the toxins they really are. This places an excessive load on our major detoxifier, the liver.

Breaking the Sugar Habit (Natural Solutions to Fight the Cravings)

Following are some supplements that should help reduce your sugar cravings and help in sugar withdrawal:

- **Vitamin C – reduces cravings for sweets**, necessary for proper nervous system function, reduces stress, enhances immune system, lowers blood pressure and cholesterol.

    Dr. Janice Keller Phelps, M.D. suggests that our greatest aid to getting through sugar withdrawal is vitamin C, and in her book *The Hidden Addiction and How To Get Free* (1986) she recommends: "*Take it every two hours during the day and whenever you crave sugar. Withdrawal will last about three to five days. **Once you eliminate the sugar from your body, you will stop craving it.** Then it will get easier. Try eating something every two hours so that you don't get ravenously hungry, which usually is caused by sugar causing an appetite for more sugar*" (p. 79).

- **Goji juice – contains 19 amino acids, 21 trace minerals, and more vitamin C than 500 oranges!**
- **The B vitamins** – necessary for proper nervous system function, in addition to assisting with the production of adrenal and stress hormones, which greatly influences metabolism. **Also necessary for formation of the neurotransmitters (i.e. serotonin and dopamine), responsible for preventing cravings.**
- **Vitamin E – reduces cravings for sweets,** as well as depression and fatigue.
- **Zinc** – promotes a healthy immune system, necessary for proper adrenal function. **Some symptoms of zinc deficiency are depression, diabetes, obesity, thyroid disorders, and compulsive cravings for sugar or alcohol.**
- **The trace mineral Chromium** – helps insulin work more efficiently at maintaining a proper blood sugar level, as well as **reducing sugar cravings and extreme fluctuations of hunger associated with hypoglycemia.**
- **The amino acid L-glutamine** – The brain can use glutamine as a source of energy, as well as water or glucose, thus **reducing cravings for sugar** as its source of energy.
- **Water – quenches your appetite naturally,** necessary for proper kidney function, promotes energy. **When the brain is dehydrated, it stimulates cravings for sugar (or carbohydrates) as its source of energy.**
- **Celtic sea salt** – an excellent source of over 80 trace minerals in their natural ionic form, **assisting the body in hydration. One of the minerals, iodine, is especially beneficial for healthy thyroid function.**

  According to Dr. E. Denis Wilson, M.D., patients with a low thyroid occasionally suffer from *"intense and previously unfamiliar cravings for sweets"* (*Wilson's Syndrome*, 1996, p. 228).
- **Mangosteen – appears to be very beneficial for eliminating the cravings for sugar. Those who had previously craved sugar discovered they no longer did.**
- *Gymnema sylvestre* – an herb well known by diabetics for reducing high blood-sugar levels, can actually **prevent you from tasting sugar.** According to an article in *Health Sciences Institute* magazine (September 2001, pp. 1-3), titled *"Overcome Sugar Addiction in 21 days with a Natural Herb,"* *Gymnema sylvestre* prevents sweet flavors from *"communicating"* with your taste buds. Because your tongue is unaware that it is eating something sweet, no signal from the brain is triggered for the release of opioid and dopamine, yet you are conquering the cycle of physical addiction by stopping.
- **Avoid Alcohol** – Just as sugar triggers eating binges, so does alcohol. **The alcoholic body has a difficult time differentiating between sugar and alcohol, and sometimes feels the need to binge on one or both substances.** This is because the body uses alcohol in much the same manner as it would use sugar. In fact, alcohol and sugar are so similar, that **when trying to give up sugar, it is suggested that alcohol be eliminated also.**

Sweet Alternatives

1. Stevia appears to be the healthiest option for a sweetener. It is a South American herb and an excellent alternative for sugar as it does not have the same effect on the body as sugar, and does not have the side effects of artificial sugar substitutes. **Stevia extract is an extremely sweet concentrated supplement that helps regulate blood sugar, and is thus especially valuable for anyone with diabetes or hypoglycemia. It is a fantastic aid to weight loss and weight management because it contains no calories.** In addition, research indicates that **it significantly increases glucose tolerance and inhibits glucose absorption, (a major benefit).** Stevia is more than just a non-caloric sweetener. **Studies show that people who consume Stevia on a daily basis often report a decrease in their desire for sweets and fatty foods.**

2. Grade B Maple Syrup is my personal first choice as a syrup, and would be a good choice for anyone who likes maple flavor. It is processed in open kettles without formaldehyde. Other grades are processed in pressurized containers with formaldehyde added. **Grade B Maple Syrup is also a lower glycemic index food, resulting in a slow, gradual rise in blood sugar levels. Remember, rapid spikes in blood sugar result in rapid plunges, which create severe carbohydrate (sugar) cravings and eventual insulin resistance.**

This just happens to be an example where grade B is actually much better than grade A. It's basically an exception to the rule. **Two critical issues: First, it still has the many minerals and enzymes in tact; and second, there is no formaldehyde added!** It can normally be found in your local health food store. Some stores carry it in bulk, which is normally the most cost effective.

3. Organic unfiltered Honey is another choice, which has a lot natural of minerals and enzymes, and is a much healthier option than sugar, if you are not a diabetic or worried about calories. It is often found in different flavors depending on the bees' diet. I personally use honey, mixed with organic unfiltered apple cider vinegar, every morning for their health benefits (as recommended by some of the ancient healers). The vinegar tends to slow the release of sugar into the blood stream. I first heat water and then dissolve ½ tablespoon of honey, and then add one tablespoon of vinegar. Honey can also be used as a syrup.

4. Xylitol actually looks, tastes and pours just like regular sugar. You can use it on your morning breakfast cereal or on anything you'd like to sweeten naturally. You can also use it for baking if you like. Discovered simultaneously by French and German chemists in 1891, Xylitol has been safely used since the 1970s as an ingredient in gums and candies. Because it can't be utilized by bacteria in the mouth Xylitol doesn't promote tooth decay, dentists and nutritionists alike encourage the use of Xylitol due to its unique and clinically proven dental benefits.

Although it is classified as a carbohydrate, Xylitol is slowly absorbed from the digestive tract, and does not cause rapid rises in blood glucose. In addition, the caloric impact of Xylitol is typically about 40% lower than other carbohydrates, making it a healthy addition to any low-carb diet.

Xylitol is a sugar alcohol that is naturally present in small amounts in various fruits and vegetables. A considerable amount of Xylitol is formed in the body every day as a result of normal metabolic processes.

For an all-around sugar replacement, Xylitol is my favorite. It comes in convenient packets, or can be purchased in bulk as well.

CHAPTER TWENTY-ONE
DIETARY RECOMMENDATIONS
FOR STABILIZAING BLOOD SUGAR

What Is A Glycemic Index?

After much research, in books and on the Internet, it soon became obvious that there are many different conclusions regarding the glycemic index, as well as glycemic ratings. In fact, just about every single source has a different opinion on the subject. To begin with, I suppose it is safe to say that **the glycemic index is a classification of carbohydrates and their blood glucose-raising potential, determined by measuring their rate of entry into the bloodstream.** While one book states that the glycemic index sets glucose at a value of 100 and compares selected foods to it (using the example of sucrose as having a glycemic index of 59), another website claims that white bread was used as a baseline set at 100 (saying that sucrose has a glycemic index of 92), and yet another source probably sums it up best by explaining that **the glycemic index was determined by** *"how fast the carbohydrate food gets into the bloodstream to glucose (=100)",* and clarified some confusion by noting that *"Some indexes are based on white bread and some on sugar so the numbers may vary"* (http://www.diabetic-lifestyle.com/articles/jul03_whats_1.htm).

The controversy became quite apparent while searching for an official glycemic index list, as it soon became obvious that no such list was ever agreed on.

Variables Regarding The Glycemic Index

The validity of testing was even in question, due to the many contributing factors that may or may not have been taken into account, which could be the reason for the extreme variation in ratings from one source to another.

✓ One important factor is **the amount of dietary fiber a carbohydrate contains** (especially soluble fiber). Fiber cannot be broken down into simple sugars, and thus will have no impact on insulin. Additionally, fiber actually cancels out some of the effects of high glycemic foods, producing balance. For example, swallowing a couple tablespoons of freshly ground flax seeds before or during a meal would be one way to reduce the potential rise in blood sugar. The fiber and good fats (EFAs) in the ground flax should attenuate the release of sugar in the bloodstream, thus reducing the insulin response.

✓ Another factor is **the amount of fat a carbohydrate contains**, as the more fat consumed with the carbohydrate, the slower the rate of entry into the bloodstream. As noted by Broda Barnes, M.D., *"There seems little doubt that a high-fat diet reduces the appetite through the slower release from the stomach of a fatty meal and by avoiding the excessive rise in blood sugar so common with carbohydrate intake"* (*Hypothyroidism, The Unsuspected Illness*, 1976, p. 267).

✓ **Sugar (or glucose)** is another factor, as is the particular form that sugar is found in. Different types of carbohydrates take different pathways in the body after digestion. The greater the amount of glucose it contains, the higher the glycemic index (the faster the rate of entry into the bloodstream). Conversely, the more fructose or lactose it contains, the lower the glycemic index. This is because both fructose and lactose are unable to enter the bloodstream without first being converted into glucose, which is a relatively slow process that takes place in the liver.

✓ And there is the issue of **mixed meals**. According to research done by Dr. Mary C. Gannon, Ph.D. at the University of Minnesota, *"Eating meals containing both carbohydrates and protein, rather than just carbohydrates alone, lowers the glycemic response in both normal individuals (nondiabetics) and subjects with Type II diabetes"* (Cheryle R Hart, M.D., *The Insulin-Resistance Diet*, 2001, p. 74). This is because the protein slows the rate at which the carbohydrates enter the bloodstream, thus the secretion of insulin is lower. Some carbohydrates, when eaten alone, without protein, fat or fiber to slow the rate of absorption, can top the glycemic index scale.

✓ **The degree of cooking and processing of food in general** is also a factor, which can often be rather difficult to evaluate. An article in *Diabetes Care* (March 1997, Vol. 20, No. 3), tells how the glycemic index (GI) values of some foods can vary markedly:

> *For example, there are many varieties of rice with different types of starch, processed in different ways that result in different GI values;* **the GI of 1-inch cubes of boiled potato can be increased by 25% by mashing them;** *subtle differences in banana ripeness can double its GI.*

Farmers soon discovered that hogs would not fatten when fed raw potatoes, but the opposite was true when they were cooked. Unfortunately, they seem to taste much better cooked.

Carrots are another example. Although they are commonly considered a high glycemic index item, according to Diana Schwarzbein, M.D. (*The Schwarzbein Principal*, 1999), when carrots are eaten raw, the intact fiber lowers their glycemic index to the point that they are not counted as a carbohydrate. However, once this fiber has been removed or broken down by either cooking or juicing, their glycemic index is considerably altered (raised).

Some foods, such as beans and other legumes, are bound by an outer layer of very complex starches, which increases the time it takes for them to be digested and turned into sugars, resulting in a lower glycemic index. However, the longer these foods are cooked, the more broken down that outer layer becomes, resulting in more rapid absorption.

We will be providing you with at least versions of the glycemic index, under Dietary Recommendations later in this chapter. Unfortunately, as noted they tend to vary, based on the source of information. I can only conclude that we have an idea, although not an entirely accurate evaluation of different foods' true glycemic index. How a food is grown, harvested, preserved, and prepared could all be influential factors.

The simple carbohydrates (devoid of nutrients) tend to be those with the highest glycemic index. For example, sugar that is normally at the top of the glycemic index has absolutely no minerals to metabolize itself. There is a considerable variation in the content of different minerals in foods, based on where, and how they were grown. For example, organically grown foods are much more nutrient dense than those grown commercially. The question is: Could that possibly influence not only their nutritional benefit, but also the foods' effective glycemic index? That might possibly be another explanation why the glycemic index tends to vary considerably at times, based on who provides it.

Just be aware that the food listed, along with their index, is basically a guide to follow (there are many varieties available on the internet). By avoiding the foods considered to be highest on the glycemic scale, and including more on the low end, you can more easily maintain a healthy blood sugar level, (as well as your weight). As you just learned, there are many factors that can come into play, which could easily influence your personal glucose response to any particular food. Also keep in mind that even stress can elevate your blood sugar, so avoid stress (especially during a meal). You can soon learn from experimentation and observation, how to most effectively control your blood sugar, and thus eventually eliminate your insulin resistance.

Dietary Recommendations For The Diabetic

The next step for anyone attempting to resolve their diabetes is a close examination of their diet. Eliminating simple sugars (especially fruit juices), as well as all starches (simple carbohydrates, white bread, pastries, rice, noodles, etc.), is an absolute must in order to effectively regulate your blood sugar.

Something else to consider regarding our diet, is that not only the food we eat, but also the way our body responds, can vary from person to person, and sometimes even from day to day. Some of us metabolize, or digest and assimilate foods more efficiently than others. How efficiently, would at least partially depend upon your stomach's ability to produce a sufficient amount of hydrochloric acid to digest proteins (which incidentally can be suppressed by acid blockers such as Zantac™). Then we also have the other digestive enzymes produced by the pancreas, which sometimes become less efficient as we age. Then our metabolism (thyroid function) will influence how efficiently all our enzymes function (including those involved in the digestion process).

Stress can also influence our blood sugar levels, causing them to vary from meal to meal. As you probably know by now, stress stimulates the secretion of glucose by the liver, which also produces a surge of insulin into the bloodstream. If a person is stressed during mealtime, it could result in an elevated level of blood sugar, although not the result of something just eaten. You can easily see why it is best to eat slowly and calmly, and avoid thinking or talking about anything stressful just before or during a meal. Try to make mealtime as relaxing as possible, in order to avoid unnecessary spikes in blood sugar and insulin production.

There are obviously many different variables that could quite easily influence your glycemic response to different foods. How well you assimilate the important nutrients in your food is also an important issue, and to a great degree something we can normally influence. Just eliminating microwave cooking, and avoiding foods inappropriate for your blood type, can quite easily improve the benefit you receive from the foods eaten. This of course should be our primary objective.

Apparently, the over-consumption of simple carbohydrates (high glycemic foods) appears to be the primary contributor to insulin resistance and diabetes. According to David Mendosa's Website (http://www.mendosa.com/wolever.htm), at least nine studies, considered well-designed, controlled, randomized trials, have been published regarding the use of a low-glycemic index diet and how it affects diabetics. In eight of the nine studies, when 127 diebetics were placed on **a low-glycemic index diet** for 2 weeks to 3 months, a significant improvement in blood glucose control was observed. Although the improvement was 10.2%, Mendosa further notes that:

Nevertheless, a 10% improvement in blood glucose control is about half that achieved in subjects with type I diabetes using intensified insulin therapy in the Diabetes Control and Complications Trial and is <u>equivalent to the effect of oral hypoglycemic agents or insulin in the treatment of type II diabetes.</u>

*The principle behind the GI [Glucose Index] is exactly the same of the x-glucosidase inhibitors [Acarbose], namely, reducing postprandial glucose responses **by reducing the rate of absorption of dietary carbohydrate.***

What We Should Eat and Why We Should Eat It

It is important to remember that everything you put into your mouth will affect insulin in some way, and all carbohydrates are definitely not created equal. Generally, it is the combination of fiber, proteins, and fats consumed during a meal, as well as the amount of each that will help reduce the elevation of the blood sugar and production of insulin.

✓ **Fiber** (also known as roughage) is the indigestible remnants of plant cells. Although it has no direct influence on insulin, as it is not broken down into sugar, it does influence how rapidly other carbohydrates are absorbed into the bloodstream. Fiber binds to carbohydrates and actually slows the rate of absorption of glucose into the system, controlling the glucose response, thus counteracting the negative effects associated with some carbohydrates. Consuming small amounts of fiber with everything you eat is an extremely effective way to manage insulin levels. According to researchers at UCLA, obese men were allowed to eat as much high-fiber, low-fat food as they wanted, combined with daily exercise, for **three weeks.** At the end of that time, they were still overweight, but *"their high blood pressure was* *reversed; cholesterol dropped 20%, <u>insulin levels dropped 46%.</u> No drug in the world can do this"* (Dr. Julian Whitaker, M.D., *Fearless Health*, pp. 29-30).

<u>Soluble fiber</u> dissolves in water and turns into gel during digestion, slowing sugar absorption from the intestines. Some soluble fibers include: pectin (found in apples, citrus fruits, legumes and certain vegetables), mucilage (found in oats and legumes), and gums.

<u>Insoluble fiber</u> does not dissolve in water, and is normally chewy. It appears to enhance the speed at which foods move through our stomachs and intestines, as well as adding bulk to the stool. Some insoluble fibers include cellulose (found in wheat bran), hemicellulose (found in whole grains and vegetables), and lignin (found in the walls of plant cells).

Although very few foods in the typical American diet provide two or more grams of soluble fiber per serving, it is possible to boost fiber levels slightly with certain raw vegetables (especially lima beans, Brussels sprouts, zucchini, and squash), fruits (especially cantaloupe, dried prunes, raisins, and papaya), seeds (especially flax), and oatmeal or oat bran. Unfortunately, the refining process removes much of the natural fiber from our foods, as well as their protective coating of fiber (as in the case of white rice).

Fiber supplements are also available. Following are a few, especially beneficial for the regulation of blood sugar fluctuations:

- *Glucomannan* is tasteless and odorless, making it an easy addition to foods. Glucomannan can expand to **sixty times** its own weight, so always be sure to drink a large glass of water when taking in capsule or pill form, as they can lodge in the throat and expand there, or result in bowel blockage.
- Guar gum is extracted from the seeds of the guar plant. The tablets must be chewed thoroughly or sucked gradually, not swallowed whole, and again should be taken with plenty of water due to the tendency to ball up in the throat when mixed with saliva.
- Lignin is a form of fiber normally found in Brazil nuts, carrots, green beans, peaches, peas, and tomatoes.
- Pectin is commonly found in apples, cabbage, and citrus fruits. I personally prefer apple pectin.

Fiber should be added to the diet slowly, and in relatively small amounts, allowing for digestive adjustments. **In order to successfully control severe insulin spikes associated with diabetes, it may be necessary to consume up to 50 grams of fiber dispersed throughout the day.** (You can get as much as 20 grams of fiber from ¼ cup of ground flax seeds!) Be sure not to take any fiber with fat-soluble vitamins (such as vitamins A, D, E, and K), as the fiber can absorb and remove them, and thus reduce their effectiveness. Excessive amounts of fiber may also decrease the absorption of zinc, iron, and calcium, thus it's best to take fiber separately from your supplements.

✓ **Protein.** Your body requires protein to repair damaged cells, or to replace them, as well as for replenishing enzymes. However, it is important to eat protein in moderation.

Protein can slow digestion and sugar absorption (as does fat and fiber), preventing insulin spikes after a meal, thus an important part of each meal. In fact, eating a small amount of protein with everything you eat can be very beneficial in maintaining stable blood sugar levels, as protein helps balance insulin. Studies have shown that people on a low protein diet commonly suffer from a selenium deficiency, which can result in hypothyroidism. And if you don't get enough protein from your diet, your body will rob it from your muscles and bones, (something we obviously must avoid).

Eggs are an excellent source of protein! In case you're the least bit concerned, although eggs do contain cholesterol, they will not increase your cholesterol level. Cholesterol is involved in many important functions, in both the body and brain. The more we include in our diet, the less the liver is required to make (normally about 80%). Our body will not produce something it doesn't require. It is also best to obtain at least some of your protein from other sources, such as nuts and vegetables, as well as fish and poultry.

However, too much protein (especially meat) can cause your body to become highly acidic (promoting the release of insulin), as well as increasing the need for additional thyroid hormone. But most importantly regarding blood sugar, in his book *The Rosedale Diet* (2004), Dr. Ron Rosedale, M.D. warns us:

> ***Protein that the body doesn't quickly use to repair or make new cells is largely broken down into simple sugars, which increases blood sugar and promotes insulin resistance.*** *Furthermore, protein itself triggers insulin production, which can worsen insulin resistance. (That is why* ***<u>diabetics should never go on a very high protein diet.</u>****)*
>
> *The more protein you eat, the more proficient you become at making glucose from the protein in your diet, and from the protein in your muscle and bone. As I tell my diabetic patients, this is something that you don't want to be good at!*
>
> ***Remember, you need to eat enough protein to replace and repair body parts, but not so much that you must burn off the excess as sugar, thus disrupting your metabolism*** (pp. 13, 23).

✓ **Good fats** not only prevent insulin receptors from becoming insulin resistant, but fat also slows digestion (as do fiber and protein), which reduces the absorption rate of sugar into the bloodstream, preventing insulin spikes after a meal.

"Good fats" are found in the omega-3 Essential Fatty Acids (EFAs), which include docosahexaenoic acid (DHA), eicosapentaenoic acid (EPA), gamma linolenic acid (GLA), and conjugated linoleic acid (CLA), and are also known as "good" polyunsaturated fats. Although the body cannot produce these fats, they can be found in cold water fatty fish, fish oil, flax seed oil, deep green vegetables, algae, and some nuts. It is important to be aware that there are numerous dietary and lifestyle factors that can decrease and even eliminate any potential benefits that may be obtained through consuming EFAs. Some examples are the consumption of sugar, alcohol, and trans (bad) fats, as well as a lack of vitamins and minerals (often depleted by medications).

EFAs perform like hormones in the body, lowering insulin resistance as well as building and maintaining healthy receptors. In fact, some scientists actually feel that diabetics may suffer in part from an EFA deficiency. Researchers from Purdue and Pennsylvania State universities found that CLA can prevent the onset of diabetes in laboratory animals, appearing to work as well as the diabetes-fighting drugs, the **thiazolidinediones**, (TZDs). Martha Belury, Assistant Professor of Foods and Nutrition and Purdue University tells us, *"If you inherit a genetic predisposition to adult-onset diabetes and you're obese and inactive, then you may well develop this disease.* ***Our study suggests that <u>CLA may help normalize or reduce blood glucose levels and prevent diabetes</u>"*** (http://www.diet-and-health.net/Supplements/CLA.html).

Other good fats are monounsaturated (omega-9) fatty acids (primarily found in olive oil, avocado, and nuts), as well other <u>healthy</u> saturated fats normally found in salmon, walnuts, olives, lamb and goat meat, goat's and sheep's milk and cheese, and other properly prepared dairy products. Saturated fats tend to be solid at room temperature, and are normally found in tropical oils such as **processed** coconut, palm and palm kernel oils. .

You should be aware that when EFAs are heated, their bonds change and they soon become trans fatty acids. Regardless of whether they started out good or not, they are irrevocably changed for the worse when heated, thus they should obviously not be used for cooking. There was one study published in an article in the June 2001 issue of *The American Journal of Clinical Nutrition*, stated that **eating too much saturated fat can worsen insulin resistance.** Unfortunately, it was not quite announced correctly, leaving the public with the wrong impression. Apparently these studies were done on **hydrogenated coconut oil.** If you recall, all hydrogenated oils produce the dangerous trans fatty acids, whether they are saturated or not. This is because hydrogenated oils are made by heating vegetable oils in the presence of metal catalysts and hydrogen, and whether they are hydrogenated or partially hydrogenated simply refers to the amount of hydrogen used in the process. Whether an oil is healthy or unhealthy depends not only on the source, but also how it was extracted and processed, which is especially true regarding coconut oil.

Extra virgin coconut oil is an excellent choice. In 1947, B. A. Houssay found that **the most protective diet against diabetes was based on coconut oil, as it provides energy to stabilize blood sugar, while protecting the thyroid system from the harmful effects of unsaturated fats** (http://www.thyroid-info.com/articles/ray-peat.htm).

Butter is a good source of fat-soluble vitamins, rich in lecithin, trace minerals, and essential fatty acids. Studies have shown that vitamins and minerals from vegetables are better absorbed when eaten with butter. However, it is best to choose butter produced from the milk of grass-fed animals free from growth hormones.

Another dairy product, milk, is quite a different story. Today's non-organic pasteurized milk that most people drink comes from cows that have been fed hormones and antibiotics, and comes from the grocery store where it is three to four weeks old. Today's commonly consumed milk no longer contains the good bacteria, the good enzymes, vitamins, minerals, or good fats that raw fresh unpasteurized milk contains.

Keep in mind that non-fat products (especially dairy) are naturally a bit higher on the glycemic index because they have had the fat removed (the fat is what slows the rate of digestion, and sugar absorption into the bloodstream).

✓ **Eat plenty of flax**. Flax seeds are both a rich source of omega-3 fatty acids (as they contain flax seed oil), as well as a good source of fiber. Flax seeds in bulk are very inexpensive. You can normally purchase a grinder for approximately $20. Just grind and take a couple tablespoons with 8 ounces of water prior to a meal. Another option might be adding a tablespoon or two of flax seeds ground into your soups, salads, or recipes. Flax seed is an easy, effective, and inexpensive way to bring more balance to blood sugar levels.

Flax seeds oxidize fairly rapidly when exposed to light or oxygen, once the seed is ground and the oil is released. Thus either grind it just before you use it, or store the ground seeds in a dark container in the refrigerator.

Flax seed oil is another option. The oil must be kept refrigerated and will stay fresh for up to 8 weeks after it is opened, or it can safely be kept frozen for at least a year. Never expose flax oil to direct heat, as it contains EFAs and will become trans fatty acids. However, flax oil works well as a salad dressing base, or added to hot cereal, soup, sauces, or dips as well. It can also be taken as a supplement in the soft gel form, if you prefer.

✓ **Raw vegetables** are generally very low on the glycemic index, as well as an excellent source of fiber. It is important to remember that cooking changes everything! Heat breaks down the fiber, changing the quality of the vegetable to a more readily available carbohydrate, thus raising the glycemic index.

Some examples of vegetables with the very lowest glycemic index are: asparagus, artichoke, cucumber, fennel, lettuce, bell peppers, tomatoes, avocados, green beans, broccoli, cabbage, kale, collards, parsley, cilantro and cauliflower.

✓ **Fresh fruit.** The body can more efficiently utilize fruit in its natural state: FRESH. There is considerably less nutritional benefit from eating processed fruit or fruit that has been altered by heat in any way. This includes canned fruit, cooked applesauce, baked apples, etc. Remember, heat breaks down the fiber in foods, necessary for controlling blood sugar levels, raising the glycemic index considerably. Cooking also alters the fruit's pH balance, leaving them more acidic, which increases insulin production.

✓ **Ezekiel 4:9™ bread** is made of sprouted organically grown grains and legumes, sea salt, water and yeast, with no added flour, and should thus be extremely low on the glycemic index. It can sometimes be found in the freezer section of your local grocery store. If not, you can call the makers, Food For Life Baking Company, at (800) 797-5090 for a location nearest you, or visit their Website at http://www.food-for-life.com/. Ezekiel 4:9™ Flourless Organic Sprouted Grain bread is the only bread I am aware of that is a complete protein, which by itself should assist in maintaining blood sugar levels. It contains 18 amino acids, including all nine essential amino acids, as well as fiber. In order to maintain freshness, it should remain frozen until eaten.

   ✓ **Eat less, more often.** A study in the *New England Journal of Medicine* reported that **frequent eaters were able to reduce insulin levels nearly 28% in only two weeks,** just by <u>dividing their meals</u> into 17 snacks per day (<u>instead of 3 large meals</u> per day), and with no change in calories or the percentages of protein, fat or carbohydrates consumed. Although this study proves a point, it's obviously not practical. Even if we ate all day, from 8:00am to 8:00pm, we would have to eat about every 45 minutes. Just don't skip meals, and eat healthy snacks, such as almonds, raw carrots, or celery between meals to help maintain healthy blood sugar levels. That is also a healthy way to lose weight. Just make sure your snacks are small and healthy.

Foods' Insulin-Producing Potential

   Considering the many variables responsible for influencing a person's individual insulin response, you might consider testing each food for yourself. See how your body responds to each, depending on your particular blood type, or the condition of your digestive system, etc.

   The following food list (obtained from Broda Barnes, M.D., *Hypothyroidism, The Unsuspected Illness*, 1976) should be a helpful guide, regarding each food's potential impact on your blood sugar levels. The more foods included in the 5 percent (low) range, the easier it will be to maintain a proper blood sugar level. Keep into consideration that as fruits ripen, their sugar content often increases, (that's especially true regarding bananas).

Percentages of Carbohydrates in Vegetables and Fruits

5 Percent Vegetables

* Asparagus	* Broccoli	* Cabbage
* Cauliflower	* Celery	* Cucumber
* Greens (beets)	* Lettuce	* Olives (ripe)
* Peppers	* Pumpkin	* Spinach
* String beans	* Tomatoes	* Summer squash

5 Percent Fruits

* Avocado	* Muskmelon	* Honeydew Melon
* Strawberries	* Watermelon	

10 Percent Vegetables

* Carrots	* Onions	* Winter squash

10 Percent Fruits

* Blackberries	* Oranges	* Peaches

15 Percent Vegetables

* Artichokes	* Peas

15 Percent Fruits

* Apples	* Apricots	* Blueberries
* Huckleberries	* Grapes	* Raspberries
* Pears	* Pineapple	* Plums

20 Percent Vegetables

* Corn or Hominy	* Potatoes	* Beans (kidney, lima, navy)

20 Percent Fruits

* Bananas	* Figs (fresh)	* Cherries (sweet)
* Grape juice	* Prunes (fresh)	

One Version of A Glycemic Index Rating Scale

As previously mentioned, glycemic index ratings can vary greatly from one source to another, and there are many factors to consider such as where and how the foods were grown, how they were prepared, as well as who they might have been tested on. However, following is a different rating of foods (by their glycemic index), according to James F. Balch, M.D., (*Thinner in 30 Days*, 2002, pp. 5-6):

Extremely High (greater than 100)

- Grain-based foods (puffed rice, cornflakes, instant rice, instant potatoes, French bread)
- Vegetables (baked russet potatoes, cooked carrots)
- Simple Sugars (maltose, glucose, honey)

High (80-100)

- Grain-based foods (white bread, whole wheat, grape nuts, corn tortilla, shredded wheat, brown rice, sweet corn, white rice)
- Vegetables (mashed potato, boiled potato)
- Simple Sugars (sucrose)
- Fruits (apricots, raisins, banana)
- Snacks (corn chips, crackers, cookies, pastry, low fat ice cream)

Moderately High (60-80)

- Grain-based foods (all bran, rye bread, white macaroni, white or brown spaghetti)
- Vegetables (yams, sweet potato, frozen green peas, canned baked beans, canned kidney beans)
- Fruits (fruit cocktail, orange juice, pineapple juice, canned pears, grapes)
- Snacks (oatmeal cookies, potato chips)

Moderate (40-60)

- Vegetables (tomato soup, lima beans, black-eyed peas, garbanzo beans)
- Fruits (oranges, apple juice, apple, pear)
- Dairy (yogurt, high fat ice cream, whole or 2% milk, skim milk)

Low (less than 40)

- Grain-based foods (barley)
- Fruits (peaches, plums)
- Simple Sugars (fructose)

Summary - What To Avoid

✓ **Sugar and simple carbohydrates.** As stated by Dr. Ron Rosedale, M.D. (*The Rosedale Diet*, 2004), ***"A bowl of cereal is a bowl of sugar, a slice of bread (with few exceptions) is a slice of sugar, and a potato is a big lump of sugar.*** *Unfortunately, these are the foods that have become the mainstay of the American diet"* (p. 77).

✓ **Bad fats (trans-fatty acids) and fried foods.**

✓ **An acidic diet**.

✓ **Overcooking your food.** Heat changes everything, and not for the better.
- When food is overcooked, fiber is lost, changing the quality of the food and allowing it to be more quickly absorbed into the bloodstream. Thus, the glycemic index of the food rises, (sometimes dramatically).
- The following important nutrients are depleted by heat and cooking: Vitamin B_1 (thiamine), vitamin B_5, vitamin B_6, folic acid, vitamin C, vitamin D, vitamin E, and bioflavonoids.
- Overcooking food can cause it to become acidic, which promotes excessive insulin production, leading to insulin resistance.
- And, overcooking food destroys the natural digestive enzymes, making digestion more difficult.

✓ **Microwave cooking**. The very worst form of cooking for nutrient depletion, as well as changing the natural structure of not only foods, but also water (which is also important).

✓ **Alcohol**. It is a carbohydrate, derived from grain or fruit or both, which are all forms of sugar. After the initial sugar rush (which rapidly raises insulin levels), extremely low blood sugar levels soon follow, resulting in hypoglycemia, as well as depleting many important nutrients.

✓ **Caffeine** – Found in coffee and caffeinated soft drinks, as well as both chocolate and some pain relievers (i.e. Excedrin™).

✓ **Limit grains.** According to an article in *The McAlvany Health Alert* (Jan 2004), **eighty-five percent of the grains we consume are refined (meaning the healthy fiber and nutrients have been removed) before they ever reach our plate.** The *"enriched grains"* that most people consume in processed food, not only contribute to insulin resistance, but they also deplete vitamins, especially the B vitamins.

CHAPTER TWENTY-TWO
RESOURCES FOR STABILIZING BLOOD SUGAR

As you can see, there is overwhelming evidence, provided by sufficient research, that substantiates the importance of reducing as many simple carbohydrates, such as sweets, pastas, and breads, as possible, and then introduce more vegetables, lean proteins, and "good fats" instead. This will go a long way toward maintaining healthy blood sugar and insulin levels. However, you may find additional supplementation extremely beneficial. Hopefully I won't overwhelm you by giving you too many options of supplements found to be beneficial for both lowering and maintaining healthy blood sugar levels, and overcoming insulin resistance. Just remember, I am providing you with different options (you don't have to take them all!).

Before attempting to resolve your diabetes, it is important to first address any thyroid issues, as they are so closely related and often experienced simultaneously. At least two different doctors found that diabetic complications disappeared when a natural thyroid hormone was administered to their patients. You may want to refer to the Hypothyroidism Chapter earlier in this book, for an in-depth discussion.

Keep in mind that we are all biologically unique, thus absolutely no one can say exactly what might work the best for you. That is something you can evaluate much better than anyone else, as your body is the very best laboratory, (so experiment). Try different foods and supplements, then evaluate how you feel, and monitor your blood sugar levels, to see how you personally are responding. Once you have determined what works the best for you, you can then stop experimenting, and follow your customized program. This can actually be a fun and very enlightening adventure, as well as a challenge to optimize and maintain healthy blood sugar levels.

Remember that although I can tell you which supplements are normally beneficial for maintaining normal blood sugar, the choice of which ones, as well as just how much of each, is a personal issue, as the most appropriate dosage tends to vary between individuals. For instance, if you are also taking medications, you will likely need more nutrients to replace those depleted. Unless you do a considerable amount of research (as I did), you won't know which nutrients are actually being depleted by your medications. As we discovered, even that amount could vary considerably, as it depends upon just how much of each drug you actually absorb. That is why getting off your medications should be your primary objective, so you can better regulate your nutrient levels. How efficient your metabolism is, and how well you digest and assimilate foods, also play a part.

Even your genetics can come into play in determining how much of a particular supplement might be appropriate for you personally. Doctors discovered years ago that one person might easily require several times as much of a particular nutrient as another might. It is likely at least partially associated with genetics. As you can see, there are many different variables involved. For instance, rats can manufacture their own vitamin C. They accomplish that task by converting glucose (sugar) to vitamin C through enzyme action. Would you believe vitamin C (ascorbic acid) is actually produced from sugar? Four hydrogen molecules are removed during a chemical process. Incidentally, rats produce as much as ten times as much vitamin C during stress, or following an injury. It was discovered from research that our body actually requires more vitamin C during the very same conditions.

It would certainly be helpful in regulating our blood sugar if we could do the same. Interestingly, according to Dr. Robert D. Milne, M.D., we just happen to have every single enzyme necessary for converting glucose into vitamin C (with one exception). Unfortunately, we are unable to produce one enzyme called Gulonolactone oxidase (GLO), necessary for completing the process. Although the human genome actually contains a gene capable of creating GLO, it is for some unexplainable reason not expressed in humans (*PC Liposomal Encapsulation Technology*, 2004, pp. 78-79). Attempting to solve this particular issue is one of my long-term goals. But first, let's concentrate on the issue at hand: Effectively stabilizing your blood sugar.

You should keep in mind **that if you are currently taking insulin or medication for lowering your blood sugar, you should carefully monitor your blood sugar level fairly often.** If you eat a proper diet and begin incorporating supplements to help reduce your insulin resistance, you should be able to gradually eliminate your blood sugar lowering medications. And don't forget, failure to compensate could result in hypoglycemia (too low blood sugar). Those on insulin sometimes find they can lower, or possibly even totally eliminate their insulin use. You will soon learn how **one woman went from 60 units of insulin (30 units, twice daily), to only 5 units daily!** She was actually able to maintain a normal level of blood sugar at **one-twelfth the dosage** that she had been taking. As the level of insulin is reduced, so is the cells' resistance to insulin. Not only is elevated insulin the underlying cause of insulin resistance, but also terribly destructive to the body in many ways.

We will now evaluate yet one more example of how the traditional approach to medicine is often not only worsening the condition being treated, but also creating others in the process, as well as providing many other natural alternatives.

1. **Mangosteen.** In his booklet *Mangosteen's Healing Secrets Revealed* (2003), Dr. Kenneth J. Finsand tells how the very first person he gave the mangosteen to was a 42-year-old Hispanic mother, with a husband and children still living at home, who was losing her eyesight due to diabetes, and suffered from neuropathy in the legs. According to her husband, **she had been receiving 30 units of insulin, twice daily,** although she had been continuing to worsen over the last few years. Dr. Finsand suggested drinking mangosteen, in addition to her current medications, and shares the following experience:

> [The husband] *tested her, and even though she had taken her first 30 units of insulin that morning, she had a blood sugar of 351, which is very high. The husband then asked her to* **drink two ounces of the juice,** *which generally if it had of been any other juice, it would have made her blood glucose rise. They tested her blood sugar levels* **a half-hour later** *and to their great delight* **her blood sugar had dropped from 351 to 150!**
>
> *One week later the husband returned to my office to tell the story and say that not only did his wife experience the drop in her blood sugar,* **she was able to cut her insulin usage dramatically.** *They continued to follow this procedure, and to date* **she is now using only five units of insulin a day,** *and she is able to keep her blood sugar at a normal level.*
>
> *I might mention that I did not tell her or her husband to cut her insulin usage down. They chose to find an alternative route on their own* (pp. 30-31).

Dr. Finsand goes on to explain that **one important amino acid helped by mangosteen is Methionine,** and notes that, *"This is extremely important, because it is through this pathway that* **the xanthones of the mangosteen are able to rid the body of diabetes so quickly in many cases.** *Impairments of methionine can result in many disorders"* (p. 27).

The essential amino acid **methionine is a precursor of the amino acids glutathione, cysteine and Taurine.** Glutathione is a powerful antioxidant that assists the immune system and slows the aging process, while **Cysteine helps in the formation of insulin. Taurine is** the building block for all the other amino acids, and is **beneficial for people with hypoglycemia, as well as hypertension.** You will learn more on the benefit of some amino acids shortly, however due to the important part that methionine appears to play in regard to mangosteen and diabetes, it makes adequate methylation a very important issue. "Methylation" is a process that will convert the rogue amino acid known as homocysteine (a well-known cardiovascular risk factor) into the very beneficial amino acid methionine.

Although homocysteine can be a serious concern (even regarding potential damage to the brain neurons), it can be easily controlled through methylation. A good vitamin B-complex formula, which includes vitamins B_6, B_{12}, and folic acid, should normally be sufficient **(unless you are taking drugs known to deplete them).** You will also learn how to resolve this issue with another supplement called tri-methyl glycine (TMG) next. If you refer to the B-vitamins listed later in this chapter (or in the Reference

Guide to Supplements provided at the end of this book), you will discover that most drugs deplete at least one B-vitamin (usually more), which could easily undermine your effort.

Incidentally, there is one more pathway for methylation, other than the conversion of homocysteine (with vitamins B_6, B_{12}, and folic acid) to methionine, and it involves vitamin B_6 only. This alternate pathway converts homocysteine into cysteine, rather than methionine. Although it would effectively eliminate elevated homocysteine, it is actually more limited as far as the potential benefits are concerned. However, if you just happen to be deficient in cysteine, the B_6 route would be the most direct approach, as it would eliminate the extra step of converting methionine into cysteine. As methionine is not only a precursor to cysteine, but also both Taurine and glutathione, it could potentially provide additional benefits. It's best to supply an adequate level of all three, and allow our body to choose the best approach (something it is very good at). As I often state, just provide an adequate supply of nutrients, and your body can very efficiently take care of the details. Unfortunately, medications not only deplete the necessary nutrients, but also intervene, and thus disrupt many normal processes (with their inhibiting actions), basically fighting our body's efforts every step of the way.

The reason I placed mangosteen at the top of my list is:
- It doesn't interact with medications.
- As you can see, it appears to be very effective at stabilizing blood sugar.
- It's perfectly safe for everyone, even nursing mothers and small children.
- Mangosteen, (with its 43 xanthones), has a very broad range of benefits throughout the body, as Dr. Templeman discovered in his practice.

2. **Goji** has been used in China for the treatment of adult-onset diabetes for many years. Its polysaccharides have been shown to help balance blood sugar and insulin response. In his first clinical trials, Dr. Victor Marcial-Vega, M.D., researcher on the effects of goji juice for years, discovered that *"blood sugar levels decrease in 64 percent of the patients with diabetes, and more than half of them decreased or eliminated their medications."* One personal experience follows:

> *I was taking 14 medications, and never anticipated the quality of my life improving. My blood sugar numbers were running in the 280s – the lowest would be approximately 250.* **After the tenth day of drinking goji juice, my blood sugar was 118, and that was not in a fasting environment, and was without any of the 14 medications that I would normally be taking.** *I'm a goji-for-life person. I can't imagine taking it out of my daily routine. -Max V., Queen Creek, Arizona*
> (*Breakthroughs In Health*, August 2006, Vol. 1, issue 1, p. 127)

3. **TMG** (**t**ri-**m**ethyl **g**lycine), an extraction of the sugar beet, is another option for methylation. I personally would recommend both a good vitamin B-complex and TMG (especially if you are taking any medications), as TMG is relatively inexpensive. Something interesting about TMG is, once it gives up a methyl donor to convert homocysteine into methionine, it then becomes **d**i-**m**ethyl **g**lycine (DMG), which itself has multiple benefits. DMG is an energy molecule the Russians gave their athletes to improve their performance (just one more benefit). **Di-methyl glycine also helps to normalize blood glucose levels,** and has been found to enhance the immune system.

Incidentally, if you also suffer from depression, then any excess TMG can be combined with the energy molecule ATP (**a**denosine **t**ri**p**hosphate) to produce SAMe, which has proven very beneficial for depression. TMG is a very versatile supplement, which I take daily (two 500 mg tablets). SAMe can also be purchased as a supplement, and for depression it appears to work even better than TMG, although it is considerably more expensive. So if you are not depressed, I would recommend TMG as an effective way to insure the methylation of homocysteine into the very beneficial amino acid methionine efficiently takes place.

4. **Chromium picolinate** appears to be the most efficient form of the mineral chromium, which is chelated with picolinate, a naturally occurring amino acid metabolite. It helps maintain more stable blood

sugar levels by promoting more efficient insulin utilization, and it helps insulin to more efficiently remove sugar from the blood and nourish the cells as intended. It is especially beneficial for anyone with diabetes or hypoglycemia.

Although chromium is responsible for the regulation of sugar, high consumption of sugar depletes chromium. And unfortunately, when you are deficient in chromium, you are more inclined crave sweets. Considering approximately 90 percent of the adult population has a chromium deficiency, which worsens each time we eat sugar, and the fact that chromium levels naturally decrease as we age, you can easily see how glucose intolerance and decreased insulin sensitivity is so prevalent.

According to one four-month double-blind study reported in *Diabetes,* **chromium picolinate significantly improved blood sugar levels in type 2 diabetics** (*American Journal of Clinical Nutrition*; 2001, Vol. 73, 753-8). Participants took 1,000 mcg of chromium picolinate per day. That is the dosage I would also recommend with diabetics. You will also find that chromium picolinate is inexpensive and readily available. It is normally found in 200 mcg capsules.

5. **Vanadyl sulfate**, a more effective form of vanadium, is an **"insulin mimic"**. In fact, **it mimics almost all known bioeffects of insulin, including the important action of transporting glucose into muscle and fat cells.** One study showed that **vanadyl sulfate could stimulate glucose uptake in cells that had lost 60 percent of their insulin receptors and were, thus insulin resistant** (*Nature's RX for Diabetes*, Balch, 2002, p. 8). Some symptoms of a vanadium deficiency include diabetes, hypoglycemia, metabolic dysfunction, and obesity. I would recommend 30 mg daily.

6. **Cinnamon** helps regulate the amount of sugars extracted from carbohydrates in the bloodstream. **Not only does cinnamon activate essential enzymes in the body thus stimulating the receptors in the cells so they will respond more efficiently to insulin, but it also inhibits the enzymes responsible for deactivating the insulin receptors, causing insulin resistance.** Cinnamon bark actually contains calcium, chromium, copper, iodine, iron, manganese, phosphorus, potassium, zinc, and vitamins A, B_1, B_2, and C, many of which are important for the prevention or treatment of diabetes. Cinnamon in capsules is also available.

Researchers from the U.S. Department of Agriculture, and Agricultural University, Peshawar, Pakistan, found that less than one-teaspoon (one gram) of cinnamon worked just as well as higher doses, at reducing blood glucose levels 20 percent on some 60 volunteers. They also found that blood sugar levels started rising when the volunteers stopped eating cinnamon (http://care.diabetesjournals.org/cgi/content/abstract/26/12/3215).

7. **Amino Acids.** Although there are nearly 30 commonly known amino acids that combine in hundreds of various ways to benefit the body, following are some that are more beneficial for maintaining blood sugar levels and insulin:

- **Alanine** – Aids in the metabolism of glucose and helps regulate blood sugar levels. Alanine levels parallel blood sugar levels in both diabetes and hypoglycemia, and alanine reduces both severe hypoglycemia and the ketosis of diabetes. As noted in the *Prescription for Nutritional Healing, 3rd edition,* (Balch & Balch, 2000), *"Research has found that for people with insulin-dependent diabetes, taking an oral dose of L-alanine can be more effective than a conventional bedtime snack in preventing nighttime hypoglycemia"* (p. 44).
- **Arginine** – Insulin production and glucose tolerance can be impaired if the body is deficient in arginine.
- **Carnitine** –Stabilizes blood glucose levels, as well as preventing nerve disease associated with diabetes. A deficiency can produce impaired glucose control and obesity.
- **Cysteine** – Helps in the formation of insulin.
- **Glutamic acid** – Aids in the metabolism of sugars and fats, and is used in the treatment of hypoglycemic coma, commonly a complication of insulin treatment for diabetes. The brain can use glutamic acid as fuel, as it is converted into glutamine, and visa versa.

- **Glutamine** – Can be used as fuel in the brain, instead of sugar, thus preventing hypoglycemia. Also assists in maintaining proper pH balance in the body. I would recommend additional supplements, to equal a total consumption of 2,000 mg daily.
- **Glycine** – Improves glycogen storage, thus making glucose available for energy needs.
- **Isoleucine** – Stabilizes and regulates blood sugar and energy levels. A deficiency can produce symptoms similar to those of hypoglycemia.
- **Leucine** – Lowers elevated blood sugar levels so effectively that it must be taken in moderation to avoid symptoms of hypoglycemia.
- **Methionine** – A precursor of the amino acids glutathione, cysteine and Taurine. Glutathione is a powerful antioxidant that assists the immune system and slows the aging process, while cysteine helps in the formation of insulin. Taurine is the building block for all the other amino acids, and is beneficial for people with hypoglycemia.
- **Taurine** – Diabetes increases the body's requirements for Taurine.

Rather than trying to take each amino acid individually, it may be more convenient to take a formula that contains a majority of the amino acids. Goji juice conveniently contains 19 amino acids, including the 8 essential amino acids, (as well as 21 trace minerals and many other nutrients). You can always take additional amounts of any particular amino acid, however it is also best to take a full amino acid complex, although at a different time, and both should be taken on an empty stomach (30 minutes before a meal, or 2 hours after). If an individual amino acid was taken with proteins in a meal, it could possibly be combined, and used for something other that the intended use.

Although there are various amino acid formulas available, one example is the Rockland Corporation's "Amino 1000" formula, which is a balanced blend of the following 20 essential and non-essential amino acids:

* L-Alanine	* L-Arginine	* L-Aspartic acid	* L-Carnitine
* L-Cysteine	* L-Glutamic acid	* L-Glycine	* L-Histidine
* L-Isoleucine	* L-Leucine	* L-Lysine	* L-Methionine
* L-Ornithine	* L-Phenylalanine	* L-Proline	* L-Serine
* L-Threonine	* L-Tryptophan	* L-Tyrosine	* L-Valine

Our body normally breaks down proteins into the individual amino acids, and then assembles them into different combinations (requiring enzyme action) for their many various uses in the body. If your digestion of proteins is in any way compromised, you could possibly be deficient, and if so supplementation might be advisable. Both strict vegetarians (vegans), and those with blood type "A", are often more prone to be deficient. A vegan diet excludes the best sources of complete proteins (meat and eggs). Then those with blood type "A" don't produce an adequate level of hydrochloric acid to efficiently digest most meat. As a result, both are also inclined to be deficient in vitamin B_{12}, so extra supplementation might also be advisable. As vitamin B_{12} is the most difficult of the B vitamins to absorb, the lozenges (1 mg) absorbed sublingually (under the tongue) should be more effective. Some people tend to respond better to vitamin B_{12} injections every two weeks (that is especially true regarding the elderly).

8. **Additional nutrients** important for regulating blood sugar, are as follows:
   Vitamins:
   ✓ **Vitamin B-complex** – I would recommend that everyone take a good vitamin B-100 complex. A vitamin B_6 deficiency is more common in those with diabetes or hypoglycemia, thus I would recommend they also take an additional 100 mg of vitamin B_6. It is involved in more important actions than any other B vitamin, and our level also tends to decrease as we age.
   ✓ **Vitamin C** is something we all need, although diabetics need it most. If you smoke, you need it even more, as smoking is well known for depleting vitamin C. Vitamin C reduces the cravings for both sugar and alcohol, and is calming to the nervous system. It is especially

important for repairing damage to the epitheal (smooth muscle) cells in the vascular system, caused by both elevated blood sugar and insulin.

Although the ascorbic acid form of vitamin C is acidic, ester-C is not, and the body also utilizes it more efficiently. The best form of ester-C also includes bioflavonoids, which help strengthen the arteries and capillaries. Vitamin C is a molecule similar to sugar, and thus insulin can escort both into the cells. Just give insulin more vitamin C and less sugar. By doing so you will begin repairing, rather than damaging your arteries.

If you are a non-smoker, and a non-diabetic, 1,000 mg twice daily should normally be adequate. If you are coming down with a virus, or just had an injury or surgery, I would recommend 10,000 mg in divided doses daily. I would recommend 5,000 mg in divided doses for a diabetic.

✓ **Biotin** – Enhances glucose utilization and is beneficial in diabetic neuropathy. **A deficiency can produce high blood sugar.** Although 100 mcg – 200 mcg of biotin is usually included in most B-complex formulas, according to *The Life Extension Foundation's Disease Prevention and Treatment, Expanded Fourth Edition* (1997/2003), the recommended diabetic dosage is considerably higher, at 8,000 mcg – 16,000 mcg daily. That is equal to 8 mg – 16 mg (1,000 mcg = 1 mg).

✓ **Vitamin D** – **Reduces insulin resistance**, as well as protecting against cataracts. A deficiency increases insulin resistance. Vitamin D also enhances the immune system. I would recommend 400 IU in the summer, and 800 IU in the winter, as our body produces vitamin D when we are exposed to the sunlight.

✓ **Vitamin E** – **Improves insulin sensitivity, and reduces blood glucose levels, often lessening insulin requirements.** It also reduces the risk of heart attack. I would recommend 800 IU daily.

✓ **Vitamin K** – Assists in converting glucose to glycogen for storage in the liver, and enhances the immune system. **A deficiency interferes with insulin release and glucose regulation.** Vitamin K also helps prevent calcification (hardening) of the arteries, as well as osteoporosis. I would recommend 10 mg daily.

Minerals:

✓ **Magnesium** – Necessary for maintaining the body's proper pH balance, as well as **maintaining stable blood sugar levels. A magnesium deficiency is often mistaken as diabetes.** Magnesium is a very important mineral, involved in 300 different enzyme actions in the body. I would recommend approximately 750 mg daily.

✓ **Manganese** – **Necessary for blood sugar regulation,** and enhances the immune system. **A deficiency can produce abnormalities in insulin secretion and impaired glucose metabolism.** 10 mg daily should normally be adequate.

✓ **Potassium** – Necessary for maintaining the body's proper pH balance. **One symptom of a potassium deficiency is diabetes.** 100 mg daily would be beneficial.

✓ **Zinc** – **Improves insulin action, and is actually one element of insulin.** Some symptoms of zinc deficiency include diabetes, obesity, and thyroid disorders. I would recommend taking 50 mg daily, (just don't exceed 100 mg).

Coenzyme: CoQ$_{10}$ – **Has proven beneficial in the treatment of diabetes, as it stabilizes blood sugar and improves circulation. A deficiency has been linked to diabetes.** I would recommend 100 mg daily. However, if you have been taking statin drugs or any other medications known to deplete this important nutrient, I would suggest taking 200 mg daily, at least for a few months. CoQ$_{10}$ also has tremendous cardiovascular benefits, and is especially beneficial for the heart.

9. *Gymnema sylvestre.* **An extract of *gymnema* leaves helps reduce blood sugar levels in those with type II diabetes.** According to studies performed at the Mayo Clinic, it appears that the

higher the initial blood sugar level, the greater the drop will be, with as much as 55% in some cases (*Journal of Ethnopharmacology*; 10(3):295-305). **Gymnema has also produced an increase in the number of beta (insulin-producing) cells in the pancreas in animal studies.** And it reduces sugar cravings in humans by blocking the taste of sugar. I would recommend 4 grams of powdered leaves as an extract or tea. **By creating more beta cells in the pancreas, *gymnema* could potentially reduce, or possibly even eliminate the need for insulin injections.** It appears that inflammation of the pancreas could also contribute to the problem (that is where goji and mangosteen would both be very beneficial).

10. **Fenugreek is an herb that slows the absorption of glucose into the bloodstream,** reducing and normalizing blood sugar levels with no side effects, and without affecting people with normal blood sugar levels. In fact, **it appears that the higher the blood sugar is, the more Fenugreek reduces it.** At the National Institute of Nutrition, Dr. R. D. Sharma reported that in clinical tests, Fenugreek reduces glucose excretion in urine by up to 54%, while also noting that none of the participants experienced low blood sugar levels. It also increases the levels of glutathione and vitamin C in the body, two important antioxidants, as well as helping to balance cholesterol. It is available in both powder and capsule form. I would recommend 2 grams (2,000 mg), three times daily with meals.

11. **Alpha-Lipoic Acid (ALA) is a universal antioxidant that has been used for nearly thirty years in Europe for controlling blood sugar levels.** It is also beneficial for treating and preventing peripheral nerve damage in people with diabetes. It enhances the utilization of glucose, as well as the utilization of other nutrients such as CoQ_{10} and vitamins C and E. I would recommend taking 1,000 mg daily

12. **Essential Fatty Acids (EFAs) – Ground Flax Seed, Flax Seed Oil, or Fish Oil.** Ground flax seeds are a good source of both fiber and flax seed oil, with many additional nutritional benefits. Fiber reduces the rate of digestion, thus slowing the absorption of sugar into the bloodstream, and preventing spikes in both blood sugar and insulin. Flax seeds in bulk are very inexpensive, and grinders are relatively inexpensive also. Refer to the Dietary Recommendation for additional information regarding flax.

Flax seed oil is another option, as it normally converts to DHA in the body. EFAs in **flax seed oil and fish oil help build healthy cell walls and receptors. This is one approach of reducing insulin resistance.** It is also beneficial for building receptors in the brain, and is thus beneficial for reducing depression. Fish oil appears to be the most beneficial regarding the brain. I personally take four 1,000 mg soft gels of flax seed oil, along with two 1,000 mg soft gels of fish oil daily. Both flax seed oil and fish oil are also available in the liquid form, so the choice is up to you. Both cod liver oil and salmon oil are beneficial.

13. **DHEA** (dehydroepiandrosterone) is a precursor to other hormones, and is the most abundant hormone found in the bloodstream. Unfortunately, DHEA decreases as we age. **It has been shown to reverse diabetes, aid in glucose regulation, and actually promote the regeneration of beta cells**, as well as prevent heart disease. Possibly both *Gymnema* and DHEA might help the beta cells in type I diabetics begin producing insulin, and thus eliminate the need for insulin injections. I would recommend taking 50 mg of DHEA in the morning.

14. **Vinegar.** Taking two tablespoons of vinegar prior to eating can considerably reduce insulin and glucose spikes in the blood that often occur following a meal. According to one study, reported in the January 2004 issue of *Diabetes Care*, blood-glucose levels were improved by 25 percent. Researchers noted that ***"Vinegar had an effect on volunteers' blood comparable to what might be expected from antidiabetes drugs, such as metformin."***

Vinegar also acts much like hydrochloric acid (HCL), and thus also assists in digesting proteins (just an added benefit). As we age, our HCL level is quite often deficient. In order to achieve the greatest benefit, I would recommend using only raw, unfiltered organic apple cider vinegar, which is available in most health food stores.

15. **MSM (Methyl sulfonyl methane)** is a special type of dietary sulfur produced from DMSO, and is beneficial for promoting the flexibility of our cells. **Sulfur is especially important for diabetics and hypoglycemics, as it is also an important component involved in the production of insulin.** You may be surprised to find that **raw garlic cloves** also contain a high amount of sulfur. As with many other nutrients, MSM levels normally decline with age.

16. **Water and Celtic sea salt.** Water is essential for healthy receptors, and dehydration causes insulin receptors to become resistant. An adequate intake of water should resolve the problem. Water is also necessary for preventing acidosis (low pH) in the body, as well as maintaining all aspects of good health. Water is an excellent solvent, and important for the effective removal of toxins.

Celtic sea salt contains 84 trace minerals, all in their natural ionic, easily assimilatable form. Two of those trace minerals are chromium and vanadium, both beneficial for maintaining stable blood sugar and improving insulin utilization. Celtic sea salt also contains both potassium and sodium, necessary for maintaining a proper pH balance, thus avoiding acidosis (which also reduces insulin sensitivity). They also function as a team in the transfer of nutrients into cells, as well as the removal of toxins.

According to Dr. Batmanghelidj, M.D., *"A low salt diet is not conductive to the correction of a diabetic's high blood sugar."* He also notes that: *"The brain is designed to resuscitate itself, when there is water and salt shortage in the body. It raises the levels of sugar in circulation. If the blood sugar is to come down, a slight upward adjustment of daily salt intake may become unavoidable"* (*Your Body's Many Cries For Water*, 1992/1998, pp. 125–127).

I recommend drinking ten 8-ounce glasses of water, along with 1 teaspoon of Celtic sea salt daily. This combination also reduces the demand for glucose, as both water and salt provide an alternate source of energy for the brain.

17. **Exercise** removes glucose from the blood, thus lowering blood sugar levels. The only time blood glucose can get into the muscle cells without the help of insulin is when your muscles are strained. Exercise also increases insulin sensitivity and lowers the blood pressure, while decreasing body fat and reducing the risk of cardiovascular disease in the process. **Regular exercise, even of moderate intensity, improves insulin sensitivity and can help prevent type II diabetes.**

However, another important fact about exercise and diabetes is: Even if you are exercising, that is not an excuse for overeating carbohydrates. There is never a reason to overeat carbohydrates, as Dr. Diana Schwarzbein, M.D. explains:

> It is true that you can burn off excess sugar as energy. However, **you cannot burn off the excess insulin that has been secreted to match the high sugar. Once insulin levels increase to a higher than normal level, damage begins to occur in your metabolism.** High insulin levels destroy the metabolism by setting off a multitude of chain reactions that disrupt all other hormones and biochemical cellular reactions. This leads to increased inflammatory responses, cellular growth, **blood clotting and insulin resistance** (*The Schwarzbein Principle*, 1999, p. 137).

According to an article in the January 20, 2003 edition of *Newsweek* magazine, **the risk of developing diabetes is 30% lower with just three hours per week of brisk walking, in addition to reducing the need for medication in existing diabetics by helping to control blood sugar** (http://www.diabetes-guide.org/diabetes-exercise.htm).

Patients who are taking medications that lower blood glucose, particularly insulin, should take special precautions before embarking on any workout program. As diabetics may have an undetected heart condition, it's always wise to check with your doctor before embarking on any vigorous exercise regimen, and especially if you have a known heart condition.

18. **GlucoVita™,** an herbal dietary formula, (sold through *Gero Vita™ International*), made from the extracts of the following 11 plants:

• ***Gymnema sylvestre*** – a common vine in the jungles of India. Studies have proven that the higher the blood sugar at the beginning, the greater the drop (as much as 55% in some cases). **It has also been discovered that Gymnema repairs or regenerates the important beta cells in the pancreas.** Clinical trials, conducted by Professor K. Shanmugasundaram at the medical school of the University of Madras in India, concluded that *"after administration of Gymnema for several months, insulin requirements go down."*

• ***Momordica charanta*** – a vegetable common to India, China and Pakistan, **has a normalizing effect and has been found to mimic insulin.** According to Dr. A. Raman of the Department of Pharmacy at Kings' College in London, ***"it reduces blood sugar and improves glucose tolerance – all without increasing insulin."*** Momordica also decreases the absorption of sugar from the food you eat and increases the amount of glycogen (stored blood sugar) kept in the liver for use by muscles.

• ***Tinospora*** – a climbing succulent shrub, **has multiple effects on diabetes.** It prevents rising blood glucose levels by inhibiting the conversion of glycogen into glucose. It is also an antioxidant.

• ***Trigonella foenum-graecum*** – a bean that grows in parts of Asia and the Mediterranean. Although it doesn't affect people with normal blood sugar levels, the higher your blood sugar, the more it is reduced. Clinical trials showed as much as a 57% decrease. No side effects have been reported

• ***Pterocarpus marsupium*** – comes from the resin and leaves of this shade tree. **Given for twelve weeks, it substantially reduces the three prime symptoms of diabetes mellitus: excessive urination, excessive eating and excessive thirst.** According to researchers at Banaras Hindu University, *"the clinical potential of this plant could provide a novel approach to diabetes mellitus since it allows you to cut down the intake of antidiabetic drugs (if not completely stop the need for them)."*

• ***Azadirachta indica*** – **normalizes blood sugar, no matter whether it is high or low.**

• ***Ficus racemosa*** – **normalizes blood sugar, no matter whether it is high or low.**

• ***Aegle marmelose*** – **normalizes blood sugar, no matter whether it is high or low.**

• ***Syzgium cumini*** – **normalizes blood sugar, no matter whether it is high or low.**

• ***Cinnamonum tamala*** – helps regulate the amount of sugars extracted from carbohydrates that get into the blood stream. No adverse side effects have been reported from any of these last five ingredients.

• ***Eugenia jambolana*** – the extract comes from the seeds of this large evergreen tree.

19. **Other Natural Supplements** exist that could assist you in your efforts to maintain stable blood sugar levels. Although not discussed in detail, following are more suggestions that you may research at your local health food store, or on the internet, and possibly test for yourself, in order to effectively choose what works best for you:

* Bitter melon (*Momordica charanta*)	* CLA (Conjugated Linoleic Acid)
* Maitake mushrooms	* Spirulina
* Aloe vera juice	* Banaba Leaf
* Curcumin (found in the spice Turmeric)	* Wheat extract alpha
* Green Tea (*Camellia sinensis*)	* Juniper (*Juniperus communis*)
* Licorice Root (*Glycyrrhiza glabra*)	* *Rhodiola rosea*
* American or Chinese Ginseng (*Panax quinquefolius*)	

Because diabetes is a major contributor to cardiovascular deterioration, if you have type II diabetes, resolving that condition should be a top priority. And, both elevated blood sugar and insulin, definitely contribute to increased vascular damage. You will now read about the many risk factors that can contribute to cardiovascular disease, and ways you can reduce potential risks.

CHAPTER TWENTY-THREE
HEART ATTACKS AND STROKES – POTENTIAL CONTRIBUTORS

Our life's balance could quite easily be contingent upon just one final straw sufficient to create a cardiovascular event such as a stroke or heart attack. Every one of those proverbial straws that we can eliminate, the greater our chance of avoiding a totally preventable premature death sentence might be. The only crime we might have committed is ignoring our body's needs, by choosing to suppress its cries for help (symptoms) with prescription medications (chemicals). If you are one of those with poor dietary habits, that will increase the potential risk. Just one minor infraction might be sufficient to tip the scale in the wrong direction. So it's important to begin reducing as many negative factors as possible, while at the same time increasing the positive ones, (our insurance policy), basically insuring a long uninterrupted lifespan. You could then have an opportunity to be a part of your children's, grandchildren's, or even great-grandchildren's lives. Incidentally, I currently have five great-grandchildren, and (God willing) I plan to be a part of their children's lives as well. I am convinced that is entirely possible, as long as I continue to remain drug-free, and consider my health as a high priority.

So, now let's take a few minutes and see just how many risk factors we can possibly avoid, in order to tip the scale in favor of the survival mode. We can thus reduce our chance of a sudden, preventable stroke or heart attack. We could quite easily be setting the stage for a heart attack, and not even be aware of the fact. For instance, at any one time something as simple as the particular foods you have just eaten during a meal, as well as the amount of each food, could easily contribute to the potential for a heart attack. We will now evaluate some potential life-threatening possibilities.

1. **Consuming Bad Fats.** One example would be consuming the wrong kind of fats or proteins, especially when consumed in excessive amounts, (as with a low-carbohydrate diet). The wrong kinds of fats, (something often overlooked) can contribute to many cardiovascular risk factors, one being an increased viscosity (thickness) of the blood following a meal. An even more serious concern in that regard, is addressed in an article by Dr. Robert Jay Rowen, M.D., in the June 2004 issue of his newsletter *Second Opinion*, when he warns that:

High levels of the wrong fats can cause all types of disease, including heart disease and cancer. **You can simply drop dead if your blood levels are too high!**

Death comes so quickly with this type of cardiac arrest that it occurs without the development of a heart attack. Instead, an electrical irritation of the heart leads to a fatal rhythm disturbance.

If this irritation happens to you, there's no chance of recovery! Death is instant.

[One study] *concluded that circulating free fatty acids is an independent risk factor for early and sudden cardiac-induced death.*

…..not all free fatty acids are the same. Omega-6 fatty acids seem to be the culprit in the damage and risk!

Omega-6 fatty acids are found in plant seed oils including corn, safflower, sunflower, and most plants that grow in more southern latitudes. [Those are the most often found on your grocery shelves and processed foods.] *The American diet has drastically altered its ratio of omega-6 to omega-3 fatty acids in the last century favoring omega 6 (pp. 1-2).*

The suggested ratio of omega-6 to omega-3 fatty acids is 1:1, however the current ratio (the American diet) is approximately 20:1 omega-6 to omega-3.

However, there just happens to be another potential contributor to the very same problem, although from a less obvious source, which stems from adhering to a very low carbohydrate diet, such as the Atkins diet, where the primary objective of the diet is to convert the body from carbohydrate to the fat burning, a process known as ketosis. Not only is consuming bad fats a critical issue, but now we also have another potential source of bad fats, those normally stored in the fat tissue that are thus broken down and released into the bloodstream as an alternate source of energy. Fat tissue stores many of the toxins from bad fats (or drugs, legal or illegal), which are released into the bloodstream along with the fat tissue during weight loss. In her book *Detoxify or Die* (2002), Dr. Sherry A. Rogers, M.D. notes that **these chemicals, when released into the bloodstream, can cause any symptom or disease, including high blood pressure, and heart failure**. So, we might possibly have identified the actual source of the electrical irritation that lead to the fatal rhythm disturbance Dr. Rowen previously alluded to.

We all have an extensive array of toxins stored in our fat tissue. Several are heavy metals such as cadmium, aluminum, mercury, antimony, lead, and even arsenic. Our heartbeat is regulated by chemically stimulated electrical impulses. Any disruption to that normal process could easily disrupt or even stop the heartbeat necessary for maintaining life. Just a deficiency of any of the important minerals, such as calcium, magnesium, sodium, or potassium, can result in an irregular heartbeat also. Unfortunately, these are the very minerals most often depleted by prescription medications, with the diuretics (water pills) being the worst in that regard. According to Dr. Rogers, **studies show that fluoride can damage the heart,** which is another toxin often stored in the fat tissue. Although we can get fluoride from several sources, the most predominant is from drinking water (in areas where fluoride is added to the water supply), or from the SSRI antidepressants. **Prozac™, for example, is a major contributor to fluoride toxicity in the body.** The reason for this phenomenon is, **every single molecule of Prozac™, actually contains three molecules of fluoride!**

As there is such a broad range of toxins normally found in fat tissue, the potential for the electrical irritation is easy to understand. Those likely to have the greatest concentration of toxins are those taking the most medications (basically toxins). Anyone who might have a low metabolism (hypothyroid condition) will find their detoxification is considerably less efficient. **Residues from alcohol, prescription or illegal drugs, as well as many environmental toxins we are all exposed to, are stored in the fat tissue.** Some are also metabolites, from partial but not complete break down, (metabolism) of toxins by the liver. A good example is acetaldehyde, which is a metabolite that results from the first stage of the metabolism of alcohol. It's even more toxic than alcohol, and at times alcohol is not broken down any further. The liver can only metabolize so many toxins at any one time, and as a result has other no other recourse than to store the excess toxins that were not completely metabolized, in the fat tissue. This is basically a temporary emergency measure by the body to place unmetabolized toxins in an inert environment. This might possibly be one reason for forming more fat tissue, thus contributing to obesity (one more cardiovascular risk factor). Basically this is an effort to provide more storage tanks for storing more toxins. As I noted, this appears to be a temporary measure only. Although the removal and utilization of this fat tissue sounds on the surface to be an excellent idea, it also poses a potential cardiovascular risk factor.

If you will just bear with me for a moment, I will present a typical scenario I can envision, that would definitely increase the risk of instant death we just discussed. First, although these toxins stored in the fat tissue create a very unhealthy toxic environment in the body potentially contributing to all disease in general, the real concern is dealing with the stored toxins that have been mobilized once the fat tissue is removed. As mentioned, this is necessary for energy production, when consuming a very low carbohydrate diet. Then, the more energy expended, such as with aerobic exercise, the more fat and toxins will be removed, and released into the bloodstream. This would greatly increase the viscosity (thickness) as well as the toxicity of the bloodstream. And we can't forget that the burning of fat tissue results in the production of a very acidic substance called ketones that must also be dealt with, potentially resulting in acidosis.

We are obviously describing an overweight individual attempting to follow a popular diet plan to lose weight. The more disciplined they might be, the greater the potential risk could be. The more a person weighs, and the longer the aerobic exercise session, the more fat and toxins will be removed to provide energy, in the absence of adequate carbohydrates. Although we have already created a hypothetical set of circumstances that could possibly lead to a sudden supposedly unexplainable loss of life, there is one more potential problem associated with the same basic issue.

I mentioned the concern regarding eating bad fats during a meal. The potential problem is: The animal fat that tastes the best is pork fat, which is the very reason that bacon is a big seller, and one reason Atkins' diet is so popular. Dr. Paul Yenick, Ph.D., who spent 30 years trying to develop a new modality referred to as Quantum Medicine, in an attempt to resolve many difficult health issues at the molecular level, said he couldn't work with anyone who ate pork. He indicated pigs' tissue is very similar to humans. They are also exposed to many of the same toxins that we are. Pigs are not very particular what they eat, and according to Dr. Yenick, they even eat their own feces. It seems logical that we would likely find that toxins are stored in their fat tissue also.

If you also ate a meal that included pork (especially bacon) just prior to or following aerobic exercise, the potential risk would be even greater. You would be basically combining the pork fat and toxins, along with your own. As you can easily see, we have so far provided a typical scenario that could possibly be life threatening, and we are just getting started!

2. **Eating the Wrong Foods For Your Blood Type.** Another potential concern would be if one or more of the foods you consumed during the meal just happened to contain the wrong lectins (a type of protein) for your particular blood type. This is an issue that Dr. Peter D. D'Adamo, N.D. discusses in his book *Eat Right For Your Type* (1996). He stresses that *"When you eat a food containing protein lectins that are incompatible with your blood type antigen, the lectins target an organ or bodily system"* (p. 23). These foods can begin agglutinating (clumping together) blood cells in one area. If the targeted organ just happened to be the heart, it would obviously be a concern, although the source of the problem would likely go undetected. The larger the portion of foods inappropriate for your blood type that you consumed during the meal, the greater the potential risk would likely be.

If you recall, we just discussed a potential problem associated with eating pork fat, and there just happens to be another opinion in that regard. After learning what Dr. Yenick had to say in regard to avoiding pork while using the Bio-com device normally used in Quantum medicine, I decided to see what Dr. Peter D. D'Adamo, N.D. (*Eat Right For Your Blood Type*) had to say regarding eating pork. I soon discovered that pork just happened to be the only meat that should be avoided for every single blood type! So, pork also contains lectins that could contribute to the agglutinating of blood cells for everyone.

3. **Elevated Insulin Levels (typical of diabetics).** When glucose levels rapidly rise and fall, it causes heart rhythms to become unstable. Excess insulin also produces high blood pressure, which further takes a toll on the heart. And there is the added problem of shrinking and hardening of blood vessels (caused by excess insulin), reducing blood flow and oxygen to the heart.

According to one study, ***"More than 80 percent of people with diabetes die as a consequence of cardiovascular diseases, especially heart attacks"*** (James Balch, *Nature's RX for Diabetes*, 2002, p. 1). And another study, from the Cleveland Clinic Department of Preventive Cardiology Department, found that **fasting blood sugar levels above 90 are consistent with a 300% increase in risk for heart disease** (*American Journal Cardiology*, March 2002(1);89(5):596-9).

A diabetes report in *Life Science Discoveries* (2001*)*, states that *"People with diabetes are 2 to 4 times more likely to have* **heart disease which is present in 75% of diabetes related deaths.** *And they are 2 to 4 times more likely to suffer a stroke"* (p. 1). This is especially a concern for diabetics who are also taking the popular oral diabetic drug **Metformin**, as studies have shown that *"**this drug can increase your chances of dying from cardiovascular problems by two-and-a-half times!**"* (p. 4).

4. **Eating a High Carbohydrate Meal.** According to Dr. Ron Rosedale, M.D., there was a "solid study" done that showed that heart attacks are two to three times more likely to happen after a high-carbohydrate meal (http://www.mercola.com/fcgi/pf/2001/jul/14/insulin2.htm). Apparently, **the immediate effects of elevated blood sugar brought on by a high-carbohydrate meal, means a raise in insulin.** This then immediately triggers the sympathetic nervous system, which causes arterial spasm (constriction of the arteries), thus increasing the potential for heart attack

5. **Smoking.** Another potential problem would be regarding people who smoke, as they often light up following a meal. This not only reduces the available oxygen to the heart, but also constricts the blood vessels resulting in an increased demand on the heart, along with the reduced blood flow. Not only does the constriction of the blood vessels by cigarettes place excessive stress on the heart, but the volume of blood reaching the heart is also reduced. When it finally arrives at its various destinations, (including the heart), it will also contain less oxygen and more carbon **monoxide** (rather than carbon dioxide).

6. **NSAIDs (non-steroidal anti-inflammatory drugs) and Cox-2 Inhibitors.** The FDA is now warning against the long-term use of over-the-counter painkillers such as Advil™, Motrin™ and Aleve™, due to an increased risk of dying from heart disease. According to an article in the *Seattle Post Intelligencer* (April 18, 2005), researchers surveyed 900 patients, who were smokers and more prone to cancer and heart problems, and discovered that those who took OTC painkillers for a minimum of six months doubled their chances of dying from stoke, heart attack, or other heart-related problems. And the risk was even higher among ibuprofen users, who were nearly three times more likely to die of cardiovascular disease than non-NSAID users.

If that straw wasn't enough, there just happens to be a fairly new class of prescription drugs known as COX-2 inhibiters that we should also be aware of (such as Vioxx™, Bextra™ and Celebrex™), which are still in the NSAID family of painkillers. They were designed to help block pain and inflammation associated with arthritis and other inflammatory conditions. But the same problem exists with the COX-2 inhibitors: They can double your risk of a cardiovascular event such as, heart attack, stroke, or angina (chest pain). This is a typical example of how drugs not only suppress symptoms, but also contribute to a potentially serious risk factor in the process.

One contributing factor may be that NSAIDs are notorious for depleting folic acid, a cofactor of the B-vitamin family. A deficiency may actually lead to elevated homocysteine, a contributing factor to heart disease. Ironically, folic acid is also a natural analgesic (painkiller).

7. **Alcohol.** If someone also had cocktails with dinner, it would result in a reduced level of oxygen in the brain, and thus place an even greater demand on the heart in order to provide an adequate supply of oxygen to the brain (a critical issue). Both our bodies' voluntary and involuntary functions are controlled by the brain, which thus requires a continuous supply of oxygen. Cigarettes and alcohol are both known to contribute to oxygen depletion. We certainly need to give alcohol its due credit for another potential contribution to the problem.

8. **Coffee.** If someone instead chose to have coffee with dinner, this would increase both homocysteine and cholesterol levels, according to a study in the *American Journal of Clinical Nutrition*. The study goes on to note that if heavy coffee drinkers (those who drink at least 4 cups a day) give up the habit, they will cut their risk of cholesterol-related ischemic heart disease by 15% and homocysteine-related ischemic heart disease by 10% (*American Journal of Clinical Nutrition* – September 2001;74:302-7).

9. **Stress.** Then, if a stressful event just happened to be encountered, (which is quite common these days), that could possibly be the final straw, as that would place an even greater demand the heart. Stress hormones not only suppress the thyroid function, but also stimulate an increase in the heart rate, resulting in an increased demand for oxygen for the heart muscle.

10. **Dehydration.** If we then take that potential scenario just a little further and add dehydration to the equation (alcohol, coffee and caffeinated soft drinks are all dehydrating), then drinking any one of these with a meal could increase the potential cardiovascular risk even more. Of course an insufficient

intake of water is the primary contributor to the problem. We are normally the most dehydrated following a meal. It takes a considerable amount of water to hydrolyze and digest the food following a meal, and the larger the meal, the more water will be required. Food must be in a liquid form before being processed by the liver.

The more dehydrated we become, the higher our blood viscosity will be (the blood basically becomes thicker). This forces the heart to work even harder to circulate the more vicious blood throughout the body and brain. Then, in an effort to preserve water and reduce its loss through the lungs (a normal process during respiration), the histamine level will become elevated. This problem can normally be avoided by drinking a large glass of water one-half hour prior to a meal.

11. **Elevated histamine** stimulates the constriction of the bronchial tubes, and the formation of mucus in the lungs to prevent any further water loss. As the blood leaves the lungs and enters the heart (a distance of only one inch), the histamine residue in the blood can also constrict the coronary arteries, thus reducing both the volume of blood, and oxygen reaching the heart muscle. We now have a greater demand on the heart, pumping thicker blood, lower in oxygen, to its own muscles. If the arteries in the heart are also partially occluded (restricted), the potential for angina pain or a heart attack increases considerably. This is also one potential cause of an asthma attack.

12. **Oral Contraceptives.** Then, if you happen to be taking "the pill", it can **double** your risk of a heart attack, according to a study published in the *New England Journal of Medicine* (December 20, 2001;345:1787-93).

13. **Elevated Estrogen.** Elevated estrogen is actually a risk factor in many different areas. For one thing, elevated estrogen suppresses the thyroid, which contributes to several cardiovascular risk factors. According to Dr. Ray Peat, Ph.D., **when estrogen levels are elevated for a prolonged period, it will cause the heart to stiffen, thus reducing its ability to pump.** He also indicates that there is some evidence that estrogen can make large arteries stiffen also, and that can take place in only a few months (http://www.thyroid-info.com/articles/ray-peat.htm).

Dr. Peat identifies two other problems associated with estrogen. One is that estrogen significantly lowers body temperature, and the other is that **estrogen consistently lowers the availability of oxygen.** I would assume that the reduction of the body temperature is likely due to estrogen's known suppression of the thyroid. Dr. Peat also noted that excess **estrogen also produces a barrier to oxygen diffusion in the lungs, and thus reduces the oxygenation of the blood.**

One contributor to elevated estrogen is **Estrogen Replacement Therapy (ERT)**, normally given to post menopausal women to prevent hot flashes. The problem is, most women already have an excess of estrogen, and Hormone Replacement Therapy (HRT) basically compounds the problem.

Soy is another source of estrogen that can lead to elevated estrogen, and also suppresses the thyroid. We are all exposed to **xeno-estrogens**, often referred to as estrogen mimics or fake estrogens, which the body mistakes for estrogen and responds accordingly. Our greatest exposure is from **plastics** that many foods and beverages are packaged in. This also includes **Styrofoam** trays meat is often placed in before the plastic wrap is applied. Studies have proven that these hormone mimics migrate from the wrap into the food. TV dinners in **plastic containers** would likely be the greatest concern. Not only has the microwave cooking been proven to destroy vitamins, and modify the molecular structure of food, but the heat would stimulate the out-gassing of the estrogen mimics from the containers into the food. A good example is the film that accumulates on the inside of the windshield from the plastic in the dash when left in the hot sun.

Even some **pesticides** and **detergents** contain xeno-estrogens. One called Atrazine is a common weed killer used on corn. Even if you don't eat corn, you will find that corn syrup is added to a surprising number of foods as a sweetener. That is particularly true in regard to most fruit juices. If you read the labels, you will find that most "fruit juices" are really water and high fructose corn syrup, with some juice or flavoring added. They will normally be found in a plastic bottle also.

So as we can easily see, **men can also accumulate excess estrogen**. As it turns out, men are also exposed from another source. They have a substance in their **fat tissue called aromatase**, which can and does convert testosterone into one form of estrogen known as estrodiol. The more fat tissue a man has, the greater the problem. This leads to the formation of more fat tissue on the chest and lower extremities (normally typical of females), obviously an undesirable problem for men.

Fortunately, there are some solutions for reducing estrogen levels. One of the many functions of the liver is to metabolize and remove excess estrogen. Earlier in the book I talked about the hypothyroid condition, and how it can be detected and resolved. The liver can't perform the function of estrogen removal nearly as efficiently when you have less than adequate metabolism (hypothyroidism). Both prescription medications and alcohol are considered as toxins by the body, and must thus be metabolized by the liver. Also, the enzymes need both vitamins and minerals, as well as the proper body temperature (98.6°), to effectively metabolize excess estrogen. So not only are medications (toxins) overloading the liver, but they are depleting nutrients important for effective enzyme action (double jeopardy). The importance of getting off your medications can't be over-emphasized, and your body will be eternally grateful.

Now for another solution: There is an important hormone called progesterone, which is incidentally made from cholesterol (mentioned in an earlier chapter)! It is very helpful in suppressing some of the negative influences of elevated estrogen. The increase of T_3 thyroid not only increases the metabolism, but also increases the conversion of cholesterol to both progesterone and bile acids in the liver. So resolving a hypothyroid condition, by increasing the production of the T_3 thyroid hormone, has many benefits. And progesterone is a hormone that both men and women can greatly benefit from.

When supplementing with progesterone cream, it is important to use **natural progesterone**, and not the synthetic progestins in tablet form usually prescribed by medical doctors for hormone replacement therapy, as they are the altered synthetic form of the hormone that are responsible for many negative side effects. **You do not need a prescription for natural progesterone cream.** Both pregnenolone tablets and progesterone cream are available from many health food stores, mail order, and even some pharmacies. *International Health* sells a natural progesterone cream called EssProL'eve™, which comes in a 3-ounce dispenser that automatically dispenses the proper amount. It is applied topically for transdermal delivery (absorption through the skin). Women's dosage is normally double that suggested for men.

We also have a couple resources available to resolve the aromatase that resides in men's fat tissue, and converts testosterone to the form of estrogen known as estrodiol. One is a bioflavonoid called Chrysin, and another is Nettle Root. They will bond to and remove aromatase, and thus prevent the testosterone to estrogen conversion. I personally use a men's formula produced by the *Life Extension Foundation* called Super MiraForte™ with Chrysin, which also contains other cofactors beneficial for men. The non-profit organization maintains high quality standards for all their products. They not only issue grants for research in various areas of longevity, but are also fighting to preserve our freedom of access to nutrients. Although many aren't aware of the fact, that is becoming more and more of a threat. Vested interests would like very much to prevent our access to vitamins in sufficient quantity to have any real benefit. The increasing interest in natural supplements is becoming a major concern of the very profitable and powerful drug industry, as well as their primary beneficiary, the FDA. This may have seemed a little off the subject, but obviously a major concern for anyone concerned about their health.

14. **Nutrient Depletion.** Following is a list of nutrients important for the prevention of a heart attack or stroke, as well as the drugs, or class of drugs, substances, and conditions (i.e. stress) that can contribute to their depletion. Incidentally, you may notice that some of the causes of nutrient depletion are also contributing factors to heart disease (i.e. smoking, alcohol, stress, caffeine, estrogen, sugar, NSAIDs), which we just discussed and listed in this section. According to a list of the top 200 most prescribed drugs, of the 180 prescription medications tested, it was also found that **every single prescription medication depleted nutrients necessary for the prevention of a heart attack or stroke!** Which isn't surprising when you consider how many different nutrients (21!) influence the condition of your heart, as follows:

✓ **Vitamin B₁ (Thiamine)** – depleted by sulfa drugs, SSRI antidepressants, smoking, estrogen (and oral contraceptives), diuretics, caffeine, antiseizure medication (i.e. barbiturates, phenytoin), **antiarrhythmic agents (i.e. digoxin),** antibiotics, antacids, alcohol, sugar, cooking (heat), food processing methods, and physical and mental stress.
  - **Needed for proper muscle tone of the heart.**
  - **Vitamin B₁ is an antioxidant, which helps to protect cells against cancer, and the degenerative effects of aging, alcohol consumption, and smoking.**
  - **Deficiency can produce heart changes, numbness of the hands and feet, weak and sore muscles, and general weakness.**
✓ **Vitamin B₆ (Pyridoxine)** – depleted by **vasodilators (i.e. nitroglycerin),** sulfa drugs, steroids and corticosteroids, smoking, sleeping pills, estrogen (and oral contraceptives), diuretics, diabetic medication, caffeine, asthma medications, antidepressants and MAO inhibitors, antibiotics, alcohol, sugar, heat (canning & roasting), and physical and mental stress.
  - **Involved in more bodily functions than almost any other single nutrient.**
  - Assists in the absorption of vitamin B₁₂.
  - **Inhibits the formation of homocysteine, thus reducing cholesterol deposition surrounding the heart.**
✓ **Vitamin B₁₂** – depleted by sulfa drugs, SSRI antidepressants, smoking, sleeping pills, proton pump inhibitors (i.e. Nexium™), muscle relaxants, mineral oil and laxatives, Histamine H₂ blockers (i.e. Tagamet™, Pepcid™, Zantac™), estrogen (and oral contraceptives), diuretics, diabetic medications, **all cholesterol-lowering drugs, including statins and bile acid sequestrants (i.e. Questran™, Colestid™),** calcium deficiency, caffeine, antiseizure medication (i.e. barbiturates), amphetamines and diet pills, antibiotics, and alcohol.
  - **Regulates homocysteine levels.**
  - **Deficiency can produce palpitations or labored breathing.**
✓ **Choline** – a cofactor of the B-vitamin family, depleted by sulfa drugs, lithium, estrogen and oral contraceptives, caffeine, sugar, and alcohol.
  - **Necessary for proper transmission of nerve impulses from the brain through the central nervous system.**
  - **Prevents and treats arteriosclerosis.**
  - **Important for cardiovascular health.**
  - **Deficiency can produce cardiac symptoms.**
✓ **Folic Acid (folate)** – a cofactor of the B-vitamin family, depleted by sulfa drugs, SSRI antidepressants, steroids and corticosteroids, smoking, NSAIDs (i.e. ibuprofen), mineral oil and laxatives, Histamine H₂ blockers (i.e. Tagamet™, Pepcid™, Zantac™), estrogen (and oral contraceptives), diabetic medication (especially Metformin), diuretics, decongestants (i.e. pseudoephedrine), caffeine, **all cholesterol-lowering drugs, including statins and bile acid sequestrants (i.e. Questran™, Colestid™), aspirin,** antiseizure medication (i.e. barbiturates), antibiotics, antacids, alcohol, food processing, heat and boiling, and physical and mental stress.
  - **Necessary for regulation of homocysteine levels.**
  - **Deficiency may lead to high levels of homocysteine, contributing to heart disease.**
✓ **Inositol** – a cofactor of the B-vitamin family, depleted by sulfa drugs, lithium, food processing, estrogen (and oral contraceptives), caffeine, antiseizure medication, antibiotics, and alcohol.
  - **Naturally reduces cholesterol levels and prevents hardening of the arteries.**
  - **Deficiency can produce arteriosclerosis.**
✓ **Vitamin C** – depleted by steroids and corticosteroids, smoking, NSAIDs (i.e. ibuprofen), muscle relaxants, estrogen and oral contraceptives, diuretics, diabetic medication, antihistamines, asthma medications, **aspirin,** anticoagulants, antidepressants (most),

antiseizure medication (i.e. barbiturates, phenytoin), antibiotics, analgesics, amphetamines and diet pills, alcohol, caffeine, cooking (heat), high fever, physical and mental stress.

- **Naturally reduces cholesterol levels.**
- **Naturally reduces blood pressure and strengthens blood vessels.**
- **Vitamin C is an antioxidant needed for more than 300 metabolic functions in the body. When combined with toxic substances (i.e. heavy metals, pollution), vitamin C can render them harmless, allowing them to be eliminated from the body.**
- **Assists the body with oxygen use.**

✓ **Vitamin D** – depleted by steroids and corticosteroids, smoking, muscle relaxants, mineral oil (laxatives), Histamine H_2 blockers (i.e. Tagamet™, Pepcid™, Zantac™), estrogen (and oral contraceptives), diuretics, diabetic medication, **all cholesterol-lowering drugs, including statins and bile acid sequestrants (i.e. Questran™, Colestid™),** asthma medications, aspirin, antiseizure medication (i.e. barbiturates, phenytoin), antibiotics, antidepressants, **antiarrhythmics (i.e. digoxin),** antacids, analgesics, alcohol, cooking (heat), light, high fever, physical and mental stress.

- **Prevents muscle weakness (the heart is a muscle).**
- **Reduces cholesterol and prevents atherosclerosis.**
- **Assists in the regulation of the heartbeat.**

✓ **Vitamin E** – depleted by NSAIDs (i.e. ibuprofen), **all cholesterol-lowering drugs, including statins and bile acid sequestrants (i.e. Questran™, Colestid™),** Orlistat™ (fat-blocking weight loss agent), mineral oil (laxatives), estrogen and oral contraceptives, **aspirin,** antibiotics, alcohol, heat, frying, oxygen, freezing temperatures, air pollution, inorganic iron, and chlorine.

- **Improves circulation and strengthens capillary walls.**
- **Naturally reduces blood pressure and assists in normal blood clotting.**
- **Prevents heart attacks. Some studies have shown that daily use of vitamin E is more protective than aspirin for prevention of heart attacks, with no harmful side effects.**

✓ **Coenzyme Q_{10} (CoQ$_{10}$)** – depleted by **vasodilators (i.e. nitroglycerin),** diuretics, diabetic medications, **all cholesterol-lowering drugs, including statins and bile acid sequestrants (i.e. Questran™, Colestid™),** phenothiazines (class of antipsychotic drugs), antihypertensive (blood pressure lowering) drugs (including ACE inhibitors, beta-blockers and calcium channel blockers), antihistamines, antidepressants (especially tricyclics), **antiarrhythmics (i.e. digoxin).**

- **Naturally lowers blood pressure and assists in circulation.**
- **Beneficial in preventing and treating cardiovascular disease and congestive heart failure.**
- **Deficiency can produce congestive heart failure, angina, mitral valve prolapse, stroke, cardiac arrhythmias, and cardiomyopathy.**

✓ **Calcium** – an essential mineral, depleted by sulfa drugs, steroids and corticosteroids, SSRI antidepressants, NSAIDs (i.e. ibuprofen), mineral oil (laxatives), Histamine H_2 blockers (i.e. Tagamet™, Pepcid™, Zantac™), high fluoride intake (Prozac™), estrogen (and oral contraceptives), diuretics, caffeine, **all cholesterol-lowering drugs, including statins and bile acid sequestrants (i.e. Questran™, Colestid™),** antiseizure medication (i.e. barbiturates), antifungals, antibiotics, **antiarrhythmic agents (i.e. digoxin), aspirin,** antacids, alcohol, high protein diet, high sugar diet, high saturated fat diet, soft drinks, excess salt or white flour, excess sweating, smoking, and emotional and physical stress.

- **Necessary for maintenance of a regular heartbeat and in the transmission of nerve impulses.**

- Naturally lowers cholesterol and prevents cardiovascular disease.
- Naturally lowers blood pressure and assists with blood clotting.
- Deficiency can produce heart palpitations, elevated blood cholesterol, and hypertension (high blood pressure).

✓ **Chromium** – an essential trace mineral, depleted by diabetic medication, excess iron, processed foods, refined carbohydrates, and sugar.
- Naturally lowers cholesterol.
- Coronary heart disease has been linked to low chromium concentrations in human tissue.

✓ **Copper** – a trace mineral, depleted by Histamine H_2 blockers (i.e. Tagamet™, Pepcid™, Zantac™), penicillamine™ (chelating agent for copper removal), excess zinc, Ethambutol™ (tuberculosis treatment), bile acid sequestrants (Questran™), antiviral HIV medication, and antacids.
- Necessary for healthy nerves and joints, and reduces the degeneration of the nervous system.
- Deficiency can produce impaired respiratory function, thickening of the heart muscle, increased blood fat levels, weakening of cells resulting in aneurysm or stoke.

✓ **Magnesium** – an essential mineral, depleted by steroids and corticosteroids, SSRI antidepressants, NSAIDs (i.e. ibuprofen), Immunosuppressants, high levels of zinc, estrogen and oral contraceptives, diuretics, diabetic medication, **all cholesterol-lowering drugs, including statins and bile acid sequestrants (i.e. Questran™, Colestid™),** antiseizure medication (i.e. barbiturates, phenytoin), antifungal medication, antibiotics, **antiarrhythmic agents (i.e. digoxin),** antacids, alcohol, antihypertensive (blood pressure lowering) drugs (including ACE inhibitors, beta-blockers and calcium channel blockers), large amounts of fats, sugar, refined flour, fluoride, soft water consumption, and physical and emotional stress.
- More than 300 enzymes are activated by magnesium.
- Necessary for healthy nervous and muscular tissues, and nerve transmission and impulses.
- Necessary to maintain normal heart rhythm and muscular contraction.
- Protects the arterial linings from the effects of stress caused by sudden blood pressure changes.
- Assists in the prevention of cardiovascular disease.
- Increases the rate of survival following a heart attack.
- Naturally reduces cholesterol and blood pressure.
- Deficiency can produce rapid heartbeat, cardiac arrhythmia (fatal), sudden cardiac arrest, and is often synonymous with diabetes.
- Low magnesium levels make nearly every disease worse.

✓ **Manganese** – a trace mineral, depleted by steroids and corticosteroids, SSRI antidepressants, diuretics, caffeine, alcohol, excess sugar, and heavy consumption of meat or dairy products.
- Promotes a healthy nervous system and immune system.
- Deficiency can produce heart disorders, high cholesterol levels, high blood pressure, rapid pulse, and tremors.

✓ **Phosphorus** – a trace mineral, depleted by ACE inhibitors, beta-blockers and other Antihypertensive (blood pressure lowering) drugs, antacids, **antiarrhythmic agents (i.e. digoxin), all cholesterol-lowering drugs, including statins and bile acid sequestrants (i.e. Questran™, Colestid™),** diuretics, mineral oil (laxatives), excess iron or magnesium, a diet high in processed cooked foods and junk food.

- **Necessary for contraction of the heart muscle and normal heart rhythm.**
- **Necessary for blood clotting.**
- **Deficiency can produce irregular breathing.**

✓ **Potassium** – an essential mineral, depleted by steroids and corticosteroids, sodium bicarbonate (Alka Seltzer™), smoking, Parkinson's disease medication, NSAIDs (i.e. ibuprofen), muscle relaxants, laxatives, immunosuppressants, diuretics, caffeine, **antiarrhythmic agents (i.e. digoxin),** asthma medication, **aspirin,** antifungal medication, antibiotics, amphetamines and diet pills, alcohol, Acetazolamide™ (a carbonic anhydrase inhibitor), ACE inhibitors and other blood pressure lowering drugs (including beta-blockers), excess sugar and refined foods, large amounts of licorice, and physical and mental stress.

- **Necessary for a healthy nervous system and the transmission of nerve impulses.**
- **Assists in regular heart rhythm and proper muscle contraction.**
- **Prevents stroke.**
- **Maintains blood pressure.**
- **Depletion can produce hypertension (high blood pressure), fluctuations in heartbeat, muscular fatigue and weakness, respiratory distress.**

✓ **Selenium** – a trace mineral depleted by steroids and corticosteroids, SSRI antidepressants, excess zinc or copper, caffeine, alcohol, food processing, high fat foods, infection, injury, blood loss, aging, and physical and mental stress.

- **Deficiency has been linked to heart disease, cancer, high cholesterol levels, and liver impairment.**

✓ **Carnitine** – a non-essential amino acid depleted by antiseizure medication (i.e. barbiturates, phenytoin), HIV medication, and valproic acid and derivatives.

- **A major source of energy for the muscles.**
- **Prevents fatty buildup, especially in the heart.**
- **Increases cerebral blood flow (blood flow to the brain).**
- **Reduces the risk of heart disorders.**
- **Reduces damage to the heart from cardiac surgery.**
- **Naturally lowers cholesterol and blood triglycerides levels.**
- **Deficiency can produce heart pain and muscle weakness.**

✓ **Glutathione** – a compound produced from other amino acids, depleted by SSRI antidepressants, narcotics (i.e. codeine), acetaminophen (i.e. Tylenol™).

- **A powerful antioxidant. Reduces some of the damage caused by tobacco smoke, ethanol, and overdoses or frequent use of aspirin or acetaminophen.**
- **Deficiency contributes to oxidative stress, which plays a key role in the worsening of many diseases including heart attack.**

✓ **Essential Fatty Acids (EFAs)** – depleted by NSAIDs (i.e. ibuprofen), estrogen (and oral contraceptives), antiseizure medication (i.e. barbiturates, phenytoin), high saturated fat diet, bronchodilators, aspirin, and food processing.

- **Naturally reduces blood pressure, lowers cholesterol and lowers triglycerides levels.**
- **Reduces the risk of blood clot formation.**
- **Beneficial for treatment of cardiovascular disease.**

15. **Statin (cholesterol-lowering) drugs.** If anything could possibly increase the potential risk for a heart attack or stroke even further, it would likely be one of the statin (cholesterol lowering) drugs, such as Lipitor™, Zocor™, and Crestor™, known to reduce the level of CoQ_{10} critical to heart health and energy. As we learned earlier, the statin drugs eventually create multiple cardiovascular risk factors including a weakening of the heart muscle, known as cardiomyopathy.

16. Over-the-counter medications. Phenylpropanolamine (PPA), an ingredient found in many common over-the-counter cough and cold medications and appetite suppressants, has been linked to an increase in the risk of stroke.

Some of the products containing PPA include drugs sold under the following names:

* Alka-Seltzer Plus	* Acutrim	* Contac
* Comtrex	* Dexatrim	* Dimetapp
* Triaminic	* Robittussin CF	

One advisory committee to the FDA is recommending that it be reclassified as unsafe, and according to Dr. Ralph I. Horwitz from Yale University's School of Medicine, *"Case reports have linked exposure to PPA to the occurrence of hemorrhagic stroke."* In fact, since 1979, more than 30 publications have reported the occurrence of intracranial hemorrhage after PPA ingestion. Researchers studied over 2000 adults aged 18 to 49, over a 5-year period, including 702 individuals who were hospitalized due to a stroke, and found that **stroke patients were 50% more likely than the control subjects to have been exposed to a PPA-containing substance within three days of their stroke** (http://64.233.161.104/search?q=cache:00QCflJKAesJ:www.fda.gov/ohrms/dockets/ac/00/backgrd/3647 b1_tab19.doc+ppa+exposure+stroke&hl=en&gl=us&ct=clnk&cd=2&client=firefox-a).

17. Low Salt Diet. Dr. Joel Wallach, B.S., D.V.M., N.D., claims that we are supposed to limit our salt intake to 1 gram a day, the Japanese actually consume from 12 to 15 grams of salt daily! On a more recent CD of his, *Have You Heard?* (2005), he discusses the fact that although the Japanese are much heavier smokers than we are, their rate of heart attacks are much lower than ours. They likely don't consume the processed salt (with only sodium) that most Americans do. Dr. Wallach also mentions that, from studies it was found that **those on a low-salt diet were six times as likely to die of a heart attack.**

Surprisingly, most doctors are still recommending their patients adhere to a low-salt diet, in spite of the fact that it can both increase the difficulty of maintaining proper blood sugar levels, and greatly increase the risk of a heart attack! The obvious question is: Why is traditional medicine totally oblivious to these very critical findings, regarding something so simple as the importance of an adequate intake of salt? My younger sister who died quite a few years ago, very faithfully followed all her doctor's recommendations, including avoiding salt. She was a diabetic, had cardiomyopathy, congestive heart failure, severe osteoporosis, suffered multiple strokes, and was on a pace maker. Just before she died, her kidneys were shutting down. The primary problem: They had "excellent insurance coverage," which as usual, conveniently excluded complimentary medicine (natural therapies) – the basic flaw in our current healthcare system. I can't help but wonder just how many in the nation are actually dying prematurely, just by following their doctor's orders.

18. Hypothyroidism. According to local retired professor Dr. Ray Peat, Ph.D., a low thyroid condition results in many conditions related to cardiovascular disease, such as heart failure, high blood pressure, and a chronic increase of lactic acid (leading to arterial damage from acidosis). One study to confirm this was addressed by Dr. Broda Barnes, M.D., in his book *Hypothyroidism: The Unsuspected Illness* (1976), as follows:

In order to run a valid scientific study…. patients were asked not to change any of their routine habits – to stop smoking, exercise more, try to avoid stress, or adopt a low-fat, low-cholesterol diet.

A total of 1,559 patients were in the study.

At the end of the twenty years, only four heart attacks had occurred. These were in men. The youngest was fifty-six; his father had died with the same disease at the age of fifty-two. The oldest was sixty-one, a man who gave little thought to his health, often trying to get by on two or three hours' sleep a night and pushing himself beyond his endurance. In these four cases, the thyroid dosage was only two grains a day; viewed in retrospect, the dosage may have been inadequate.

*Of the 1,569 patients observed for **a total of 8,824 patient-years, 844 were women; there were no heart attacks among them*** (pp. 178-179).

All participants in the study received two grains of natural Armour™ thyroid daily, and the statistics unquestionably speak for themselves. **A total of <u>8,824 patient years, with only four heart attacks,</u> is quite incredible!** So, in light of the evidence, wouldn't supplementing with a natural thyroid hormone seem much more responsible than resorting to the potentially dangerous cholesterol lowering medications. Incidentally, elevated estrogen has historically been associated with a low thyroid condition, thus the thyroid hormone would often also stabilize the cholesterol level if it were elevated.

19. **Selenium Deficiency**. Not only is selenium necessary for healthy thyroid function, but it is also necessary for the production of antioxidant enzymes, which remove toxins formed from oxidation. Selenium actually binds to heavy metals (such as mercury), reducing toxicity. Apparently, one of the greatest risks for those with a selenium deficiency appears to be heart disease. Unfortunately, the level of selenium in foods depends on the levels of selenium in the soil where the food was grown, thus actual concentrations are unpredictable. In his book *The Antioxidant Miracle*, Lester Packer states that research by Dr. Raymond Shamberger of the Cleveland Clinic has shown *"that **people who live in states with the lowest selenium content were <u>three times more likely to die of heart disease</u> than those who lived in states that were more selenium rich"*** (Mark Stengler, *The Natural Physician's Healing Therapies*, 2001, p. 414). He goes on to list the states that were found to have selenium-deficient soil include Connecticut, Illinois, Ohio, **Oregon**, Massachusetts, Rhode Island, New York, Pennsylvania, Indiana, Delaware, and District of Columbia.

Selenium is also depleted by steroids and corticosteroids, SSRI antidepressants, excess zinc or copper, caffeine, alcohol, food processing, high fat foods, infection, injury, blood loss, aging, and physical and mental stress.

20. **Depression.** If you also happen to be depressed, keep in mind that emotional depression affects physical health. It has been proven that depressed individuals are more likely to die from cardiovascular disease (a heart attack contributor), compared with non-depressed individuals, as follows:

*[One] report sheds light on how emotional depression affects physical health. It seems that **depressed individuals are more likely to die from cardiovascular disease, compared with their non-depressed peers.***

*The 54-month observational study, which involved 2,847 participants in the Netherlands (aged 55 to 85 years), found that **among those without cardiac disease at the study's onset, heart disease deaths <u>nearly quadrupled</u> in participants with major depression. In those who had cardiac disease when the study began, deaths from heart disease tripled in subjects with major depression.*** (*Archives of general Psychiatry*, March 2001; 58:221-7 <u>http://archpsyc.ama-assn.org/</u>)

If depression is something you are dealing with, be sure and read the chapter in this book on Depression, as you now have more than one reason for effectively resolving depression if it is an issue. Incidentally, depression can easily be eliminated without drugs.

One Example Of A Stroke Caused By Dehydration

On his series of audiotapes titled *WATER: Rx for a Healthier Pain-Free Life* (1997), Dr. F. Batmanghelidj, M.D. recounted an incident regarding his sister who suffered a stroke from dehydration, which he claims is one potential cause of a stroke. I assume that it would be especially true when the brain becomes dehydrated. He attributed her dehydration to an insufficient water intake, and lying in the hot sun too long, while also drinking alcohol. Alcohol can easily cross the blood-brain barrier and is very dehydrating to the brain. He indicated that she had also taken up smoking, so we have one more risk factor involved. Smoking causes a constriction of the arteries, while also increasing the level of **carbon monoxide** and decreasing the level of oxygen reaching the brain, (a very bad combination).

Then as we learned, when we become dehydrated, the viscosity of the blood increases (the blood thickens). There just happens to be a potential indirect result of dehydration that would also increase the viscosity of the blood, which is elevated low-density cholesterol (LDL) in the bloodstream. I want to stress that although the concentration of the LDL in the bloodstream may at times be elevated, thus thickening your blood, it is just doing its job, and that is an unavoidable byproduct.

We already discussed one function of LDL, that of sealing a potential leak due to a lesion from a weakened artery wall. But in this case, another function of LDL is sealing the cell wall of the cells at greatest risk, in order to prevent further dehydration. In other words, while the LDL is just doing its job, an unavoidable temporary condition is the increased viscosity of the blood.

Then, when you add alcohol to the equation, not only is it very dehydrating to the brain, but alcohol is also a solvent, which tends to destabilize the fat tissue in the brain cells. We could also be dealing with an additional substance considered to be even more toxic than alcohol. It is actually a metabolite of alcohol called acetaldehyde, produced by the liver during the first phase of alcohol detoxification. Until alcohol has been completely metabolized and converted to the relatively benign acetylic acid and water (which takes place in the second phase), either alcohol or acetaldehyde would likely continue circulating through the brain.

Another function of LDL that we just alluded to is temporarily stabilizing the brain cells, to assure that the receptors will be properly aligned, so they can begin communicating more efficiently. In other words, so someone who is intoxicated can begin to function normally, (no more staggering and slurred speech). I believe that passing out from excessive consumption of alcohol at any one time is an important defense mechanism, which helps prevent destroying the brain entirely. It allows the liver time to detoxify the alcohol, and it allows the LDL time to shore up the cell walls and receptors. It appears that LDL has many temporary although critical emergency functions, as a sealant and stabilizer, and is obviously not an enemy that must somehow be suppressed at all costs by the dangerous statin drugs, (as promoted).

So we have another typical scenario that can lead to an unsuspected serious life-threatening (or at least life-changing) stroke. And dehydration appears to be at least a major contributor to the problem. Also, anything that can in any way restrict oxygen flow to the brain should be our primary concern and avoided at all costs. I'm not sure if Dr. Batmanghelidj's sister was taking any medications, but as we learned, the class of blood pressure medications called calcium channel blockers was proven to cause neuron shrinkage in the brain, and thus another potential contributor to the problem.

Pathologists conducting autopsies evaluating the condition of various brains discovered that alcoholics' brains were not only shriveled, but also very unstable, and thus difficult to dissect. This basically confirms the theory regarding the influence of alcohol on the stability of the brain. Although LDL can help deal with the temporary emergency so a person can still function, if they continue drinking the body can't possibly restore the damage. If a person suffers from a stroke, the potential for damage would be even greater if the brain had already suffered damage from either drugs or alcohol.

The good news is, contrary to previous theory, the brain surprisingly has considerable restorative capability. This is an issue I will cover in detail in a forth-coming book on dementia and Alzheimer's disease. I will show you how the risk of such degenerative diseases can be greatly reduced (if not entirely eliminated). You will discover ways that existing brain damage can often be repaired. I will also explain ways that I have been able to greatly improve both my retention and recall.

Finally, it appears that Dr. Batmanghelidj might have discovered another emergency therapy for preventing, or at least reducing, brain damage if the stroke was induced by dehydration, as was the case regarding his sister. He had her begin drinking water every few minutes. He claimed that the paralysis in her left side began to subside, and she gradually regained her sensation and mobility. He noted that following that rather scary experience, she stopped drinking and smoking, and began drinking water daily.

I would also suggest taking a teaspoon of Celtic sea salt (daily), as well as drinking eight to ten 8-ounce glasses of water daily. As we learned, the combination provides an excellent source of energy for the brain. This could possibly be an adjunctive (additional) therapy, although our Heart Attack and Stroke emergency kit appears to have the greatest overall potential, regardless of what might have contributed to a heart attack or stroke.

As you will learn in the following chapter, cayenne will not only rapidly dissolve a clot, but it will also stop an Aneurysm, (which would result in leakage of blood in the brain)! Only Our Creator could possibly create something with that kind of potential, yet few are even aware of its tremendous benefit. It even stops blood loss during surgery, yet doctors still continue injecting the very expensive, "highly dangerous" drug Trasylol™, instead of cayenne tincture, (liquid cayenne). Although it has been responsible for thousands of deaths, from kidney failure, or strokes or heart attacks, the FDA still allows Trasylol™ to remain on the market! The question is, why? The answer should be obvious, (corruption in the FDA).

Few are aware of some of the most valuable drug-free resources, and cayenne is just one example. Many are unnecessarily suffering with a lifetime of brain damage caused by a stroke, which could have been easily prevented, just with cayenne alone, (what a crime)! Cayenne "rapidly" resolves the problem, (be it a clot or an Aneurysm), normally in five minutes or less, and according to the well-known and highly respected herbalist, Dr. John Christopher, has never once failed. That knowledge alone could easily prevent a tremendous amount of brain damage that most stroke patients normally experience, and are thus forced to live with for the remainder of their lives! Spread this valuable information to everyone you know! You can rest assured that the pharmaceutical giants are not about to, in spite of the fact that millions are at risk. To them, it's all about their bottom line, and the CEO's salary, and annual bonuses.

The Conclusion –
Regarding Contributors to Strokes and Heart Attacks

As we can easily see, the wrong combination of events, (which we are ultimately in control of), could quite easily set the stage for a cardiovascular event such as a heart attack or stroke, something we obviously want to avoid. Fortunately, all these risk factors are quite easy to avoid or remedy, and without the use of drugs. Just eliminating both the statin drugs and blood pressure medications that deplete the critical CoQ_{10} would go a long way toward reducing the cardiovascular risk factors. A common saying is: Knowledge is power. If this knowledge is properly applied, it could easily save many lives (including yours) that would otherwise be unnecessarily lost by sudden unsuspected cardiovascular events. Our potential lifespan could quite easily be prematurely shortened, sometimes by decades, just from one totally avoidable cardiovascular event, such as a heart attack or stroke. There is a good explanation why so many people in their 30's and 40's are currently dying unexpectedly of a heart attack. This occurrence is becoming more and more common. In my opinion, a major contributor to the problem, other than the increased battle with diabetes, is the continued promotion and prescribing, of cholesterol and blood pressure lowering medications. The cholesterol medications especially, are placing people at increasing and unnecessary risk.

CHAPTER TWENTY-FOUR
HEART ATTACKS AND STROKES -
SOME WARNING SIGNS & EMERGENCY SOLUTIONS

The information in this chapter could very well be the most important of all, as it could possibly save your life, or prevent a permanent (often major) disability. You will soon learn exactly how you personally can easily prevent either a stroke or heart attack. Most people's first response would be to immediately call the emergency number 911, although depending on the circumstances, it might possibly be too late by the time you finally receive help. You will learn how you can immediately apply safe emergency measures that could easily save your life or someone else's in the interim.

In medicine today, we tend to resort to very expensive high-tech solutions for potentially serious, yet easily preventable problems. There are many variables that could influence the total response time to an emergency call, such as: Availability of an ambulance, traffic and weather conditions, distance to the hospital, and how many other patients are also awaiting for emergency care once you finally arrive. These are all conditions that you have absolutely no control of. So what's the solution?

First, it would be helpful if you learn how to detect the typical symptoms associated with a pending stroke or heart attack. Anyone who has previously experienced a heart attack or stroke is more than likely already familiar with the normal symptoms associated with each. For those unfamiliar, the following might be helpful.

HEART ATTACK –
What Normally Happens When a Heart Attack Occurs

The medical term for a heart attack is *myocardial infarction* (death of cardiac tissue). When the supply of blood to the heart is sharply reduced or cut off, the heart is deprived of needed oxygen. If blood flow is not restored within minutes, portions of the heart muscle begin to die, permanently damaging the heart muscle.

Some Basic Scenarios of a HEART ATTACK

In the first heart attack scenario, the roughening of arterial walls by deposits of plaque not only narrows the arteries, but also makes it easier for blood clots to form along their inner surfaces.

In the second heart attack scenario, an arrhythmia may set in, so that the heart is no longer pumping enough blood to ensure its own supply.

In the third, a weak spot in a blood vessel, called an aneurysm, may rupture, causing internal bleeding and disrupting normal blood flow.

Typical HEART ATTACK Symptoms

With the onset of a heart attack, the primary symptom is a consistent deep, often severe, pain in the chest that can spread to the left arm, neck, jaw, or the area between the shoulder blades. The pain may be present for up to twelve hours.

Other possible symptoms include shortness of breath, sweating, nausea, and vomiting. In addition, a heart attack can cause abnormal heartbeat rhythms called arrhythmias.

Many people complain of intermittent angina, shortness of breath, and/or unusual fatigue in the days or weeks leading up to a heart attack. Like a heart attack, angina is pain in the chest, caused by a lack of oxygen in the heart muscle, although the extent of oxygen deprivation is normally not sufficient to actually damage heart tissue.

STROKE – What Normally Happens When a Stroke Occurs

The primary difference between a stroke and heart attack depends on where the obstruction of blood flow, and thus oxygen, occurs. Although heart attacks are much more common, unless it results in sudden death, the potential problems associated with a stroke can be much more debilitating, and life changing.

The eventual outcome normally depends on what part of the brain was deprived of oxygen, and how much time lapsed before oxygen was finally restored. The time element is a critical factor that will not only determine how extensive the damage might be, but also how permanent. For that very reason, our primary focus will be early detection of typical symptoms, and then either removing the obstruction, or reducing the blood loss.

Due to the stress and typical hassle associated with the ambulance and hospital emergency procedures, and the potential that it might just be a false alarm, some tend to procrastinate and postpone making the 911 call. Amazingly, 42% of stroke patients wait as long as 24 hours before presenting for medical treatment. This time lapse can be critical regarding the eventual outcome, and might very well be the reason strokes are currently the leading cause of disability in the United States, as well as the third leading cause of death.

Typical STROKE Symptoms

According to the National Stroke Association (1999), strokes more often occur abruptly, with the following symptoms, which often develop suddenly:
- Difficulty standing or walking, dizziness, loss of balance, loss of coordination
- Numbness in the face, arm or leg weakness, particularly on one side of the body
- Confusion, difficulty speaking or understanding
- Vision difficulty in one or both eyes
- Severe headaches that have no known cause

Other important, but less common stroke symptoms include:
- Nausea, fever, and vomiting that is different from a viral illness in the speed of onset (begins in minutes or hours instead of over several days)
- A brief loss of consciousness or a period when there is a reduced level of consciousness (sudden fainting, increased confusion, convulsion, or coma)

HEART ATTACKS AND STROKES: An Emergency Solution

At the very first sign of any of the previously mentioned symptoms associated with a stroke or heart attack, there just happens to be what I will refer to as your "**Stroke / Heart Attack Emergency Kit,**" which you should use immediately upon recognition of any of the common symptoms noted. First, drink a large glass of water along with your emergency kit (supplements). Then, either sit or lie down, and take slow deep breaths while trying to relax. You will likely find your symptoms will begin to subside in a matter of minutes. Even if you decide to call 911 (at times that might be advisable), you should still take your own emergency measures also (the "Stroke / Heart Attack Emergency Kit"). It includes safe and natural substances that I personally have taken for years as a preventative measure, and at 75 I have never experienced any side effects, or cardiovascular concerns.

Cayenne Pepper Capsules – The basis of our emergency kit. The late well-known herbalist Dr. John Christopher discovered that cayenne pepper would stop either a stroke or heart attack in a matter of minutes. He said that in hundreds of cases, he never found it to once fail. I also found it to hold true in many cases of heart attacks. In my opinion, this is an emergency measure that all paramedics should implement in order to more effectively save lives. Although like many other natural and very effective therapies, it will likely never happen. Maybe together we can begin to bring about a change, and finally make a difference.

This emergency kit is a prime example of a simple, inexpensive, safe, yet very effective, life-saving solution that everyone should be aware of. Instead, an expensive ambulance trip to the hospital Emergency Room is normal procedure. At times, the time element can be a critical factor. From the time the emergency call is made, the ambulance arrives to pick you up, and you finally arrive at the hospital, and are processed in the Emergency Room, it might possibly be too late. If not, either you or your insurance company will normally be faced with a sizable bill (often easily avoidable). The most expensive options are those that medicine normally tends to promote, and are unfortunately those most often considered as standard approved procedures. Just one more reason our current healthcare costs are completely out of control, and unnecessarily so.

Cayenne Tincture – An alternative to the cayenne capsules. Although swallowing a couple cayenne capsules with water will normally work, there is an even more effective delivery system. Cayenne is also available in a tincture (liquid) form. If water is not readily accessible, or you have eaten within the last couple hours, that can be a critical issue! The cayenne liquid tincture doesn't require water, and bypasses the digestive system. One dropper full can be squirted under the tongue and absorbed sublingually, directly into the bloodstream. If you have eaten recently, food will still remain in your stomach. The time necessary for digestion can vary from 2 hours to as long as 8 hours, and all depends upon: (1) Your level of digestive enzymes; (2) The amount of food consumed; (3) The combination of foods eaten. Improper food combining is discussed later in the chapter on "Acid Reflux Disease" (actually not really a disease).

I probably should clarify something you might have wondered about. Cayenne cannot only eliminate blood clots, but also an aneurysm (internal hemorrhage) in the brain. Although they appear to be opposing conditions (clotting or lack of clotting), cayenne is basically multi-talented, and very adept at effectively resolving either condition.

Another potential use of cayenne, due to its ability to stop internal hemorrhaging, is its ability to normally eliminate the necessity of a blood transfusion following surgery. I once not only helped a friend stop a heart attack following a particularly stressful event, by using cayenne, but another time avoid a blood transfusion from major surgery. He was anemic at the time, and his doctor assumed that a transfusion was eminent. I told him to take cayenne just prior to his surgery, which he did. His doctor was totally amazed that there was no loss of blood, and wondered what he had done. When he told him, his doctor said, *"I am going to have all my patients do that!"* The obvious question is: Why is this not standard procedure? It would save the necessity of many blood transfusions that could easily be avoided. It could also prevent the unnecessary loss of blood following a serious injury, which could easily be life threatening, yet totally avoidable, (one more reason to always have cayenne on hand).

You might say that cayenne is an amazing herb with tremendous life-saving potential. You can now better appreciate the importance of carrying a small bottle of tincture, to assure rapid absorption and thus benefit. Just keep in mind that cayenne capsules, taken with water, are easily accessible and normally sufficient.

Following are four other supplements that would also work synergistically with cayenne, plus a fifth if you might possibly be experiencing any stress:

1. Coenzyme Q$_{10}$. A major energy molecule for the heart muscle is CoQ$_{10}$, which works synergistically with the cayenne. I would suggest two 100 mg capsules.

2. L-Arginine. The amino acid L-Arginine then causes a dilation (widening) of the arteries. This increases the flow of blood, and thus the availability of oxygen to both the heart muscle and the brain (our major focus). Normally 1,000 mg should be adequate.

3. Magnesium. The mineral magnesium helps relax the muscles in the arteries. 1,000 mg should normally be sufficient

4. Calcium. The mineral calcium may reduce your risk of stroke and heart attack in more ways than one! Calcium not only helps excrete more saturated fat (another contributing factor), but it also decreases the absorption of cholesterol, thus lowering blood cholesterol levels. **Remember to take twice as much magnesium as calcium.**

5. Valerian Root. If the heart attack might possibly have been precipitated from some stressful event (quite common), Valerian Root is one herb that would be very beneficial. It, like cayenne, is very inexpensive, and readily accessible. It is a very calming herb, perfectly safe, and relatively fast acting. It won't make you drowsy, but is excellent for helping you relax. Reducing stress, (if present), will normally help resolve one common contributor to a heart attack.

If in doubt, just take a couple capsules of valerian root anyway, as they are perfectly safe, and definitely can't hurt. I would recommend just including them in your emergency kit, as the possibility of a pending stroke or heart attack can be rather stressful. So, just take a couple and relax, while your symptoms subside and you get back to normal. As far as dosage is concerned, two 500 mg capsules are normally adequate.

Keep in mind that the well-known and respected herbalist Dr. John Christopher claimed that just cayenne alone was able to stop either a stroke or heart attack hundreds of times, and never once failed. If we then use the fastest absorbing form (cayenne tincture) and add a natural supplement important for heart energy (CoQ_{10}) along with magnesium and the amino acid arginine, in order to dilate the arteries and increase the blood flow, we now have a winning combination.

This emergency kit would be especially beneficial for those who tend to procrastinate, and avoid calling 911, as about 42% of stroke patients apparently do. I actually take 4 capsules of cayenne, and 100 mg of CoQ_{10} every morning, and calcium and magnesium each evening. L-arginine is just one of several amino acids I take on occasion. I personally prefer prevention, rather than disease and emergency situations, which I have so far managed to avoid.

You must remember that both strokes and heart attacks can occur unexpectedly, and not only any time, but also anywhere. I would recommend making up at least three emergency kits, and carry one in your pocket or purse, another in the glove compartment in your car, and at least one at home. It would be wise to carry a small bottle of drinking water in your car. If you use cayenne in the capsule form, along with the arginine, magnesium, CoQ_{10}, and valerian root to reduce stress (normally two capsules each), you should have a total of ten capsules, which should fit in a relatively small container. It would also be helpful to carry a small bottle of cayenne tincture, in case you have just eaten, and would prefer a faster response. Keep in mind, you might also be able to save another life, if you happen to have your emergency kit with you. It is also a good idea to make sure your family and friends are aware of what it is, and where it can be found.

I can't help but wonder how many there are with various disabilities that resulted from a stroke that possibly might have been avoided, had they only known. Our objective is to reduce that risk as much as possible in the future. But first, it is very important that you are aware of the various symptoms that normally precede both a stroke and heart attack. This is what I refer to as our body's early warning system, and something that should never be ignored. Once you have your early response emergency team, your "Stroke / Heart Attack Emergency Kit," standing by, the potential threat is now greatly reduced.

CHAPTER TWENTY-FIVE
HYPERTENSION – OVERCOMING THE RISK FACTORS

What Is Considered High Blood Pressure?

The heart is responsible for pumping the blood through miles of arteries and small capillaries, such as those found in both the kidneys and eyes, as well as those supplying the extremities such as the hands and feet. Forcing blood against gravity, to the highest point in the body (the brain), can at times require considerable pressure. Especially when there is a blockage in the kidneys, more pressure will be required to adequately supply oxygen and nutrients to the cells throughout the body, thus the blood pressure must increase in order to meet the body's demands.

Just artificially lowering the blood pressure with anti-hypertensive (blood pressure-lowering) drugs will not solve the basic underlying problem (the restriction). That approach would just make it impossible to get an adequate supply of oxygen and nutrients to some cells where the greatest restriction exists. This is especially critical regarding the brain, because brain cells can begin to die from an insufficient supply of oxygen (one contributor to dementia and Alzheimer's disease). It is similar to a stroke where cells in a particular region of the brain die from lack of oxygen. The basic difference is, during a stroke a specific area of the brain is damaged and cells die, based on where a blood clot or aneurysm occurs. The damage can at times be extensive, but normally localized (in just one area). Insufficient blood pressure to adequately supply oxygen to all the brain cells is not as easily detected, as it is basically systemic (throughout the brain) and thus not as dramatic. Unfortunately, it can be very insidious, and to many the cause is often not normally apparent. Although the deterioration is a gradual process, it is none-the-less very serious, and will eventually take its toll.

Our body has an extremely efficient regulatory system built in. We absolutely must stop forcing it to do what we somehow think it should be doing. If we instead provide it with the natural resources it needs in order to do the job it was designed to do, we soon would begin experiencing much more success. Our objective should be working with our body in order to achieve optimum health, and that is the only way that goal can be accomplished.

The very first question we must ask ourselves is: Is there such a thing as an ideal blood pressure level for everyone, or might we possibly be overlooking some critical deciding factors? One basic flaw in medicine is the assumption that there is one particular blood pressure that is normal or appropriate for everyone. Absolutely nothing could be further from the truth! I believe our blood pressure will adapt to the body's needs, by taking into account any restrictions, be they in the kidneys, or possibly the carotid arteries that supply the brain.

One example is that diabetics normally experience higher blood pressure than non-diabetics. Their insulin and blood sugar levels typically run higher, which often results in the excessive accumulation of plaque in the arteries. The most common form of diabetes (type II) is normally due to an excessive amount of simple carbohydrates and inadequate proteins and fiber in the diet, which produces elevated insulin. This results in a more rapid heartbeat, along with a constriction of the arteries, which combined with the existing plaque, causes the blood pressure to soar even further. Many diabetics are overweight, which also makes the heart work harder, and thus an increase in the blood pressure. Diabetics often develop kidney damage, further restricting the blood flow. If the blood pressure is lowered with drugs, without resolving the underlying conditions, an oxygen deficiency will result (especially regarding the brain). And often, just a dietary change or drinking more water can have a positive influence on lowering the blood pressure.

I have talked with many who indicated that their blood pressure had typically ran high for years, with no apparent problem. Another factor may be your age, and according to an article in his *Alternatives* newsletter (Summer 2004, Volume 9, No. 29), Dr. David G. Williams, M.D. tells us that:

As we age, our blood vessels lose some of their elasticity, *which often leads to higher systolic (top number) blood pressure. So, while a systolic pressure of 140 or even 120 may be characterized as risky for a very young person,* ***it's perfectly healthy for someone 60 years or older to have a systolic blood pressure of up to 160*** (p. 28).

At one time, anything from 139/89 and under was considered as normal. Borderline hypertension was anywhere from 140 to 159 systolic, and 90 to 94 diastolic. And at that time, anything from 160/95 or above was classified as hypertension. It was when the new lower levels were "**arbitrarily**" established regarding both blood pressure and cholesterol, that an increasing number of blood pressure medications were being prescribed, (the obvious objective). It is now considered borderline hypertension to have a blood pressure of 120/80!

The aggressive advertising of drugs on TV just compounded the problem. Most doctors soon responded to the new recommendations, with more medications or increased dosages. It appears that doctors are also watching the commercials on TV, and the end result is more prescriptions. And as if the new lower guidelines weren't enough, it has been discovered that patients are often the unknowing victims of improper blood pressure testing. Researchers at the VA Medical Center in Long Beach, California, estimate that **20 to 30 percent of patients diagnosed as hypertensive actually have normal blood pressure** (*JAMA*, 1987;2258:14, 1909-15). Let's now find out how we can help assure that our blood pressure reading is truly accurate.

What Can Influence Your Blood Pressure Reading?

1. **Stress.** Just being in the doctor's office often raises people's blood pressure.
2. **A Cold Room.**
3. **The Need To Go To The Bathroom.**
4. **Changing positions** can often cause blood pressure to skyrocket.
5. **The wrong size cuff (there are different sizes!)**
6. **Naturally occurring biological rhythms** cause blood pressure to normally be higher in the afternoons and evenings, and lower in the mornings.

Additional ways to assure accurate blood pressure readings, from Dr. David G. Williams, M.D.:

✓ Do not exercise or eat for 30 minutes before having your blood pressure taken.
✓ Rest at least five minutes before having your blood pressure taken.
✓ Be comfortable and relaxed in the surroundings.
✓ Remove all clothing from the waist up. Just rolling up a shirtsleeve can act like a tourniquet and cause false readings.
✓ Your elbow should be at the same level as your heart. An elbow that is even a couple of inches below the heart can make the reading as much as 17 points higher than it should be.
✓ Have your blood pressure taken three times with at least one minute's rest between each one.

Blood vessels can easily sense any restriction in the flow of blood, and at first it is considered as a blockage. This stimulates an increase in blood pressure to address the perceived problem. It is instead the result of the temporary blockage from the inflated cuff, necessary for assessing the systolic (highest) reading. That is why Dr. Williams recommends three readings. The autonomic nervous system soon gets the message, and stops stimulating the increased heart rate, and thus the abnormally elevated blood pressure. This is the body's way of assuring that you have an adequate supply of oxygen to all cells, (especially the brain).

Additional Influences On Your Blood Pressure Reading

An announcement made on CBS in the segment they call *TimeLine*, where brief health announcements are sometimes made, claims that **your blood pressure could vary up to 40%, depending upon the time of day and season!** That is a major variation potential. Our hormone levels often vary during the day, so that could possibly be one connection. Both the thyroid and serotonin levels seem to vary seasonally, and both tend to run lower in the winter months.

A prime example of how many are unnecessarily placed on blood pressure medications due to a temporary fluctuation, is regarding a neighbor. She had apparently parked several blocks from her doctor's office, and was running late for her appointment. As she walked fast, her heart rate, and thus her blood pressure, became elevated. Then she was also stressed, as she was concerned about running late for her appointment. Stress also causes elevated blood pressure. Her doctor never even considered the extenuating circumstances that would contribute to elevated blood pressure, or that it might be temporary, and thus not a concern. He instead decided to add "another" blood pressure medication, even though her reading had been perfectly normal during her prior visit. Under the circumstances, you would assume some evaluation would obviously be in order, although that might possibly have taken a couple more minutes, (and of course, time is of the essence).

This is just one more example of instances where people could easily have been needlessly placed on medications that were entirely inappropriate. Even our thoughts can influence our blood pressure. For example, one day a friend of mine was discussing some very troubling experiences he dealt with as a child. I then had him check his blood pressure, and it was considerably elevated. Next I asked him to relax, think of something more pleasant, and again test his blood pressure. Within five minutes there was an amazing 22-point difference! If you just take into account the many variables that could easily influence a person's blood pressure, and that in some cases lower is not necessarily better, I believe that is an issue that should receive serious consideration.

If these factors are not taken into account, a false reading is quite possible. That wouldn't be such a concern, if it wouldn't lead to unnecessarily taking potentially dangerous blood pressure medications for years. If you consider the "one size fits all" theory, along with the new lower acceptable levels, and then add the inaccurate inflated reading, you have a perfect way to promote the unnecessary prescribing of potentially dangerous blood pressure medications. That is usually where many health problems begin to develop, due to insufficient circulation, and thus an inadequate supply of both oxygen and nutrients to many cells (especially the brain).

Once you are certain that your blood pressure is truly a concern, you can then address the underlying problem, and not just add another drug!

What Conditions In The Body Cause High Blood Pressure?

There are basically three primary conditions in the body that can contribute to high blood pressure. One is a restriction in the kidneys, where scar tissue builds up on the glomeruli inside the kidneys. This basically reduces the total surface area where blood filtration can take place. The resultant restriction means more pressure is required for filtration, and the removal of anything the body currently has no need for, which we call urine. We can easily see that by forcing the blood pressure lower, we would obviously reduce the effectiveness of the filtration process, resulting in excessive fluid retention. So our primary objective should be to reduce the source of the problem (in this case, the restriction in the kidneys).

Another cause of high blood pressure is a buildup of plaque, or restriction in the vascular system. When the blood vessels loose their elasticity, or are reduced in diameter from the accumulation of plaque, more pressure is required to force the blood through smaller openings. Thus, another objective should be the removal of plaque.

The third contributor to high blood pressure is regarding the viscosity (thickness) of the blood, which would influence how easily it can pass through all those little capillaries, as well as the kidneys.

As there are so many risks associated with blood pressure medications, which are not actually addressing the underlying problem and can even cause it to worsen, I would recommend trying some of my recommendations for using natural solutions to effectively lower your blood pressure. Once you read the following explanation of different prescription blood pressure medications, with a complete evaluation of each, I believe you will likely agree. So, read on.

Your Medications Could Be A Major Contributing Factor To Your High Blood Pressure

Resolving hypertension (or any other condition) can be rather difficult due to a little known negative influence that can easily undermine your effort. We find that many different medications can cause elevated blood pressure. Even some seemingly unrelated and widely prescribed medications, such as antidepressants and pain medications, as well as oral contraceptives. **The cholesterol-lowering medications appear to be the worst class of medications of all for contributing to elevated blood pressure, in addition to cardiomyopathy and congestive heart failure.**

On a list of the top 200 most prescribed drugs, a total of **83 different prescription medications (41.5%) actually listed <u>"high blood pressure"</u> as a potential side effect.**

Not only prescription medications, but over-the-counter medications can also contribute to elevated blood pressure. For instance, frequent use of non-steroidal anti-inflammatory drugs (NSAIDs) may block the production of prostaglandins, which are known to dilate blood vessels. This causes blood vessels to narrow, which can lead to hypertension. Following are results from one study, as noted in the *Archives of Internal Medicine* (October 28, 2002;162:2204-2208):

> *The study followed more than 80,000 women between the ages of 31 and 50 years who were initially hypertension-free. Frequency of use (in days per month) of aspirin, NSAIDs, and acetaminophen was recorded and compared with the number of cases of physician-diagnosed hypertension two years later. Of women who used NSAIDs 22 days or more per month, the risk of high blood pressure increased some 86 percent.*
>
> *Additionally, women who used acetaminophen 22 days or more per month were almost twice as likely to have high blood pressure as those who did not.*
>
> *When researchers removed other factors that could lead to hypertension, such as obesity, from the equation, the increased-risk remained.*

Another major problem with any medication is their nutrient depletion. **On the previously mentioned list, of the 180 prescribed medications that were tested for nutrient depletion, we found that <u>every single prescription depleted nutrients that, when deficient, contribute to high blood pressure!</u>**

The depletion (or a deficiency) of the following nutrients can result in high blood pressure. Also listed are the drugs, or class of drugs, and substances, as well as conditions (i.e. stress) that can contribute to each nutrient's depletion. How each nutrient specifically affects blood pressure, is also noted:

1. **Vitamin B$_2$ (riboflavin)** – depleted by sulfa drugs, steroids and corticosteroids, muscle relaxants, mineral oil and laxatives, estrogen and oral contraceptives, **diuretics,** diabetes medication, antidepressants (SSRI and tricyclics), antiseizure medication (i.e. barbiturates, phenytoin), antibiotics, alcohol, antacids, sugar, ultraviolet light, physical and mental stress.
   - **Deficiency can produce high blood pressure.**

2. **Vitamin B$_3$ (niacin)** – depleted by sulfa drugs, SSRI antidepressants, steroids and corticosteroids, sleeping pills, estrogen (and oral contraceptives), caffeine, antibiotics, alcohol, sugar, and physical and mental stress.
   - **Needed for proper circulation.**
   - **Reduces blood pressure and lowers cholesterol.**

3. **Vitamin B$_6$ (pyridoxine)** – depleted by vasodilators (i.e. nitroglycerin), sulfa drugs, steroids and corticosteroids, smoking, sleeping pills, estrogen (and oral contraceptives), **diuretics,** diabetic medication, caffeine, asthma medications, antidepressants and MAO inhibitors, antibiotics, alcohol, sugar, heat (canning & roasting), and physical and mental stress.
   - **Diuretics and cortisone drugs block the absorption of this vitamin.**
   - **Acts as a diuretic, yet maintains sodium and potassium balance (pH).**
   - **Deficiency can produce high blood pressure.**

4. **Choline** – depleted by sulfa drugs, lithium, estrogen and oral contraceptives, caffeine, alcohol, and sugar.
   - **Important for cardiovascular health.**
   - **Deficiency can produce high blood pressure.**

5. **Vitamin C (Ascorbic acid)** – depleted by steroids and corticosteroids, smoking, NSAIDs (i.e. ibuprofen), muscle relaxants, estrogen and oral contraceptives, **diuretics,** diabetic medication, antihistamines, asthma medications, aspirin, anticoagulants, antidepressants (most), antiseizure medication (i.e. barbiturates, phenytoin), antibiotics, analgesics, amphetamines and diet pills, alcohol, caffeine, cooking (heat), high fever, physical and mental stress.
   - **Lowers blood pressure and strengthens blood vessels.**
   - **Assists in the production of anti-stress hormones.**
   - **Protects against abnormal blood clotting.**
   - **Deficiency can produce tissue swelling (edema).**

6. **Vitamin E (tocopherol)** – depleted by NSAIDs (i.e. ibuprofen), **all cholesterol-lowering drugs, including statins and bile acid sequestrants (i.e. Questran™, Colestid™),** Orlistat™ (fat-blocking weight loss agent), mineral oil (laxatives), estrogen and oral contraceptives, **aspirin,** antibiotics, alcohol, heat, frying, oxygen, freezing temperatures, air pollution, inorganic iron, and chlorine.
   - **Improves circulation and strengthens capillary walls.**
   - **Reduces blood pressure.**
   - **Assists in normal blood clotting.**
   - **Assists in the prevention of cardiovascular disease.**
   - **Prevents heart attacks.**
   - **Deficiency can produce blood clotting.**

7. **Calcium** – depleted by sulfa drugs, steroids and corticosteroids, SSRI antidepressants, NSAIDs (i.e. ibuprofen), mineral oil (laxatives), Histamine H$_2$ blockers (i.e. Tagamet™, Pepcid™, Zantac™), high fluoride intake (Prozac™), estrogen (and oral contraceptives), **diuretics,** caffeine, **all cholesterol-lowering drugs, including statins and bile acid sequestrants (i.e. Questran™, Colestid™), aspirin,** antiseizure medication (i.e. barbiturates), antifungals, antibiotics, antiarrhythmic agents (i.e. digoxin), antacids, alcohol, high protein diet, high sugar diet, high saturated fat diet, soft drinks, excess salt or white flour, excess sweating, smoking and emotional and physical stress.
   - **Lowers blood pressure.**
   - **Assists with blood clotting.**
   - **Deficiency can produce high blood pressure and heart palpitations.**

8. **Magnesium** – depleted by steroids and corticosteroids, SSRI antidepressants, NSAIDs (i.e. ibuprofen), Immunosuppressants, high levels of zinc, estrogen and oral contraceptives, **diuretics,**

diabetic medication, **all cholesterol-lowering drugs, including statins and bile acid sequestrants (i.e. Questran™, Colestid™),** antiseizure medication (i.e. barbiturates, phenytoin), antifungal medication, antibiotics, antiarrhythmic agents (i.e. digoxin), antacids, alcohol, **antihypertensive (blood pressure lowering) drugs (including ACE inhibitors, beta-blockers and calcium channel blockers),** large amounts of fats, sugar, refined flour, fluoride, soft water consumption, and physical and emotional stress.

- **Reduces blood pressure.**
- **Necessary to maintain normal heart rhythm and muscular contraction.**
- **Assists in maintaining the body's proper sodium and potassium balance (pH) and body temperature.**
- **Increases the rate of survival following a heart attack.**
- **Assists in the prevention of cardiovascular disease.**
- **Deficiency can produce high blood pressure, rapid heartbeat, cardiac arrhythmia (fatal), sudden cardiac arrest, and is often synonymous with diabetes.**

9. **Manganese** – depleted by steroids and corticosteroids, SSRI antidepressants, **diuretics,** caffeine, alcohol, excess sugar, and heavy consumption of meat or dairy products.
    - **Assists vitamin K in the regulation of blood clotting.**
    - **Deficiency can produce heart disorders, high blood pressure, and rapid pulse.**

10. **Potassium** – depleted by steroids and corticosteroids, sodium bicarbonate (Alka Seltzer™), smoking, Parkinson's disease medication, NSAIDs (i.e. ibuprofen), muscle relaxants, laxatives, immunosuppressants, **diuretics,** caffeine, antiarrhythmic agents (i.e. digoxin), asthma medication, aspirin, antifungal medication, antibiotics, amphetamines and diet pills, alcohol, Acetazolamide™ (a carbonic anhydrase inhibitor), **ACE inhibitors and other blood pressure lowering drugs (including beta-blockers),** excess sugar and refined foods, large amounts of licorice, and physical and mental stress.
    - **Assists in regular heart rhythm and proper muscle contraction.**
    - **Prevents stroke.**
    - **Maintains blood pressure.**
    - **Depletion can produce high blood pressure, edema (swelling), fluctuations in heartbeat, heart malfunction and respiratory distress.**

11. **Sodium** – depleted by narcotics, muscle relaxants, laxatives, **diuretics, beta-blockers (blood pressure lowering drugs), aspirin,** antigout medication, antifungal medication, antidepressants (especially SSRI antidepressants), Acetazolamide™ (a carbonic anhydrase inhibitor), **ACE inhibitors and other blood pressure lowering drugs,** dehydration (fever, heat, diarrhea, vomiting).
    - **Assists in the regulation of blood pressure.**
    - **Assists in making the cell walls permeable.**
    - **Necessary for maintaining proper water balance and blood (pH).**
    - **Deficiency is most common in people who take diuretics.**
    - **Deficiency can produce dehydration and heart palpitations.**

12. **Essential Fatty Acids (EFAs)** – depleted by NSAIDs (i.e. ibuprofen), estrogen (and oral contraceptives), antiseizure medication (i.e. barbiturates, phenytoin), high saturated fat diet, bronchodilators, **aspirin,** and food processing.
    - **Reduces blood pressure.**
    - **Reduces the risk of blood clot formation.**
    - **Beneficial for treatment of cardiovascular disease.**

13. **Coenzyme Q_{10} (CoQ_{10})** – depleted by vasodilators (i.e. nitroglycerin), **diuretics,** diabetic medications, **all cholesterol-lowering drugs, including statins and bile acid sequestrants (i.e. Questran™, Colestid™), ACE inhibitors, beta-blockers, calcium channel blockers and**

other antihypertensive (blood pressure lowering) drugs, phenothiazines (class of antipsychotic drugs), antihistamines, antidepressants (especially tricyclics), antiarrhythmics (i.e. digoxin).

- **Lowers blood pressure.**
- **Assists in circulation.**
- **Beneficial in preventing and treating cardiovascular disease and congestive heart failure.**
- **Deficiency can produce congestive heart failure, high blood pressure, angina, mitral valve prolapse, stroke, cardiac arrhythmias, cardiomyopathy, and has been linked to diabetes.**

SUGAR – Another Major Contributing Factor To High Blood Pressure and the Creation of Plaque

Sugar is one of the most commonly accepted contributors to high blood pressure (often unknowingly), by its depletion of nutrients. Because sugar has absolutely no nutrients of its own, it robs nutrients from your body for its own metabolism. Sugar is responsible for the depletion of calcium and magnesium (the most important minerals regarding blood pressure regulation), as well as depleting vitamin B_2 (riboflavin), vitamin B_3 (niacin), potassium, manganese, and choline, which are also necessary for maintaining normal blood pressure. When you consider that **out of the 13 nutrients necessary to control blood pressure, sugar depletes EIGHT (more than half!), which is comparable to the damage prescription drugs do!** Sugar consumption also contributes to elevated insulin, leading to diabetes and insulin resistance, as well as obesity (all contributors to high blood pressure).

An excessive level of sugar (a molecule similar to vitamin C) in the bloodstream also weakens the arterial walls, sometimes leading to lesions. I might add that the common form of vitamin C, known as ascorbic acid, is actually made from sugar. It goes through a chemical process that removes four hydrogen molecules. Although similar in molecular structure, sugar is destructive to the vascular system, while vitamin C (especially when combined with bioflavonoids) is important for building a protein known as collagen that helps heal, and thus strengthen the vascular wall. Once the arterial wall is sufficiently healed, the high-density cholesterol (HDL) then does it s job of removing the LDL cholesterol. Interestingly, the LDL cholesterol is not really the bad guy it was somehow made out to be, but is actually preventing the possibility of internal hemorrhage or leakage from a lesion (basically scurvy). The LDL cholesterol is not really a cardiovascular risk factor unless it becomes oxidized and thus hardened.

A high intake of sugar greatly increases the incidence of cardiovascular disease, and the resultant strokes and heart attacks. This is the reason diabetics are much more prone to die from strokes and heart attacks than non-diabetics. The way to reverse the process is to reduce the consumption of sugar and increase the intake of vitamin C. Once you do, you will soon discover that your level of LDL will decrease and the HDL will increase accordingly. Also, **once the level of vitamin C is increased, more LDL cholesterol will be converted to bile acids and then excreted, due to the body's decreased demand.**

Now How Can We Remove The Plaque In The Arteries?

Incidentally, vitamin C and bioflavonoids not only assist in healing the arterial wall, but are also antioxidants that help prevent the oxidation of the LDL cholesterol. This would help explain why relatively high doses of vitamin C lowers the level of LDL cholesterol, while also increasing the HDL. Once the healing begins, less LDL is required for the temporary shoring up and sealing process, while more HDL would be required for its removal once its job is complete (both good guys just doing their job). The late Dr. Linus Pauling recommended supplementing with 2 grams (2,000 mg) or more of vitamin C daily, along with the amino acid lysine. First, I might add that many doctors consider lipoprotein-A to be a greater risk factor for heart disease than LDL cholesterol. With that in mind, Dr. Pauling discovered that when extra lysine molecules were in the bloodstream, something important took place. The lysine entered into competition with the LYSL residues on the arterial wall, preventing the lipoprotein-A from being deposited. He also discovered that it could actually help break down and remove the plaque. It was later discovered that adding the amino acid proline to the vitamin C and lysine, actually potentiated the benefit even more.

So, we now have one oral chelation (removal) process for the prevention and removal of arterial plaque. There are also several oral chelation formulas available, which normally contain the chelator **e**thylene**d**iamine **t**etracetic **a**cid (EDTA), along with various combinations of other synergistic cofactors. Translated means: Something that grabs hold of and helps remove arterial plaque (chelator). Cofactors are other nutrients that help in the process, and synergistic basically means they work together as a team to support each other in one common effort. In this case, it is the effective removal of plaque from the arteries.

A newer chelation process that has proven successful is goji. According to studies, drinking goji can reduce the blockage in arteries by 30%, which is an unbelievable reduction (Dr. Eddie Rettstatt, *Goji – Listen To What Doctors Are Saying*, CD). That benefit, combined with Dr. Victor Marcial-Vega's discovery that in less than 36 hours after ingesting goji there is a major improvement in the oxygen delivery to the cells, should definitely help the circulation, and reduce the risk of blood clots as well. Two things that many could definitely benefit from, (especially anyone who had prior bypass surgery). To read about the full benefits of goji, see the chapter in this book titled "A Few of Nature's Miracles".

There is one form of chelation that must be performed by a doctor familiar with the therapy. Although normally faster than oral chelation, it is more expensive and less convenient. EDTA is also utilized, although it is administered in a doctor's office or clinic by an IV drip, and several sessions are normally required. It also helps remove heavy metals that also accumulate in the plaque.

Chelation, in any form, should eventually assist in lowering the blood pressure while also reducing the risk of a stroke or heart attack. This approach will assure that more oxygen (rather than less) will reach the brain, thus reducing the loss of brain cells from an oxygen deficiency.

The basic difference between this approach, and the many different blood pressure medications normally prescribed, is that it is natural and thus free of side effects, and rather than suppressing symptoms, actually attacks and resolves the underlying problem. This approach is preventative as well, by reducing the potential for future problems. This approach seems much more logical, and should in my opinion be standard procedure in medicine. Until it is adopted and fully implemented, many will continue to suffer and die needlessly.

Likely the most important issue is, avoiding heart bypass surgery. This particular surgery is in my opinion, (as well as some **honest cardiologists**), by far the most abused surgeries of all. It is also one of the most expensive and invasive. The profit potential appears to be the primary driving force. Heart surgeons normally become very wealthy, usually at the expense of their patients, not just financially but also physically.

There are many ways to not only prevent the accumulation of plaque in the arteries, but also remove the existing plaque, and without drugs or surgery. As the surgery normally lasts from 7 to 10 years, many are required to repeat the surgery (if they live long enough). What a terrible thing to look forward to, for a surgery that is seldom (if ever) necessary.

The Cardiovascular Risk Factor - Acidosis

The class of blood pressure medications known as beta-blockers reduce the heart rate, as well as available oxygen, which is just one cause of acidosis. Even aerobic exercise can contribute to acidosis, but especially when taking beta-blockers. Although it is termed aerobic exercise, it soon becomes anaerobic (oxygen deficient) leading to the increased level of the lactic acid produced. Beta-blockers do an excellent job of assuring that you will soon experience an oxygen deficiency during any kind of physical exertion, as they suppress the normal increased heart rate during physical exercise.

For anyone who also has a **hypothyroid** condition, the normal metabolizing and elimination of lactic acid will be much less efficient. The more intense the exercise and the longer the duration, the more lactic acid will be produced. Although we all need exercise, we can easily see how, under the wrong set of circumstances, we could easily be creating a very acidic condition in the body.

Sugar, soft drinks, common table salt, and most processed foods, are acidic. Both stress and anger also contribute to an acidic environment in the body, as does dehydration. **Coffee, alcohol, tobacco, and <u>most prescription and over-the-counter medications</u>, as well as illegal drugs, are all acidic.**

An overly acidic (low pH) environment in the body actually results in oxygen depletion. **An unhealthy low pH condition contributes to** an increased risk of cancer, obesity, **high blood pressure, an excessively elevated level of low density lipoprotein (LDL) cholesterol, and cardiovascular disease (CVD) in general. Acidosis tends to be especially corrosive to the arteries,** and stimulates the removal of calcium from the bones (contributing to osteoporosis), in order to help alkalinize the bloodstream, and maintain the critical pH balance. **An acidic pH stimulates the binding of both LDL cholesterol and lipoprotein-A to the arterial wall.** This is the result of an increase in the electrostatic potential caused by the acid pH, which **stimulates the bonding of the infused calcium, and heavy metals to the arterial wall, and even contributes to the oxidation of LDL cholesterol. Thus, some of the calcium removed from the bones could very well end up in your arteries (obviously not our objective).**

Excess Fibrin and Vitamin K Deficiency – Both Contributors To Plaque

There are a couple more contributors to the accumulation of plaque that I am aware of. One is fibrin, which the body normally produces in order to form temporary scaffolding for tissue to adhere to until a lesion can be repaired. We normally have protolytic (protein digesting) enzymes, whose job is to digest and remove any excess fibrin after the healing process is complete. The problem is, after about age 30, our level of protolytic enzymes gradually decreases, and thus we eventually lack an adequate supply to effectively remove the excess fibrin. This creates a rough surface of fibrin in the arteries, which provides a perfect framework for solid fats and calcium to form. This is particularly a problem when acidosis is also present as we just discussed, or when taking medications such as the blood thinner Coumadin™, or statin drugs such as Zocor™ or Lipitor™, as they all deplete vitamin K. If we have an influx of calcium from the acidosis, combined with the electrostatic potential along with a vitamin K deficiency, the deposition of calcium into the arterial wall (calcification) is very likely. Just one more example of multiple ways that medications prescribed for preventing CVD, actually contribute to the problem instead. These medications are not only unreasonably expensive, but are all too often very counter-productive.

Solving The Excess Fibrin and Vitamin K Deficiency Issues

Rather than leave you hanging on the excess fibrin issue, I believe a solution is in order. There just happens to be a few protolytic enzyme formulas on the market today that can help resolve that particular issue. The one I use as a preventative measure (I passed age 30, over forty-five years ago) is called Vitalzyme™. Although there are other protolytic enzyme formulas, according to Dr. William Wong, N.D., who has done a great deal of research on enzymes, Vitalzyme™ is in his opinion the very best. He claims to have tried most enzyme formulas on the market, with his patients in his practice, as well as on himself. Vitalzyme™ also helps reduce inflammation, which can contribute to a blockage in the arteries as well.

Dr. Wong also refers to Vitalzyme™ as the poor man's chelation. Taking magnesium along with Vitalzyme™ actually assists in the removal of calcium along with the underlying fibrin. Magnesium will not only bond to and assist in the removal of calcium, but also helps the muscles in the arteries relax and dilate, and thus assist in lowering the blood pressure. It will also help prevent muscle spasms in the arteries, as this is normally the result of too much calcium, along with insufficient magnesium. Calcium causes the muscles to contract, while magnesium in turn stimulates their release. Although both are important, magnesium is the one most people are normally deficient in. It becomes a particular concern when you get two or more contractions (a muscle spasm) without the normal release that magnesium is responsible for. A major contributor to a magnesium deficiency is again many medications. The diuretics (water pills), often prescribed in combination with other blood pressure medications, appear to be one of the worst offenders regarding magnesium depletion.

Several herbs are natural diuretics, although they do not deplete nutrients as drugs do. Again, diuretics are one more class of medications designed to treat CVD that contribute to multiple problems instead. First, magnesium can lower the blood pressure, basically the same way the dangerous calcium channel blockers do although in a safe way (and won't shrink your brain in the process!). According to Sherry A. Rogers, M.D., that is one problem associated with the calcium channel blockers. Then, a magnesium deficiency is not only the cause of spasms in the vascular wall, but also an irregular heartbeat, (for which your doctor might recommend a pacemaker implant). Both conditions can easily contribute to an unsuspected heart attack.

And finally, regarding the vitamin K also depleted, you can either begin withdrawing the medications known to deplete vitamin K, or take a vitamin K supplement (or both). One function of vitamin K is escorting the calcium to the bones where it belongs, rather the arteries. You can thus promote stronger bones and more flexible arteries, basically preventing one problem, while solving others.

Thyroid's Influence on Blood Pressure

One common cause of excessive fluid retention in the body is the low body temperature, associated with a hypothyroid condition. In the book *Wilson's Syndrome* (1991/1996), Dr. E. Denis Wilson, M.D. explains the reason why, as follows:

*I believe that **abnormal body temperature patterns (especially low temperatures) cause the muscular tone of the vessels to decrease, making blood vessels more leaky, which results in tissue fluid retention.** Proper thyroid hormone treatment can be used to normalize the temperature patterns, causing them to be closer to 98.6 and causing them to be more steady. When this is accomplished, it improves vascular tone of the blood vessels in the body causing them to be less leaky and enabling them to more effectively prevent too much fluid from leaking into the tissues and to more effectively carry tissue fluid back into circulation. I believe that this one aspect of Wilson's Syndrome itself, had profound physiological consequences when one considers how it can influence so many other symptoms* (pp. 173-174).

In case you wondered, the Wilson's Syndrome that Dr. Wilson referred to is just a hypothyroid condition associated with an inadequate level of the active T_3 thyroid hormone. Dr. Wilson just chose to name the condition after himself, although his predecessor, the late Dr. Broda Barnes, did the majority of the pioneering research in that area, and thus likely deserves the majority of credit for identifying the problem.

Unfortunately, a common source of fluid retention is hypothyroidism, which is seldom ever considered, and thus resolved. A typical response by most doctors is a prescription for a nutrient depleting, dehydrating diuretic, which will never address the true cause of edema. This is a prime example why people are not only placed on, but also normally left on drugs for an entire lifetime. I know an 80-year-old lady who claims she has been taking diuretics most of her adult life. Incidentally, she has very poor health, is on oxygen, and goes to her doctor about once a week. Fixing the thyroid problem would help resolve many other conditions in the process. Doesn't that make much more sense to you? It certainly does to me.

A low thyroid condition can also reduce the strength of the heartbeat, as well as the amount of blood pumped with each beat. According to Broda Barnes, M.D. (*Hypothyroidism: The Unsuspected Illness*, 1976):

> ***In severe hypothyroidism, studies have shown that the blood circulating per minute through the body may be reduced by as much as 40 percent, thus the effective oxygen-carrying capacity of the blood is only 60 percent of normal.***
>
> *Yet even mild reduction of circulation, despite the presence of adequate hemoglobin and adequate red cells, can mean that less than normal amounts of oxygen are reaching the tissues which are always anemic to a degree* (p. 60).

Dr. Barnes also notes that studies proved that: *"Among the patients placed on thyroid during the ten-year period, ninety-five had been hypertensive in varying degrees. **Of the ninety-five, only five had failed to show satisfactory declines in pressure after being placed on thyroid therapy"** (p. 147).

Seems like we keep coming back to the thyroid. It is amazing how many things our thyroid influences! You will find more information in the Hypothyroidism chapter of this book. In case you didn't notice, **diuretics deplete FIVE of the TEN nutrients listed as being necessary for healthy thyroid function.**

Incidentally, another less-common cause of excessive fluid retention in the body is congestive heart failure, normally caused by cardiomyopathy or a weakened heart. This is just one of several side effects associated with statin (cholesterol lowering) drugs, primarily due to their CoQ_{10} depletion.

The Importance of Water

Water like oxygen, is an extremely important resource for the body. In fact, according to Dr. Batmanghelidj, water is the best diuretic there is. And although water is something we all can afford, the majority of people in the nation are actually dehydrated, (some more than others). Those that substitute caffeinated soft drinks, or coffee, or possibly even alcohol (or a combination thereof) would experience the worst water depletion of all, as these beverages are very dehydrating.

Due to the extreme importance of water in the body, dehydration is considered as a stress, and thus the body basically goes into a panic mode and begins hoarding water. Thus, dehydration leads to fluid retention. This process takes place in the kidneys. The constriction in the kidneys, necessary for that retention, leads to an elevation of the blood pressure. This also results in more concentrated (thicker) blood, which also contributes to elevated blood pressure. The body's ability to efficiently remove toxins is also reduced. So as we can see, dehydration is a major contributor to both hypertension and a toxic acidic environment in the body, which in turn depletes our oxygen level.

Water should be our primary source of liquid. If not, and dehydration is allowed to continue, the constant stress on the kidneys can eventually lead to kidney damage. This would then make it even more difficult to control the blood pressure in the future. Those at the greatest risk of all would be anyone who drank mostly dehydrating beverages, and also took statin (cholesterol lowering) medications. They can cause congestive heart failure, which would result in excessive fluid retention, due to a weakened heart. Plus, they are also very damaging to the kidneys. And Crestor™ appears to be the worst statin drug in that regard, sometimes leading to kidney failure. The problem should worsen in the future, due to the change in recommended guidelines (that most doctors appear to be following). The recommendation is to double their patients' dosage of statin drugs to meet the guidelines for lower cholesterol levels. Aren't drugs exciting? It's rather like going to a horror movie, and you just hope the main character learns where the danger lies before it's too late. But I guess in this case, I just gave away the plot.

CHAPTER TWENTY-SIX
BLOOD PRESSURE MEDICATION Vs. NATURAL SOLUTIONS

Evaluating Your Blood Pressure Medications

Now let's see what the well-known and respected Dr. James Balch has to say regarding all blood pressure medications in general. In his booklet *Healthy Tips For The Mature Heart* (1999), he states that ***"Anti-hypertensive drugs can lead to serious health problems!"*** He explains that *"Since all of these methods interrupt normal bodily functions, **they all have negative side effects.**"* Most importantly, according to Dr. Balch points out that:

***Studies prove these drugs are not effective in extending life!** We have yet to see convincing proof that these medications do anything to improve survival rates in those with mild hypertension. Moreover, they make you feel worse – not better.*

A comparison of diuretics, beta-blockers and calcium channel blockers shows that ALL these drugs have very serious side effects...and that NONE of them actually reduces the likelihood of death.

The 1995 Multicenter Isradipine Diuretic Atherosclerosis Study showed that calcium channel blockers caused an increase in cardiovascular complications including angina, stroke, and cardiac arrest. Even worse, the drugs increased the risk of cancer.

We are clearly on the wrong track with these drugs (pp. 24-27).

I most heartedly agree with Dr. Balch, and his assessment of all blood pressure medications. As he noted, these drugs work by interrupting normal bodily functions (which is unfortunately true regarding all prescription medications). Only by a cooperative approach, and working with our body, rather than suppressing important natural processes with toxic chemicals, can we possibly expect to truly resolve any health issue. We must become our body's best benefactor, rather than its worst enemy, as traditional medicine has insisted on doing for far too long, by depending upon drugs as a first line of defense.

Anyone who had been taking blood pressure medications, and were thus forced to deal with the many associated side effects, assuming they would somehow extend their life, find that excuse is no longer valid, now that the real truth has been exposed. That issue becomes especially apparent once we evaluate the problems associated with each class of blood pressure medication, and then provide a natural approach to effectively accomplish the reduction of elevated blood pressure. You will likely be quite amazed at just how simple, yet effective these safe natural therapies can actually be. Once you learn the following, you must then ask yourself: How can I, in any way, justify continuing these medications (possibly for a lifetime)? I believe the answer will soon become quite obvious.

As each different class of medication uses a different approach in order to force the reduction of blood pressure, in spite of the body's attempt to regulate important bodily functions, we will evaluate each class individually. We will begin by evaluating the diuretics.

Prescription Diuretics (Water Pills)

A major concern regarding the diuretics prescribed for eliminating excess fluid in an attempt to lower blood pressure, is the extensive list of critical vitamins and minerals that are depleted in the process. We will now evaluate one commonly prescribed diuretic and the important nutrients it depletes, as well as listing some of the more important functions associated with each nutrient depleted.

Hydrochlorothiazide (generic name)

A thiazide diuretic (water pill), used to lower blood pressure and decrease edema (swelling).

1. **Vitamin B$_1$ (thiamine)**
   - **Needed for proper muscle tone of the intestines, heart, and stomach.**
   - **Important for healthy nervous system functioning. Reduces stress and anxiety.**
   - **Assists in blood formation and enhances circulation.**
2. **Vitamin B$_2$ (riboflavin)**
   - Necessary for red blood cell formation and normal cell growth.
   - **Deficiency can produce high blood pressure.**
   - Promotes healthy skin, nails and hair.
   - **Strongly influences how well the thyroid gland synthesizes its hormones.**
   - Assists in converting protein into energy.
3. **Vitamin B$_6$**
   - **Involved in more bodily functions than almost any other single nutrient. It affects both physical and mental health.**
   - **Acts as a diuretic, yet maintains sodium and potassium balance (pH).**
   - **Deficiency can produce high blood pressure.**
   - Required by the nervous system (stress resistance) and needed for normal brain function.
   - Enhances the immune system and antibody production.
   - **Assists in the prevention of arteriosclerosis.**
   - **Inhibits the formation of homocysteine, thus reducing cholesterol deposition surrounding the heart.**
4. **Vitamin B$_{12}$**
   - **Assists in cell formation, prevents nerve damage, and promotes normal cell growth.**
   - Assists in memory, concentration and learning.
   - **Maintains a healthy nervous system.**
   - Prevents insomnia by enhancing normal sleep patterns and REM sleep.
5. **Folic acid**
   - Is considered a brain food, and is needed for energy production.
   - **Helps control the cardiovascular risk factor (homocysteine) level.**
   - Assists in the formation of blood cells and tissue functions.
   - **Prevents and treats anemia to improve oxygen delivery.**
   - A natural analgesic or painkiller.
6. **Vitamin C**
   - **Reduces cholesterol and prevents atherosclerosis.**
   - **Lowers blood pressure and strengthens blood vessels.**
   - Necessary for the growth and repair of body tissue cells.
   - Assists in the production of anti-stress hormones.
   - Enhances the immune system.

- **Is an antioxidant, needed for more than 300 metabolic functions in the body.**
- **Protects against abnormal blood clotting and bruising.**
- **Assists the body with oxygen use.**
- **Deficiency can produce tissue swelling (edema)**

7. **Vitamin D**
   - Prevents muscle weakness
   - **Reduces cholesterol and prevents atherosclerosis.**
   - **Assists in the regulation of the heartbeat.**
   - Enhances the immune system.
   - **Assists in normal blood clotting.**
   - **Necessary for healthy thyroid function.**

8. **Coenzyme Q_{10}**
   - Is a powerful antioxidant.
   - **Plays a critical role in energy production.**
   - Enhances the immune system.
   - **Lowers blood pressure.**
   - **Assists in circulation and increases tissue oxygenation.**
   - **Beneficial in treating diabetes.**
   - **Beneficial in preventing and treating cardiovascular disease and congestive heart failure.**
   - **Deficiency can produce congestive heart failure, high blood pressure, angina, mitral valve prolapse, stroke, cardiac arrhythmias, cardiomyopathy,** fatigue, decreased immune system.

9. **Calcium**
   - **Necessary for the maintenance of a regular heartbeat** and in the transmission of nerve impulses.
   - **Lowers cholesterol and prevents cardiovascular disease.**
   - Necessary for muscular growth and the prevention of muscle cramps.
   - **Lowers blood pressure and assists with normal blood clotting.**
   - Assists in neuromuscular activity and the entire nervous system.
   - **Deficiency can produce elevated blood cholesterol, hypertension (high blood pressure), heart palpitations.**

10. **Magnesium**
    - **Low magnesium levels make nearly every disease worse.**
    - **More than 300 enzymes are activated by magnesium.**
    - Responsible for the production and transfer of energy.
    - Necessary for healthy nervous and muscular tissues, and nerve transmission and impulses.
    - **Necessary to maintain normal heart rhythm and muscular contraction.**
    - Is a natural tranquilizer, known as the anti-stress mineral.
    - **Protects the arterial linings from the effects of stress caused by sudden blood pressure changes.**
    - **Necessary for the prevention of calcification of soft tissue.**
    - **Assists in the prevention of cardiovascular disease,** osteoporosis, and certain forms of cancer.
    - **Increases the rate of survival following a heart attack.**
    - **Reduces cholesterol.**
    - **Reduces blood pressure.**
    - **Deficiency can produce high blood pressure and rapid heartbeat.**

11. **Manganese**
   - **Assists vitamin K in the regulation of blood clotting.**
   - Enhances the immune system.
   - Assists in energy production.
   - **Assists with blood sugar regulation.**
   - Assists in proper digestion and utilization of food.
   - **Necessary in the syntheses of thyroxine, the principal hormone of the thyroid gland.**
   - **Deficiency can produce high cholesterol, high blood pressure, heart disorders, rapid pulse, tremors, abnormalities in insulin secretion, impaired glucose metabolism and pancreatic damage.**

12. **Phosphorus**
   - **Necessary for normal blood clotting.**
   - **Necessary for contraction of the heart muscle and normal heart rhythm.**
   - **Necessary for kidney function.**
   - Assists the body in utilization of vitamins and the conversion of food to energy.
   - Deficiency can produce irregular breathing.

13. **Potassium**
   - **Assists sodium to neutralize acids and restore alkaline salts to the bloodstream, thus controlling the body's water balance (pH).**
   - **Assists in regular heart rhythm and proper muscle contraction.**
   - **Prevents strokes.**
   - **Maintains blood pressure.**
   - **Depletion can produce hypertension (high blood pressure), salt retention and edema (swelling), fluctuations in heartbeat, high cholesterol levels, muscular fatigue and weakness, heart malfunction, and respiratory distress.**

14. **Sodium**
   - **Necessary for maintaining proper water balance and blood pH.**
   - Necessary for nerve and muscle function.
   - **Assists in the regulation of blood pressure.**
   - Assists in making the cell walls permeable.
   - **Deficiency can produce heart palpitations and muscle weakness.**

15. **Zinc**
   - **Reduces cholesterol deposits.**
   - **Necessary for collagen formation.**
   - Enhances the immune system.
   - Is a natural antioxidant.
   - **Zinc is a constituent of insulin.**
   - **Deficiency can produce high cholesterol levels,** decreased immune system, and **propensity to diabetes.**

If we just take a moment and consider just how important every single one of the nutrients depleted by diuretics actually are to our cardiovascular health, as well as our overall health, one can't help but wonder if there is any possible justification for a doctor to prescribe this drug, just to remove a little excess water. The problem is, all too often the water excreted by diuretics is not actually excess, but instead critical to our overall health, as are the nutrients they are known to deplete in the process.

Another concern is some of <u>the more serious potential side effects</u> <u>associated with the use of the diuretic Hydrochlorothiazide</u>, which are as follows:

- **Weak or irregular heartbeat**
- Muscle pain or cramps
- **Anemia**
- **Blood disorders**
- **Changes in blood sugar**
- **Difficulty breathing**
- Dizziness
- **Fluid in the lung**

- **Inflammation of the lung**
- **Inflammation of the pancreas**
- Risk when exercising in hot weather
- **Kidney failure**
- Muscle spasms
- **Weight Gain**
- **Impotence**
- Vision changes

How Diuretics Can Cause An Oxygen Deficiency

Although diuretics are quite often prescribed in combination with blood pressure medications to lower blood pressure, they can actually contribute to hypertension, in at least two different ways. As you just learned, one is by depleting minerals important for controlling hypertension. The other is by causing dehydration. This leads to a constriction of the capillaries in the kidneys, discussed under the ACE inhibitors. By forcing the excretion of salt and water, as well as many important nutrients, diuretics not only contribute to hypertension, but also an overall unhealthy condition throughout the body and brain (dehydration).

Anything that can contribute to dehydration (such as diuretics) can create an oxygen deficiency, which increases the risk of angina pain, heart attack, and stroke. Once the body becomes dehydrated, not only does the constriction in the kidneys take place to retain the much needed salt and water, but the lungs are influenced also. Dehydration is considered by the body as stress, which then causes elevated histamine. This results in a constriction of the bronchial tubes in the lungs, as well as the formation of mucus. This is the body's attempt to reduce the loss of water through the lungs. The dehydration is often exacerbated following a meal, as the body requires a considerable amount of water for digestion. This is one common cause of an asthma attack, and can also contribute to a heart attack.

During dehydration, the blood viscosity is higher (the blood becomes thicker). Then, due to the bronchial constriction and the coating of mucus, less oxygen will be absorbed in the lungs. And now a third factor comes into play. Some of the histamine residue in the blood also results in the constriction of the coronary arteries supplying the heart with oxygen. So we basically would have thicker blood with less oxygen feeding the heart muscle through constricted (basically smaller) coronary arteries. This same blood must also supply the entire body, as well as the brain with oxygen.

Although few drink an adequate amount of water, or get a sufficient supply of complete sea salt, the diuretics and ACE inhibitors that many are placed on, are among the most serious contributors to dehydration. It appears that far too many medications actually contribute to, rather than resolve, the very condition they are **supposed to be** controlling.

Natural Diuretics That Really Work - Safe and Simple Solutions to Edema (Fluid Retention)

I believe you will be quite amazed at just how easily excess fluid can be effectively removed (with absolutely no nutrient depletion!). Natural diuretics should be every bit as effective and would **"First do no harm,"** as Hypocrites, the father of medicine, once stressed. If we took his advice seriously, we would never consider using the toxic chemicals known as prescription medications. There is always a natural solution that in my opinion makes taking any chemical symptom-suppressant drug totally unnecessary.

- **Check your thyroid.** A hypothyroid condition should be your very first consideration, as it contributes to fluid retention, among other things. That is especially true regarding women, as they are ten times as likely as men to experience a low thyroid condition. Both identifying the problem (if one exists), as well as an effective solution, is discussed in detail in the Hypothyroid Chapter of this book.

- **Water and Celtic sea salt.** Another important issue is to drink at least ten 8-ounce glasses of water daily, along with 1 teaspoon of Celtic sea salt, to avoid dehydration, and to remove any excess water retention (edema) if necessary. As we noted earlier, according to Dr. Batmanghelidj, water is the best diuretic there is.

- **Herbal combinations.** There are several herbal combinations that are known to be effective diuretics, and are available in most health food stores. For example, one herbal formula contains the herbal diuretics **parsley**, **uva ursi**, and **juniper berry.** You will find they are perfectly safe and **far less expensive** than your nutrient depleting prescription diuretics.

- **L-Carnitine.** If you also might possibly be suffering from a condition known as congestive heart failure due cardiomyopathy (a weakened heart), we also have a natural solution. Dr. Jonathan Wright tells us of a natural amino acid called L-carnitine. He claims that taking 250 mg three times daily will normally resolve congestive heart failure, which results in an excess build-up of fluid. He notes that L-carnitine enables the heart muscle to utilize its energy sources more effectively. I would also recommend **adding 200 mg of CoQ$_{10}$ daily,** especially if the congestive heart failure was the result of statin (cholesterol lowering) medications. The heart requires more CoQ$_{10}$ than any other organ, and the statin drugs are notorious for its depletion.

Calcium Channel Blockers

Calcium channel blockers are another class of hypertension (blood pressure) lowering medications. Studies announced in the *Journal of the American Medical Association* (*JAMA*, December 15, 2004, 292:2849-2859), involving almost 20,000 women between the ages of 50 and 70 proved that **women taking calcium channel blockers had twice the risk of dying from heart disease,** thus contributing to a heart attack risk. Although this study involved only women, I would expect the same to apply to men also.

I assume you are aware by now that God obviously doesn't make mistakes, (although man is continuing to do so). Some of the so-called scientists who design these drugs seem to either be unaware of, or are totally disregarding, the important functions these drugs are suppressing. Have you ever noticed that many drugs are referred to as inhibitors, or blockers? They are basically overriding critical functions in the body just to come up with some number, such as a cholesterol or blood pressure level, considered as acceptable, although it somehow mysteriously continues to change. The newer acceptable numbers always seem to change in favor of the requirement for either higher levels, or additional medications in order to control. Have you ever wondered why? I believe the answer is quite obvious, although you are unfortunately the ones paying the price. You will also be forced to deal with more unnecessary side effects, as well as a worsening of health from additional nutrient depletion, something drugs are well known for.

Calcium Channel Blockers' Influence On The Body

It might be helpful if we better understood just how these drugs actually lower the blood pressure, as well as some very critical functions being compromised in the process. There are two important minerals that stimulate muscles in the body, (calcium and magnesium). The two have opposing, yet important functions. The function of calcium is muscle contraction, and magnesium is responsible for muscle release. They basically work together as a team, and are important for regulating the distribution of both oxygen and water throughout the body and brain. Our body has a very efficient distribution system that is responsible for diverting the resources to the areas of greatest demand.

Unfortunately, the calcium channel blockers attempt to override this critical process by preventing the flow of calcium to both the nerves and muscles. This tends to relax the arteries and thus reduces the blood pressure. If their only function was to lower the blood pressure, that might not necessarily be a concern, but unfortunately there is much more to the story. The question is: Are we possibly ignoring some very important functions in the body that are being unnecessarily suppressed? Any time we focus strictly on a particular number such as "ideal" blood pressure, without any consideration of what might be compromised in the process, that approach is obviously seriously flawed.

The important function that is being suppressed, and totally ignored, is the body's ability to divert blood, and thus oxygen, to the area of greatest demand. This can only be accomplished by the constriction of muscles in the arteries in the area of least demand (calcium's responsibility), along with the dilation in some other area of greater demand, (magnesium's responsibility). One example would be following a meal, when more water is required to hydrolyze (liquefy and break down) the food in the stomach, as well as by the pancreas in order to produce digestive enzymes, which are in liquid form. More blood is also always diverted to the stomach following a meal. The larger the meal, the greater the requirement. The water also hydrates the mucosa lining in the stomach in order to prevent damage to the stomach, from the hydrochloric acid produced to digest protein. This dilutes the action of the acid on the stomach lining, and thus helps prevent the formation of ulcers. This is just one example of how calcium channel blockers prevent important everyday functions from naturally occurring in the body.

This now takes us to the brain. If you recall, we found that there is a serious concern associated with the calcium channel blockers, regarding the potential neuron damage, and shrinkage of the brain. I believe we will soon discover a good explanation for this mysterious phenomenon, which is not really a mystery after all. Our brain, like our heart, never rests. Different parts of the brain assume different responsibilities, and every single one is critical to our overall welfare, both physically and mentally. So, let's evaluate what the calcium channel blockers' influence on the brain might be.

Calcium Channel Blockers' Influence On The Brain

The brain, due to its extreme importance, receives preferential treatment (has top priority), as it obviously should. Our body was designed with that in mind, and the priority system has proven very efficient when allowed to function as intended. It should be obvious that when the neurons begin dying prematurely, something is drastically wrong with a drug that creates the problem. One major concern, regarding the importance of getting off this dangerous drug, is its potential for brain damage. According to Dr. Sherry Rogers, M.D., *"Calcium channel blockers cause shrinking of the brain and function loss within a few short years. Not to worry, this is casually dismissed as 'normal aging' or later, Alzheimer's"* (*Detoxify or Die*, 2000, p. 188).

Although we seem to be concerned about the increasing incidence of dementia and Alzheimer's disease in the nation, we somehow tend to ignore the evidence. The evidence that many in the nation are continuing to take a medication recommended by their doctor, that has been proven by brain scans to be contributing to brain deterioration! . Elevated blood pressure is actually a minor concern in comparison. Also, as Dr. Balch noted, **75% of those placed on medication actually have only marginally elevated blood pressure.** The unnecessary destruction of the brain that many are unknowingly experiencing, (often for years), is obviously a major concern and totally unnecessary. So, if you are currently taking a calcium channel blocker, and you value your brain, you might seriously consider making a change before it's too late!

Another important function that calcium channel blockers prevent, is the body's ability to divert water to the brain in sufficient supply during time of need. Dr. Batmanghelidj stresses the importance of water in the brain. In his opinion, the primary cause of Alzheimer's disease is brain cell dehydration. He states that *"In prolonged dehydration, the brain cells begin to shrink"* (*Your Body's Many Cries For Water*, 1992/1998, p. 33). He also discusses a couple important functions of water in the brain. According to Dr. Batmanghelidj, the brain uses water (along with sodium & potassium), to generate electrical energy. And when the supply of water is insufficient, the many functions of the brain that depend upon this particular form of energy become inefficient. He also notes that an adequate supply of water is also necessary for transporting neurotransmitters throughout the brain. The extreme importance of water in the brain is evidenced by the fact that the brain cells are considered to be 85% water.

Dr. Batmanghelidj also emphasized that dehydration in the brain is interpreted as stress by the body, thus leading to the production of stress hormones. Then, according to Dr. David Perlmutter, M.D., stress hormones are also known to damage neurons in the brain. As we can easily see, just the inability of the body to adequately divert water to the brain, in sufficient supply when needed, is a major contributor to brain deterioration, as evidenced by brain scans.

Now let's see what some of the important resources necessary for efficient brain function might be. Oxygen is obvious, as is glucose. Others are vitamins, minerals (especially sodium and potassium), and amino acids necessary for creating neurotransmitters. And of course both calcium and magnesium are normally important for diverting critical resources. We are often utilizing different parts of the brain based on what we might be doing at any particular time. For instance, we sometimes utilize the visual right brain, and at other times it might be the left, our logical side (the part I tend to overwork). Cholesterol is also a major component of the brain, (something statin drugs can force to dangerously low levels).

Regarding the glucose and oxygen issue, any time there is an increased demand for either, more blood is normally diverted to the area. One established priority system is controlled by selective insulin sensitivity. It's thought that dehydration also contributes to insulin resistance. Interestingly, although the body relies on the beta cells in the pancreas for producing insulin, it was discovered that the brain produces its own insulin. Possibly the resultant insulin resistance in the body might ensure that an adequate supply of glucose would be made available for the brain for energy, (especially when there is a deficiency of water).

Incidentally, there's an added concern, which I failed to mention. According to Dr. James Balch, M.D., the calcium channel blockers also increase the risk of cancer (*Healthy Tips For The Mature Heart*, 1999, p. 27). It is likely due to an insufficient supply of oxygen to cells, as cancer hates oxygen. I believe this particular class of blood pressure medication tops my list as the worst of the worst (most potentially dangerous), and here I thought the diuretics were bad. In regards to drugs in general, I would say the cholesterol lowering drugs are at least right at the top of the list. Regarding the brain, the calcium channel blockers appear to pose the greatest risk, although with the statins, it's the heart and kidneys.

A Closer Look At The Calcium Channel Blocker – Norvasc™

Below you will find additional proof that calcium channel blockers can be potentially dangerous, which is reflected in the following **40 of the <u>more than 100</u> potential side effects** attributed to the use of just one of the most commonly prescribed calcium channel blockers:

<u>Norvasc™ / generic name = amlodipine</u>

- **Dizziness**
- Flushing
- **Fluttery or throbbing heartbeat**
- Agitation
- **Anxiety**
- Back pain
- **Depression**
- Difficult or painful urination
- General feeling of illness
- **Inability to sleep**
- **Inflamed blood vessels**
- **Irregular pulse**
- **Joint pain or problems**

- Fatigue
- **Fluid retention and swelling**
- **Either slow or rapid heartbeat**
- Allergic reactions
- Apathy
- Chest pain
- **Difficult or labored breathing**
- Frequent urination
- **Heart failure**
- Indigestion
- **Inflamed pancreas**
- **Pain**
- Lack of coordination

- Lack of sensation
- **Loss of sense of identity**
- Muscle weakness
- Stomach inflammation
- **Tremor**
- **Vision problems**
- **Weight gain**

- **Loss of memory**
- Muscle cramps or pain
- Nervousness
- Sexual problems
- Twitching
- Weakness
- Hair loss

Additional warnings:

- **Elderly people may be especially sensitive to the effects of amlodipine. This may increase the chance of side effects during treatment.**

- Make sure you tell your doctor if you have any other medical problems, especially congestive heart failure, as there is a small chance that amlodipine may make this condition worse.

- Although very rare, **if you have severe heart disease, you may experience an increase in frequency and duration of angina attacks, or <u>even have a heart attack</u>,** when you are starting on amlodipine or when your dosage is increased.

Replacing Calcium Channel Blockers With Something Much Safer

After uncovering the serious potential for brain damage associated with calcium channel blockers, a different solution should be apparent. The threat of loosing mental function is the number-one concern of most seniors, and the primary reason people are placed in nursing homes in increasing numbers. We must begin making those critical decisions, such as eliminating potentially dangerous drugs, while we still have the mental capacity to do so. If not, your doctor might very well decide that you are no longer capable of making rational health decisions, and thus assume that responsibility for you. A scary thought, as once that happens, you will be like the majority of those in nursing homes today, needlessly placed on many unnecessary medications, such as the calcium channel blockers we just discussed. As the pharmacist Armon Neel stressed, almost 100% of the seniors he evaluated were placed on at least twice as many medications as they should have been.

The good news is, the use of calcium channel blockers for dilating the arteries to control blood pressure is totally unnecessary. Natural alternatives to accomplish the same thing are surprisingly simple, as well as inexpensive.

1. Sufficient Magnesium. One simple solution is sufficient magnesium, known as **"Nature's calcium channel blocker"**, as it **helps relax and dilate the arteries.** Magnesium is a critical mineral that most people are deficient in. One reason is, many medications deplete magnesium (especially diuretics). A magnesium deficiency is often the cause of muscle spasms, and irregular heartbeat. Another reason for a widespread magnesium deficiency is the standard dietary recommended ratio of two-to-one calcium-to-magnesium. The truth is, the ratio should actually be reversed. Research has shown that **our body needs at least twice as much magnesium as calcium.** Magnesium is important for the activation of over 300 enzymes in the body. When we were young, our level of magnesium was approximately 3 times our level of calcium.

Dr. James Balch, M.D. tells us that *"A low magnesium level makes nearly every disease worse"* (*Prescription for Nutritional Healing, 3rd edition,* 2000, p. 30) and that *"magnesium deficiencies are at the root of many cardiovascular problems."* He even claims that *"A magnesium deficiency can be synonymous with diabetes."* And as we are aware, diabetes is a major contributor to not only damage to the cardiovascular system, but many other serious complications.

Insufficient magnesium is also one primary cause of calcification of soft tissues, as both calcium and magnesium are needed to form bone tissue. Another is a deficiency of vitamin K, which escorts the calcium into the bone where intended. Unfortunately, many medications also deplete vitamin K. Two of the worst drugs for vitamin K depletion are Coumadin™ and the statin (cholesterol lowering) medications. The very last thing we want to do is to deprive our body of calcium, or in any way suppress its normal function of artery constriction when necessary to distribute resources such as oxygen or water. If the constriction somehow results in a temporary slight increase in blood pressure, it shouldn't really be a concern. Also, while some arteries or capillaries might be constricted, others would in turn be dilated, so the net result would likely be very little if any variation in blood pressure.

2. L-Arginine. Another inexpensive resource proven to **dilate the arteries** is just a common amino acid, which as usual has multiple benefits. One function of L-arginine is increasing the level of nitric oxide (NO), in the bloodstream. Nitric oxide is best known as a vasodilator. In my opinion, the combination of 400 mg of magnesium twice daily, along with 500 mg of L-arginine twice daily away from meals, would likely be considerably more effective in lowering the blood pressure, than the calcium channel blockers. Most importantly, they will not only do so safely, but will also provide additional important benefits in the process.

Other benefits of L-arginine include reducing body fat and increasing muscle mass, strengthening the immune system, as well as **the production of insulin.** This is typical of natural solutions. They have **many side <u>benefits</u>**, versus the **multiple side effects** associated with prescription medications. The best option should be obvious.

3. Increasing Nitric Oxide. If we're real serious about dilating the arteries even further, there are products that specialize in increasing the level of nitric oxide, which dilates the arteries. One such formula is called NOX-3, and is produced by Universal Nutrition. Stimulators of nitric oxide such as NOX-3 are often used by body-builders to provide more oxygen and nutrients to the muscles during workout. It would seem logical that the same would also apply to increasing oxygen to the brain. The ingredients include synergists that result in more effective forms of the amino acids arginine and orthinine. One source that sells NOX-3 is Nutrition Express, and the current discounted price is $27.89 for a one-month's supply. Normally, magnesium and L-arginine should be sufficient.

Best of luck with your calcium channel blocker withdrawal, and in successfully maintaining healthy brain function (obviously a major concern), before it's too late.

ACE Inhibitors

The full name is "**A**ngiotensin **C**onverting **E**nzyme Inhibitor." The ACE inhibitor attempts to suppress the renin-angiotensin (RA) system. The RA system regulates kidney function, and is initiated once the body recognizes a deficiency of fluid volume, or dehydration. The body is constantly attempting to maintain an adequate level of both water and salt, but when a deficiency is recognized, a tightening of the capillary bed (especially the tufts of capillaries in the kidneys called glomeruli) takes place. This tightening (vascular constriction) can at times result in hypertension.

There are several things that can potentially lead to the stimulation of the RA system, and the subsequent vascular constriction. The first, and most likely is obviously **dehydration.** One all too common practice in medicine that makes absolutely no sense, is combining a diuretic with a blood pressure medication, such as the ACE inhibitors, as they both can contribute to dehydration.

Vascular constriction is also a problem associated with a **sodium deficiency.** The body uses sodium to retain an adequate level of water. Unfortunately, many doctors advise their patients to avoid salt, which complicates the problem even further.

One more condition that stimulates the tightening of the capillary bed in the kidneys (or vascular constriction) is insufficient blood pressure for effective filtration, and thus the secretion of urine. The body attempts to make up for the low blood pressure, by increasing the vascular pressure in order to assure that sufficient urine removal takes place. The more restriction there is in the kidneys, the more pressure is required for filtration. Unfortunately, many are needlessly placed on blood pressure medications, when their blood pressure is only marginally high to begin with. As a result, the blood pressure is often insufficient for effective kidney function, which would then stimulate vascular constriction out of necessity, resulting in an increase in blood pressure. This is a prime example of how forcing the blood pressure below what is an adequate level for a particular individual, is actually counter-productive.

A Closer Look At The ACE Inhibitor - Lisinopril

Now before we look at some natural ways to lower your blood pressure, it might as usual, be helpful to look at some of the more serious potential side effects associated with another class of medication for hypertension. We will be evaluating one of the most common ACE inhibitors, called Lisinopril, or Prinivil™. Although not included in the list below, **pain in twelve different areas of the body** was included in the complete list of **over 100 potential side effects** (we will just list forty). This drug appears to be a real pain, I would say. Following are our forty selections:

- **Anemia**
- **Blood clot in lungs**
- Bronchitis
- **Coughing up blood**
- **Diabetes**
- Fainting
- Feeling of illness
- **Fluid retention or swelling**
- Heart burn
- Incoordination
- Indigestion
- **Irritability**
- Lung cancer
- **Memory impairment**
- Painful breathing
- **Pneumonia**
- Sinus inflammation
- **Stroke**
- Urinary Tract infection
- Weight loss

- **Asthma**
- **Blurred vision or changes in vision**
- **Confusion**
- **Dehydration**
- Double vision
- Fatigue
- **Gout**
- **Heart attack**
- Impotence / Decreased sex drive
- **Inability to sleep / Insomnia**
- **Irregular, rapid, or flutter heartbeat**
- **Kidney trouble or failure**
- Lung inflammation
- Nervousness
- Painful urination
- **Respiratory infection**
- Arthritis
- Tremor
- Weakness
- **Weight gain**

I don't know about you, but I find it hard to understand why a drug would be designed to suppress such an important function in the body in the first place. Dr. F. Batmanghelidj, M.D., in his book *Your Body's Many Cries For Water* (1992/1998), stresses the importance of proper hydration. If you noticed, dehydration is just one of the many problems listed, and yet it can contribute to many diseases and unhealthy conditions in the body. **The brain is especially dependant upon an adequate supply of water. One contributor to insulin resistance in the receptors is dehydration.** A leading contributor to back pain is dehydration. **It can even contribute to strokes and heart attacks,** as well as angina pain. And the list goes on, as do the potential side effects (over 100) associated with this drug, which we just discovered.

Any drug with the potential to create such an extensive list of major side effects has to be creating a considerable amount of chaos throughout the body. If we then combine the diuretics, as many doctors all too often do, you should expect to experience even more of the side effects on our list. If you recall, Mary Lou was placed an ACE inhibitor, along with a diuretic (which is not recommended), which is unfortunately common practice in medicine today. This is especially a concern if we consider Dr.

Batmanghelidj's theory regarding the importance of adequate hydration of the body and brain. As we just discussed, many doctors also recommend a salt-free diet, which just compounds the problem even further. The body depends on both sodium and potassium (found in natural sea salt) for many of its important functions. They are both responsible for the transfer of nutrients into the cell, as well as removal of toxins. The body also depends upon sodium to maintain an adequate supply of water, and to produce the hydrochloric acid necessary for digesting proteins. The brain can actually generate energy when an adequate level of natural sea salt and water are available.

Fixing The Problem Without ACE Inhibitors

First, let's review for a moment, what the ACE inhibitors are actually attempting to accomplish. As we just discussed, there is a natural and very important process in the body called renin-angiotensin (RA), which regulates the kidney function. The only time this system is activated is when we become dehydrated. Therefore, if we never become dehydrated, these ACE inhibitors have absolutely no purpose in the body, except possibly creating a very extensive list (over 100!) of potential side effects. This is a typical example of another drug that is inhibiting an important function in the body, (to prevent further dehydration), although it is actually contributing to dehydration instead. All in an effort to arrive at a particular lower number (blood pressure), and to do so at all costs, and often without any real benefit.

The question is: What were all those other drugs actually doing? Obviously nothing, other than depleting important nutrients and creating dozens of side effects in the process. Quite often, the blood pressure medications prescribed have absolutely no influence on the blood pressure, although many patients remain on them for years. And all too often, the medications are not even addressing, (or should I say suppressing), the actual cause of hypertension.

The obvious drug-free solution would be to resolve, or prevent, dehydration, rather than contributing to the problem. This is remarkably easy to accomplish, as well as the least expensive of all our solutions for hypertension. It's just a matter of drinking ten 8-ounce glasses of (chlorine-free and fluoride-free) water, along with one teaspoon of Celtic sea salt daily. It's just that simple!

Things you should avoid that normally contribute to dehydration are:
- Coffee
- Caffeinated soft drinks
- Alcohol
- Diuretics
- Smoking
- Stress (yes, even stress contributes to dehydration)

I can see absolutely no reason to take a medication that would just make a bad situation (dehydration), even worse. Can you?

Beta-Blockers

We now come to the beta-blockers, whose primary function is suppressing any increase in the heart rate. The theory is that by keeping the heart rate low, we can also keep the blood pressure low. Although that might be true, it's a terrible price to pay if you consider the potential damage caused by oxygen deprivation. As we learned in Al's story, that is especially a concern for anyone who exercises, (which we should all be doing). The more intense the exercise, the worse the problem will become. During exercise, or any physical activity for that matter, unless the heart rate increases, you will soon begin experiencing an oxygen deficiency, followed by extreme fatigue. Our heart rate increases for a very good reason, and suppressing it could be potentially dangerous. An oxygen deficiency results in the production of lactic acid, leading to a very acidic state (low pH), which is a contributor to cardiovascular damage, as well as cancer. Also, any time the brain is deprived of oxygen (which would be the case), the cells will begin to die.

As we discussed earlier, another class of blood pressure medication (the calcium cannel blockers) also suppress the body's ability to divert the available oxygen, water, and nutrients to where the greatest demand exists. When the calcium channel blockers are combined with the beta-blockers, you end up with an insufficient supply of oxygen in the bloodstream combined with an ineffective distribution system (double jeopardy). If you then add dehydration, caused by the diuretics many are also placed on, the risk of brain damage is even greater (triple jeopardy).

We constantly hear of the increasing incidence of Alzheimer's disease in the nation today, although some of the major contributors to Alzheimer's disease are obviously being ignored. From the information I have uncovered the past several years, I am convinced I could establish an effective protocol for greatly reducing the rate of Alzheimer's disease in the nation. I can't help but wonder why some doctor or scientist hasn't discovered the solution to preventing Alzheimer's disease by now. Scientists are always looking at the DNA as a possible cause, or looking for some drug as a solution. In my opinion, the solution will not be found in any drug, but instead a lack thereof, along with some important nutrients. Although I'm aware of a few other things we can do to avoid Alzheimer's disease (and possibly even repair some of the damage), just eliminating these medications, in my opinion, would likely have the most benefit when you consider their potential for damage.

A Closer Look At The Beta-Blocker Atenolol

One commonly prescribed beta-blocker is Atenolol. As is all too often the case, the very important CoQ_{10} along with some of the most important minerals magnesium, phosphorus, potassium, sodium, and zinc, are all depleted by Atenolol. Another problem is:

*After you have been taking a beta-blocker for a while, it may cause unpleasant or even harmful effects if you stop taking it too suddenly. **After you stop taking this medicine or while you are gradually reducing the amount you are taking, <u>you may experience chest pain, fast or irregular heartbeat,</u> general feeling of discomfort or illness or weakness, headache, shortness of breath (sudden), sweating or trembling.***

This class of blood pressure medication appears to be the most difficult to withdraw from, due to the uncomfortable, and rather scary side effects often experienced during withdrawal. I believe that gradually reducing the dosage for approximately one month could possibly help. Just by reducing the pill by ¼ each week might help your body adjust. Be sure to check your blood pressure every day to assure you are staying in the safe range.

Another reason for eliminating this drug is the common side effects that include:

*…Breathing difficulty and/or wheezing, cold hands and feet, **mental depression, shortness of breath,** slow heartbeat (especially less than 50 beats per minute), swelling of ankles, feet, and/or lower legs, decreased sexual ability, dizziness or lightheadedness, drowsiness, **trouble in sleeping,** vertigo, **unusual tiredness or weakness, weight gain.***

I would assume that the symptoms from withdrawal are likely the result of the over-production of adrenalin by the adrenals. When the normal action of the adrenalin on the beta-receptors has been suppressed by the Atenolol, the tendency would be for the adrenals to produce even more adrenalin. This is similar to what happens with a diabetic when the insulin receptors become increasingly resistant (the pancreas produces more insulin). As you begin the withdrawal from the beta-blockers, it's as though the beta-receptors are suddenly turned on, and the heart thus goes into overdrive, which would explain the rapid heartbeat. That would be especially true anytime you might be experiencing stress, or during physical exercise, when the natural release of adrenalin would be the most pronounced. By gradually reducing the level of Atenolol, you are in theory, gradually opening the valves (the beta receptors).

The majority of the side effects associated with Atenolol are also typical of those associated with low thyroid function. And, according to Dr. David Brownstein, M.D., in his book *Overcoming Thyroid Disorders* (2002), **beta-blockers inhibit the production of T_4 to T_3, (referring to thyroid hormones).** This basically results in suppressed thyroid function, and thus reduced metabolism. If you also take into consideration the beta-blockers' depletion of the major energy molecule CoQ_{10}, you now have a perfect combination for extreme fatigue, depression, and weight gain, as well as the many other symptoms associated with low thyroid function.

The more closely we evaluate the wide range of potential problems associated with these medications, the more serious concerns we can identify. If we also consider the broad range of potential side effects associated with each individual drug, it should be obvious that there is even more potential for creating major problems when multiple medications are combined, as is all too often the case.

It appears that the primary function of beta-blockers is the suppression of the normal increase in the heart rate during stress or physical exercise. **This is a normal response that should not be suppressed!** When it is, a serious oxygen deficiency could easily result. For that very reason, my only recommendation would be to take two capsules of the safe yet effective stress-reducing herb, Valerian Root, when experiencing stress. Suppressing the heart rate during exercise makes absolutely no sense, so that should not even an option to be considered.

Summary Of Blood Pressure Medications

1. **Your medications could very well be the cause of your high blood pressure.** First, every single one of the medications evaluated for nutrient depletion, actually resulted in the depletion of nutrients important for maintaining healthy blood pressure. A total of 83 (out of 200) also listed **"high blood pressure"** as a potential side effect.

2. Dr. Balch's conclusions: *"**Anti-hypertensive drugs can lead to serious health problems!** Since all of these methods interrupt normal bodily functions, they all have negative side effects. **Studies prove these drugs are not effective in extending life!**"* (*Healthy Tips For The Mature Heart*, 1999, pp. 24-27).

3. **Prescription diuretics:** Often prescribed indiscriminately, and can easily lead to serious dehydration. **Diuretics deplete 7 vitamins, 7 minerals, and the critical molecule CoQ_{10}.** Every one of the nutrients depleted provides multiple benefits for cardiovascular health. **Seven of the nutrients depleted are known to help lower blood pressure naturally!** Diuretics could very easily cause elevated blood pressure, from both their nutrient depletion, and dehydration, which results in a constriction in the kidneys in order to retain salt and water.

According to Dr. Batmanghelidj, *"**Water itself is the best diuretic**"* (*Your Body's Many Cries For Water*, 1992/1998, p. 76). As well as ten 8-ounce glasses of water daily, I would recommend 1 teaspoon of Celtic sea salt daily (which contains both sodium and potassium). If that's not sufficient, you can always try an herbal diuretic, which won't deplete important nutrients or lead to dehydration.

4. **Calcium channel blockers:** According to Sherry Rogers, M.D. *"**Calcium channel blockers cause shrinking of the brain and function loss within a few short years.** Not to worry, this is casually dismissed as 'normal aging' or later, Alzheimer's"* (*Detoxify or Die*, 2000, p. 188). **Calcium channel blockers place women at twice the risk of dying from heart disease.** They suppress the body's ability to divert resources such as oxygen, water, and nutrients to the areas in greatest demand. Just the mineral magnesium, along with the amino acid L-arginine, will accomplish the same thing, as well as providing additional benefits.

5. **ACE Inhibitors: These have the most extensive list of potentially serious side effects of all the blood pressure medications.** The only time ACE inhibitors could have any influence on the blood pressure, is when the body is dehydrated, or the blood pressure is too low to effectively filter the blood in the kidneys. Both problems could easily be caused by other medications prescribed for controlling blood

pressure, thus producing a vicious circle. For instance, diuretics are the most likely cause of dehydration. Then, blood pressure medications attempt to lower the blood pressure at all costs, which can force the pressure too low for normal kidney function.

The solution should be to eliminate the dehydrating, and nutrient depleting diuretics. You should then drink ten 8-ounce glasses of water (as we just discussed under #3), along with 1 teaspoon of Celtic sea salt to avoid dehydration. And remember, using the natural approach to regulate the blood pressure will not force it too low. This should then prevent the activation of the enzyme that the ACE inhibitors are attempting to suppress, which would otherwise lead to even worse dehydration, (an obvious unhealthy condition).

6. **Beta-blockers:** The primary function of the beta-blockers is to suppress another important function. They stop the heart rate from increasing when it obviously should. This **results in a serious oxygen deficiency,** along with extreme fatigue, during exercise or any physical exertion. They also suppresses the thyroid function, which leads to even worse fatigue, as well as increasing other cardiovascular risk factors. The rather scary side effects associated with stopping the beta-blockers, make their withdrawal more difficult than the others. But it's definitely worth the effort, so just withdraw slowly and allow your body time to adjust.

Next we will look at some natural ways we can effectively lower our blood pressure. As controlling the heart rate in any unnatural way is just one of many serious flaws in medicine, that is something we will not even attempt to duplicate. If you can find any possible justification for continuing to use any of these blood pressure medications, I suggest you seriously consider re-reading this chapter.

Natural Solutions For Lowering Blood Pressure

Following are many natural solutions for effectively lowering your blood pressure to choose from. Keep in mind that these are just options, so just pick the ones that fit your budget, and work the best for you personally:

1. Vitalzyme™. There just happens to be a product that I use as a preventative, which should address three important issues. It is a protolytic (protein-digesting) enzyme formula called Vitalzyme™. According to Dr. William Wong, N.D., Ph.D., it will eat away at the fibrosis buildup in the blood vessels, as well as the scar tissue accumulation in the tufts of capillaries in the kidneys (glomeruli). He also claims it will digest any excess fibrin in the bloodstream, thus reducing the chance of a blood clot, which could contribute to a stroke or heart attack. This would also assist in the removal of any abnormal protein in the bloodstream, which would clean the blood, thus reducing the viscosity and lowering blood pressure.

2. Water And Celtic sea salt. The more dehydrated we become, the higher the viscosity of our blood will likely be, so an adequate intake of water would obviously be beneficial. Celtic sea salt contains many important ionic minerals, and thus has many benefits over common table salt, which contains only sodium chloride and aluminum, (and sometimes iodine). It contains both sodium and potassium (a major issue), and thus won't cause the fluid retention associated with common table salt. It also has more than 80 minerals in the ionic easily-assimilable form. Many of the minerals are important for maintaining healthy blood pressure. Although common table salt can solidify and harden in the kidneys, Celtic sea salt won't. Another distinction is although regular salt is acidic, Celtic sea salt is instead alkaline. That is an important issue also, as when the body is too acidic it can cause damage to the arteries, as well as depleting oxygen. I would recommend drinking ten 8-ounce glasses of water, along with 1 teaspoon of Celtic sea salt daily.

3. Vitamin E is important for the heart function, as well as thinning the blood. Use the natural D-alpha tocopherol form. I personally use 800 IU daily.

4. Omega-3 fatty acids, such as flax seed oil or fish oil, help lower the blood pressure and improve the circulation. According to Jordan S. Rubin, N.M.D., C.N.C, **more than 60 double-blind studies show that** *"either fish oil supplements or flaxseed oil [both rich in omega-3 fatty acids] are very effective in lowering blood pressure,"* **as well as significantly reducing the risk of**

developing heart disease (*Patient Heal Thyself*, 2003, p. 136). Take four 1,000 mg soft-gels daily of either flax seed oil or fish oil, (or both).

5. Garlic helps reduce clotting and lowers blood pressure. According to the *Prescription for Nutritional Healing, 3rd edition* (Balch & Balch, 2000), **garlic actually dilates blood vessels, and aids in preventing heart attacks.** You can purchase tasteless, odorless powdered garlic in capsule form (however, raw is best). Be sure to read the label when buying garlic supplements though, as some in the soft gel form can be as much as 99 percent vegetable oil with just a touch of garlic. Take 3 capsules, twice daily.

6. Cayenne improves circulation, as well as acting as a catalyst for other herbs. Cayenne may also help to "clean out" the arteries and reverse the effects of atherosclerosis, as well as benefiting the heart and entire cardiovascular system. **Cayenne is especially beneficial for preventing strokes or heart attacks, thus it is the main ingredient in our "Emergency Kit",** and is pretty well covered earlier in the chapter on HEART ATTACKS AND STROKES. Cayenne is readily accessible, inexpensive, but a very versatile and valuable herb. Be aware that cayenne is a natural blood thinner.

7. Magnesium, Calcium and L-arginine. We have discussed the fact that magnesium and L-arginine help relax and dilate the arteries, and lower blood pressure. Be sure to take calcium with your magnesium, and just remember: **The ratio should be twice as much magnesium as calcium (contrary to what you likely were told).** This is something many nutritionists are still unaware of.

8. Vitamin C and Lysine. Taking vitamin C and lysine will help with the chelation (removal of plaque). Vitalzyme™ is beneficial in that regard also. The oral chelation takes time, although it's definitely worth the effort.

9. Lecithin granules. Lecithin is inexpensive, helps emulsify fat (keeps them in a liquid form), and helps lower blood pressure. Lecithin is also beneficial for healthy liver and brain function, and very inexpensive. It is available in the soft gel capsules, although the granules are the most cost-effective form. Two tablespoons daily is normally sufficient.

10. Vitamin B-complex. The B vitamins are beneficial for many important functions. They help lower blood pressure, and control the major cardiovascular risk factor homocysteine. B vitamins are also very important for supporting healthy brain function. I would recommend taking **50 mg of each major B vitamin (or a B-50 complex), <u>twice daily</u>.**

11. Extra vitamin B$_6$. I would also suggest taking 100 mg of vitamin B$_6$, twice daily. This helps work as a mild natural diuretic, removing excess fluid retention. This will also help resolve carpal tunnel syndrome, as well as preventing the formation of kidney stones, and reducing homocysteine. A hypothyroid condition contributes to the excessive accumulation of fluid in the tissues, so this issue may need to be resolved also. Additional information can be found earlier in the Hypothyroidism chapter of this book.

12. Coenzyme Q$_{10}$ (CoQ$_{10}$). Increases circulation and is beneficial for the entire cardiovascular system. **Deficiencies of CoQ$_{10}$ have appeared in most patients with high blood pressure, and researchers in Osaka Japan concluded that CoQ$_{10}$ was often the only thing needed to return blood pressure to normal, in patients with mild or even moderate hypertension.** In fact, CoQ$_{10}$ has been approved in Japan for use in treating congestive heart failure. This very important nutrient is depleted by many medications, but especially by the statin drugs used for lowering cholesterol.

13. Alfalfa. Sometimes referred to as the king of herbs, and rightly so. The roots of an alfalfa plant can extend as far at 130 feet into the earth. For that very reason, alfalfa is one of the most mineral-rich herbs. One important issue is that the minerals in alfalfa are balanced, and in the natural form that is more effective at lower dosages. Alfalfa is easy to find and very inexpensive. It is beneficial for anemia and asthma, as well as high blood pressure, meaning it could possibly help increase our oxygen level. One more way it can improve your oxygen level is due to the alkalizing benefit of alfalfa. When our body is more alkaline, less oxygen is depleted. As you can see, alfalfa is definitely a beneficial and multi-talented herb.

14. Sunlight. Studies have shown that exposure to UV rays causes a release of endorphins in the brain, which are linked to both pain relief and euphoric feelings, thus reducing stress and lowering blood pressure. Additionally, other studies have shown that the vitamin D obtained through sunlight is actually a negative inhibitor of the renin-angiotensin (RA) system and thus serves to lower the blood pressure (*Hypertension*. 1997;30:150-156).

15. Control insulin levels. In her book *The Schwarzbein Principle* (1999), Dr. Diana Schwarzbein points out that:

High insulin levels result in high blood pressure in two ways:

1. Insulin causes an abnormal increase of salt retention at the kidney level. Increased salt in the system increases water retention. More overall fluid means higher blood pressure.

2. Insulin overstimulates the nervous system, which increases blood pressure. The amount of blood pumped out by each contraction of the heart is increased, and the artery wall becomes stiffer.

Avoid grains and sugars. As grain breaks down to sugar and raises insulin levels, sugar and all sweets are even worse. Continually elevated insulin levels results in insulin resistance. One job of insulin is to store magnesium, but if the cells become resistant to insulin, they can't store magnesium as efficiently. And without sufficient magnesium (which relaxes muscles), your blood vessels constrict, normally resulting in high blood pressure. For more detailed information on controlling blood sugar levels, you may want to refer the Diabetes Chapter earlier in this book.

16. Goji. Dr. F. G. Nicley spoke on a goji marketing CD titled "Goji – Listen To What Doctors Are Saying", about one woman who had an elevated blood pressure level of 158/98, and was taking two medications to control her blood pressure. After taking goji, was able to get off both medications, once her blood pressure normalized. Dr. Nicley states that in his 45 years of practicing medicine, he never encountered anything that paralleled the many benefits of goji.

17. Noni contains more than 140 important vitamins, minerals, and other nutrients. One powerful ingredient found in noni is Scopoletin, which has been found to reduce blood pressure by naturally dilating blood vessels.

18. Oral chelation formulas. There are oral chelation formulas that combine EDTA with various combinations of amino acids. It won't happen overnight, but they do work, and the long-term benefit is definitely well worth the effort.

19. IV Chelation provided by some doctors, is considered as faster, although more expensive and less convenient. It is definitely a much better option than heart bypass surgery, (which I wouldn't recommend to anyone). If you live long enough, you will likely need more than one surgery, and sacrificing more veins would be mandatory.

If your cardio blockage were fairly serious, I would recommend the IV chelation, along with incorporating some of the other options listed here. Taking 200 mg of CoQ$_{10}$, along with 5 capsules of Vitalzyme™, three times daily would also be highly recommended. And definitely don't forget the Celtic sea salt and water, which according to Dr. Batmanghelidj, was normally sufficient to eliminate angina pain, (a sign of an oxygen deficiency in the heart muscle).

20. Holistrol™. Although Dr. Wong often stresses the benefits of Vitalzyme™ in attacking the source of elevated blood pressure, it appears that he might have discovered what appears to be a real find, for lowering blood pressure fairly rapidly. He poses the question: *"What if there was a way of lowering blood pressure that was also life enhancing? One that, after a while, also made you feel good!"* He was referring to a formulation of ancient Chinese herbs called Holistrol™, tested by University of New Hampshire. According to Dr. Wong:

Holistrol's' double blind placebo controlled research was highlighted by the American Heart Association at the 2003 Inter-American Society for Hypertension conference. During this 12-week study patients with mild to moderate hypertension were given either Holistrol or a placebo for 8 weeks. Afterward blood pressure monitoring continued for another 4 weeks. The FDA approved clinical trial found that:

- *Holistrol treated subjects showed a quick response:* **most of the patients' blood pressures were back to normal in 2 to 4 weeks.**
- *Holistrol subjects reported improved energy and mood.*
- *Holistrol subjects' blood pressures remained stable and in the normal range even 4 weeks after not taking the product.*
- *Holistrol's natural ingredients were shown safe for long term use.*

Holistrol works by decreasing resistance to blood flow (Central and Peripheral Vascular Resistance), this action:

- **Improves blood flow to the heart.**
- **Increases blood flow to the brain.**
- **Increases elasticity of blood vessels.**
- **Decreases pressure in the pulmonary artery and all arteries in general.**
-

It does this all naturally using time proven and safe herbs from Chinese Medicine.
"Holistrol safely and effectively helps reduce high blood pressure within 4 to 8 weeks. While at the same time improving mood and energy level."

Physicians who have tested the product on their patients report similar findings with **one doctor saying that: "Holistrol is as effective as and better than ANY hypertension medicine."**

Some other good points: **Holistrol does not force blood pressure to lower as the drugs do.** *It supports the body in maintaining normal blood pressure. There's difference there.* **Holistrol's mechanism of action actually seems to make blood vessels healthier!** *That's why when the test subjects went off the herbal product their blood pressure did not shoot back up as would have happened if they had been on any of the current crop of blood pressure medications.* **One of the reasons BP medication is so dangerous is that there is a rebound effect if you ever stop using the meds.**

One of the root causes of high blood pressure is the lack of elasticity in the arteries. The ingredients in the Holistrol have been used for centuries to improve arterial health (http://www.drwong.us/ArchivedBloodPressure.html).

Wouldn't it be a terrific feeling just knowing we would not only be lowering, and managing our blood pressure in a natural way, but also be restoring our vascular health in the process? An added benefit is: These nutrients also have many positive benefits in both the body and the brain (which is typical of herbs). What a sharp contrast compared to the very risky prescription medications, with their serious nutrient depletion, and outright scary side effects, as well as their associated risk of drug interactions.

CHAPTER TWENTY-SEVEN
CARDIOMYOPATHY & MITRAL VALVE PROLAPSE (MVP)

The Causes, The Deception and Solutions

Tens of thousands each year are diagnosed with either cardiomyopathy or Mitral Valve Prolapse (MVP), or both. The latter is the result of the former. Once the heart muscle becomes weak and enlarged, both the heart and the valve soon become distorted. Any valve, be it in your engine, a pump, or your heart, will not function as efficiently when distorted. The more the distortion, the greater the leakage would become.

Although cardiomyopathy and MVP are both diagnosed by cardiologists as diseases, they are not actually diseases but instead conditions caused by nutritional deficiencies. This is another example similar to the cardiovascular risk factor homocysteine, conveniently suppressed from the public for decades. As a result, the cholesterol-lowering medications (for a non-disease) are still being aggressively promoted, while the true risk factor continues to be ignored. Although every adult that goes to a doctor, or watches TV, knows what a terrible threat elevated cholesterol is "**supposed to be**", few have even heard of **the true risk factor (homocysteine).**

Due to the pharmaceutical industry's tremendous influence on medicine, our doctors are taught, and we are often led to believe, that vitamins are not really necessary. Although I don't want to detract from the subject at hand, of resolving both cardiomyopathy and MVP, there's an important issue we need to become aware of: The unbelievable deception involved. So if you don't mind, I would like to discuss that critical issue first.

In order to sufficiently validate my claim regarding the broad influence of the very powerful pharmaceutical industry, it might be helpful if we take a look at the evidence. The problem is, their strongest ally just happens to be their regulatory agency the FDA, which will soon become quite obvious. This appears to be a dichotomy, as most regulatory agencies seldom maintain such a close relationship. For example, the Environmental Protection Agency (EPA) is seldom best friends with the industries they regulate, as industries are often imposed fines for non-compliance. The basic problem is the way the FDA is structured. The majority of their revenue comes from the 100's of millions of dollars paid directly to them, by the company seeking their approval of a new drug. Then the companies seeking drug approval are allowed to conduct their own studies, (a very bad idea). It provides an opportunity for manipulating or controlling the results of a study. They are truly "controlled" studies!

Following are some excerpts from the newsletter *Nutrition & Healing* (March 2005, p. 6), by Dr. Jonathan V. Wright, M.D. They fall under the heading: **"A Century of FDA Scandals."** Keep in mind that the following quotes are from an FDA commissioner, a U.S. senator, and from the FDA dietary supplements task force. They read as follows:

"[We are fighting] the good fight against dried vegetables, mineral mixtures, and similar products." -Dr. George Larrick, FDA Commissioner.

"The FDA...[is] actively hostile against the manufacture, sale, and distribution of vitamins and minerals as food or food supplements. They are out to get the health food industry and drive the health food stores out of business. And they are trying to do this out of active hostility and prejudice." -United States Senator William Proxmire.

And the FDA isn't shy about its motives for it's anti-vitamin and natural health stance:

"...the task force considered many issues in its deliberations including: to insure [that] the existence of dietary supplements on the market does not act as a disincentive for drug development." FDA Dietary Supplements Task Force Final Report, June 1992

Just keep in mind that this is just a small part of a major conspiracy, to not only suppress the obvious value of natural supplements, but also to eventually restrict your access to vitamins and minerals in quantities sufficient to prevent or resolve disease. The movement is being promoted by multinational corporations (Big Pharma) under the World Trade Organization (WTO). Their primary objective is to take over, and completely control the supplement industry. Several doctors, including Dr. Jonathan Wright, M.D., and Julian Whitaker, M.D., both of whom I highly respect, have expressed this major concern regarding the serious threat to our access of nutrients. And as I previously mentioned, 87% of the doctors who determine what will be covered by your medical insurance are tied to the pharmaceutical industry. It's not just a coincidence that all natural supplements just happen to be excluded. By including them, they would be recognizing their value. That would pose a serious threat to drug manufacturers, (something they can't allow).

But that's only half of the story. The other half involves the promotion of drugs, through agencies funded by the Federal Government (our tax dollars), and through private donations. I'm referring to agencies such as the National Institutes of Health (NIH). From a congressional probe into the ethics at the NIH, prompted by the *Los Angeles Times*, hundreds of unreported consulting payments to NIH researchers from private industry were uncovered. For example, it was discovered that **one doctor, while employed by the NIH, also received $517,000 in fees by the pharmaceutical giant Pfizer!** This organization (the NIH) is an agency that makes decisions that doctors normally follow. They were the ones responsible for the announcement on TV (free advertising), from what appears to be a credible source, that it was discovered that acceptable cholesterol levels should now be lowered, due to the increased risk of strokes and heart attacks. They stated that more people should now be taking cholesterol medications, and that dosages should possibly be doubled, or additional medications added. Most doctors responded immediately to their recommendation. If you consider the side effects associated with statin drugs, it's quite obvious the true cardiovascular risk factors are the cholesterol medications themselves, rather than any lack thereof. The higher the dosage, the greater the risk will be.

Why is this particular issue such a serious concern? I believe I stressed the major cardiovascular problems associated with this particular class of drugs called statins (for a non-disease). The worst problem associated with statins is the terrible muscle wasting caused by the CoQ_{10} depletion. We can easily see why one of the serious problems associated with statins is cardiomyopathy, as the heart is the most important muscle in the body with the highest CoQ_{10} demand of all.

If you recall the true story of our poster boy, (my friend Al), who is a retired professor, and had been a dedicated body builder most of his life, and how he had gone from solid muscle, to hardly any muscle in just a couple years, in spite of his continued exercise regimen. He also went from a bright professor to an absent-minded professor in the process, obviously a major concern for anyone. It all began with a 20 mg dose of Simvastatin (Zocor™) prescribed by his doctor. The dosage was then doubled to 40 mg a few months later, along with the addition of another drug for elevated blood pressure (just one side effect of Zocor™). The blood pressure medication was Atenolol, a beta-blocker, which does not allow the heart rate to increase (even though an oxygen deficiency would result), especially during exercise, which Al continued to do. In a few more months, his doctor again doubled his dosage of Zocor™ to 80 mg (four times the original dosage of 20 mg). Then, following the major announcement by the NIH we referred to, his doctor decided that another cholesterol-lowering drug was in order. Al soon began experiencing terrible muscle pain as well as extreme fatigue. Fortunately, he discussed his concerns with me, and was relieved to discover there was a good explanation, as well as a viable solution. His statement was ***"You saved my life,"*** but a more accurate description might be, **his doctor nearly took his life!**

The question is: How many other doctors are unknowingly doing the very same thing? Al is now steadily making progress, and again building muscle, as well as regaining both his energy and memory. All he did was get off his medications, and start taking 200 mg of CoQ_{10} daily to restore his level of an extremely important nutrient.

We could soon be experiencing a major epidemic of degenerative heart disease throughout the nation, like nothing in the history of medicine. For that very reason, I feel compelled to devote every waking hour to the completion of this book. This terrible corruption of medicine absolutely must be stopped. The best possible way to rebel against such injustice is to say, **"We no longer need your highly inflated potentially dangerous medications!** If others were able to safely get off their medications, there is no reason I can't also." Just be cautions when doing so, and check your appropriate levels, such as blood sugar or blood pressure (if necessary). Some, who possibly have diabetes and are overweight, might possibly be required to continue taking some blood pressure medication, (at least for a while). In my opinion, absolutely no one needs cholesterol-lowering medication, and everyone who stopped were glad they did, (especially the professor, Al). He was so impressed with the improvement he made following the drug withdrawal, that he is continually spreading the word.

Modern Medicine's Approach

Anything capable of wasting muscle tissue in the body, will especially influence the heart, which is mostly muscle. Conversely, anything that will build muscle tissue throughout the body will do the same for the most important muscle in our body, our heart. Contrary to other muscles, the larger the heart, the weaker the muscle. The heart basically has chambers surrounded by muscle. As the heart muscles weaken, they loose their strength and tone. The muscles atrophy and stretch as well as weaken, thus the heart gradually enlarges.

According to cardiologists, there is no known cure. If you choose to exclude nutrients as a viable solution, as traditional medicine has stubbornly continued to do for decades, there would be no possible cure. Fortunately, you will soon discover there is a very effective solution, but as usual the solution involves only nutrients.

But first, let's evaluate the typical approach currently employed by most cardiologists (heart specialists). Unfortunately, they are only trained to treat symptoms or conditions with either medications or surgery. We will first discuss the symptoms normally associated with cardiomyopathy, and then we will evaluate the traditional approach for a solution.

In the August 2004 issue of his *Health Alert* newsletter, Dr. Bruce West states that *"Thousands upon thousands of people are diagnosed with leaky heart valves. Many are subjected to a lifetime of powerful drugs. Many more suffer through open heart surgery to have a pig or other heart valve implanted in their chest – followed by a lifetime of rat-poison drugs to thin the blood"* (referring to the drug Coumadin™). Quite blunt and to the point, but unfortunately true.

Dr. West goes on to share his experience with one of his patients, regarding her diagnosis, and the recommended therapy proposed by her cardiologist, followed by his approach to resolving her condition using only phytonutrients as follows:

Most cases are similar to the following – one of my own patients. Before coming to me, she got an abnormal reading on a heart scan and was referred to a cardiologist.

She wrote to me, "I am so anxious to know about a protocol to help my heart. I am 75 years old and in good health. I have no weakness or chest pain. Was referred to a cardiologist following an abnormal heart scan. The cardiologist told me I have atrial fibrillation and mitral valve prolapse. He also told me I had a valve problem that was causing an enlarged heart. He prescribed Coumadin, Cardizem, Lotensin, and a diuretic.

He wants to do an angioplasty right away with valve surgery as soon as possible thereafter. I never knew I had a heart problem."

In this case the cardiologist was almost right, he just had things reversed. The valve problem did not cause the enlarged heart. Rather the enlarged (weak and flaccid) heart caused the valve problem. Luckily, and thankfully for phytonutrients therapies, the entire set of problems was resolved in six months with the right nutritional treatment. You can rest assured that since the underlying cause of the entire problem was beri-beri of the heart, all the drugs and all the surgery combined would not have done much for this wonderful lady. In fact, none of the treatments prescribed by the doctor was ever needed in the first place.

Had she taken her cardiologists advice, she would have unnecessarily had two surgeries, and been placed on four different medications!

Many live a life of restricted activity, and die prematurely from this debilitating condition. Others take their doctor's advice and resort to a heart transplant, along with a lifetime of immune suppressant medication. Some later acquire cancer, (usually following any organ transplant), due to the immune suppression medication required following transplant surgery.

Another problem is an overall deterioration of health following a transplant, as all the nutrients important for strengthening the immune system must be avoided. Anything that could strengthen the immune system and improve overall health, could easily stimulate the body to reject the organ. This is basically a catch 22, as the immune suppression caused by these medications is very similar to acquiring the HIV virus, and quite often leads to cancer.

Most transplants, (including heart transplants), are in my opinion, totally unnecessary. So our focus will be to restore, rather than replace your heart. You will learn how to not only strengthen your heart muscles, but also restore its conformation (size and shape) back to normal! This is something cardiologists never attempt, as it can only be accomplished by supplementation with the proper amount and form of nutrients. Although this very effective therapy costs a fraction of the costs associated with a heart transplant, and would not require a lifetime of expensive and potentially dangerous immune suppressant medications, you can rest assured, it won't be covered by your insurance, and thus you have likely never heart of it.

The three organs most often transplanted are the heart, kidneys, and liver. All three are very resilient, and thus have tremendous restorative capability. The basic problem is: The solution involves eliminating toxic medications, along with incorporating natural nutrients. Unfortunately this type of therapy, (along with prevention), is never taught in medical school (as nutrients are apparently not worth mentioning). For that very reason, restoring and thus saving organs is considered impossible by traditional medicine. The good news is, you will soon discover that it is actually is **very possible**. This is in my opinion, when **not healing is a crime!** Especially when **the solution is already known, readily available, and obviously much less expensive.**

And now, back to the subject at hand:

Safely and Effectively Dealing With Cardiomyopathy and MVP

✓ **Check your thyroid!** Although cardiomyopathy can eventually lead to other conditions, those conditions can only be effectively treated and resolved by addressing the underlying problem (restoring the health of the heart). One seemingly unrelated contributor to cardiomyopathy might be the thyroid. In his book, *Hypothyroidism: The Unsuspected Illness* (1976), Dr. Broda Barnes, M.D. tells how a German physician named Dr. H. Zondek, in 1918, had many patients under his care that were bedridden with heart failure, and *"when he tried thyroid therapy their response was remarkable. Their enlarged hearts shrank to normal size, their edema disappeared, and they were able to resume normal* *activities"* (p. 186). Just remember to use the natural hormone Armour™ thyroid, (not Synthroid™). If you have a hypothyroid condition, that should be your very first focus (explained in detail in the Hypothyroidism chapter of the book).

✓ **Phytonutrients, usually in the form of Cardio-plus™ and Cataplex-B™.** Interestingly, one doctor that appears to have achieved the greatest success in regard to resolving cardiomyopathy (Dr. Bruce West), is actually not a cardiologist, in fact he's not even an M.D! As it turns out, he's "only a chiropractor" (as if it really matters). I have always contended that results, and not title or credentials, is what really counts. A doctor's motivation and sincere desire to look for and utilize the very best therapy, is the most important criterion for selecting a doctor to place your trust in. Although in theory cardiologists should be your best resource for resolving any heart or cardiovascular concern, unfortunately that is not always the case. Any doctor that continues to resort to surgeries or medications as the only available solutions will seldom experience the kind of success that Dr. West, and other natural practitioners such as Jonathan Wright, Julian Whitaker, and James Balch have. Just remember, there are many other natural practitioners in the nation today. All three doctors mentioned are actually M.D.s, taught to use drugs while in medical school. The same applies to Dr. Frederic Templeman, M.D., who continues conducting research on the many benefits of the different xanthones in the mangosteen fruit. After 20 years of prescribing medications, he finally discovered that much better natural solutions are available. He continually poses the question: *"Why would anyone take a medication when a food works better"* (referring to the mangosteen juice).

So now let's see what Dr. West has to say regarding cardiomyopathy and MVP. In an issue of his *Health Alert* newsletter, (Vol. 21, Issue 8), Dr. West explains that:

> *When heart muscle loses tone, it is very similar to any other muscle in the body that loses tone, it begins to sag, droop, and stretch. When the heart muscle is weakened because of a vitamin B deficiency, the entire heart will sag, droop, enlarge, and stretch. This stretches the heart valves out of their normal shape and position and can even make them seem deformed, as in mitral valve prolapse. This allows for heart valve leaks and murmurs.*

He also indicates that he has resolved thousands of similar cases with the right kinds of phytonutrients, usually in the form of Cardio-plus™ and Cataplex-B™, by Standard Process™, Inc. I just happen to use both, as a preventative. Although the company's products are perfectly safe and are high quality, they can only be purchased through a doctor. Dr. West seems to use their products almost exclusively. Their products are the ones he normally suggests for various other conditions also in his monthly newsletter, (one of several I have subscribed to over the years). Dr. West notes that:

> **With this nutrition, heart conditions begin to clear up. Murmurs disappear. Leaks suddenly seal up. Enlarged hearts shrink and shed excess water. And the heart actually repositions higher and more normally in the chest cavity. All of this means that tens of thousands of other folks have had open-heart surgery with valve replacement and drugs, all of which was never needed.**

> **The average time before a response can be seen is 90 to 120 days. And the response is easy to measure with standard medical diagnostics. The murmurs disappear, the leaking seals up, and the heart on x-ray is seen shrinking and repositioning in the chest. These are the kinds of changes that no surgeon, no drugs, and even no synthetic vitamins and minerals can produce.**

Quite amazing if you just compare it with the traditional therapy of bypass surgery, or transplants and a lifetime of immune suppressing medications. The reason Standard Process™ only sells their products through doctors is because they have a fairly extensive line of products, which can be confusing when determining which ones might be the most appropriate for a particular condition. As doctors, we are provided a lot of excellent information in that regard. Unfortunately, the FDA will not allow a company selling nutrients to state their benefits. This is normally a deterrent (their primary objective), as few are actually aware of the benefits of most supplements. The only options are to either take the time to learn, or find a doctor or nutritionist knowledgeable in nutrition. The more knowledgeable the doctor, or the more knowledgeable you become, the better.

Dr. West often stresses that synthetic vitamins and minerals will not produce the same results as those derived from natural sources. I recall that in the past he has mentioned that Cataplex-B™ contains vitamin B_4, which won't be found in synthetic vitamins, although it is apparently important in this regard. **I would also recommend employing both the CardioPlus™ and Cataplex-B™ that Dr. West employs, as well as the following additional nutrients that should not only speed up the recovery, but also strengthen the heart even more.**

✓ **Goji.** On a goji marketing CD titled "Goji – Listen To What Doctors Are Saying", Dr. Eddie Rettstatt tells an outstanding story of one of his patients, a 67-year-old gentleman, who had two prior triple-bypass surgeries, and also had considerable restriction in his carotid arteries. Surprisingly, in only a few months of drinking goji, (he didn't specifically how long or the amount), but the blockage in his carotid arteries went from 43% flow to an amazing 73%, an unbelievable reduction. I'm not aware of any therapy, (even IV chelation), that could possibly remove plaque that rapidly. To read about the full benefits of goji, see the chapter in this book titled "A Few of Nature's Miracles".

✓ **Mangosteen.** The Xanthones in mangosteen increase circulation and improve overall cardiovascular health.

✓ **Coenzyme Q_{10} (CoQ_{10}).** As we learned, a B-vitamin deficiency isn't the only deficiency associated with cardiomyopathy. A CoQ_{10} deficiency caused by statin drugs, as well as many blood pressure medications, can lead to cardiomyopathy as well. We also know the highest level of CoQ_{10} (when available) is found in the heart. For that reason, CoQ_{10} should also be part of our regimen. For anyone who has **not been taking** cholesterol-lowering or hypertension medications, (or any of the other 88 drugs that also deplete CoQ_{10}), 60 mg might be sufficient. For anyone else who has unfortunately been taking medications responsible for depleting CoQ_{10}, I would recommend 200 mg of CoQ_{10} to restore the level back to normal, and to help strengthen the heart. In regard to the amount of CoQ_{10}, more is better if you can afford it.

✓ **Magnesium.** Not only can cardiomyopathy result in MVP, but it often leads to the condition known as congestive heart failure (CHF) as well. The result is an excessive accumulation of fluid in both the body and lungs. This condition, along with any MVP (or valve distortion), should begin resolving once the heart is again strengthened. In the interim, for CHF, Dr. Jonathan Wright has some good suggestions, which should also strengthen the heart in the process. As he is an M.D., Dr. Wright suggests that magnesium frequently works better when given by a series of IV injections initially. I personally feel there might possibly be an effective approach for rapid absorption that would be less invasive, less expensive, as well as more convenient. It is liquid magnesium that can be purchased in pints, quarts or gallons, from a company called Water Oz, in Grangeville, Idaho. They can be contacted at (800) 547-2294 for more information. Their liquid magnesium is in an ionic form that rapidly absorbs, due to the super-small molecule size. For instance, magnesium can at times resolve a headache. When in this ionic form, I have seen it at times resolve a headache in a matter of five minutes or less, (depending on the cause). Taking a bath in Epsom salts (which is magnesium) might also be helpful, as would drinking a large glass of cold water.

✓ **Dr. Jonathan Wright recommends three other nutrients**, which I would also recommend, and ones I personally take as a preventative (as well as taking 100 mg of CoQ_{10} daily, which I already discussed). Following are Dr. Wright's recommendations:

- **L-carnitine,** *250 milligrams three times daily. This takes care of congestive heart failure all by itself sometimes. It enables the heart-muscle cells to use more sources of energy and to burn them all more efficiently.*
- **Taurine,** *another naturally occurring amino acid like L-carnitine. It's <u>the most abundant amino acid found in the heart</u> and is known to <u>keep the electrical activity of the heart flowing smoothly.</u> Take 1,500 milligrams twice daily between meals. The other supplements can be taken at any time.*
- **Hawthorn** *(the solid extract; take either ½ teaspoon twice daily or 250 milligrams of the standardized 10 percent proanthocyanidin extract three times daily. <u>Hawthorn improves energy production in heart-muscle cells</u> and <u>improves heart-muscle contraction. It dilates coronary arteries, providing more blood flow. It also acts as a mild diuretic,</u> <u>can lower cholesterol,</u> and can slow and possibly even reverse atherosclerosis a bit* (Dr. Wright's New Secrets for Repairing Your Heart & Arteries, 2000, p. 9).*

While a good multi-amino acid complex containing all essential amino acids should be taken, it is best to take additional individual supplements (such as the L-carnitine and Taurine just mentioned) at a separate time.

✓ **Several inexpensive herbal formulas** are also available that contain herbs such as parsley, Uva Ursi, and juniper berry, (all natural diuretics). Most importantly, they won't deplete critical minerals, such as the diuretics produced by the pharmaceutical industry are well known for.

Bypassing Bypass Surgery With EECP Therapy

There is a very promising new alternative to heart bypass surgery and angioplasty for those experiencing vascular constriction in the coronary arteries with the accompanying angina pain. The therapy is called **E**xternal **C**ounter**P**ulsation (ECP), or you might also find that it is sometimes referred to as EECP, which simply stands for **E**nhanced **E**xternal **C**ounter**P**ulsation. This is a non-invasive drug-free treatment that was actually approved by the FDA in 1995 for the treatment of angina pectoris and coronary heart failure (CHF), which is even currently covered by Medicare. It's quite amazing to me that we seem to have a safe yet effective therapy, which would actually be covered by your insurance. That is a rather rare occurrence in medicine today. And best of all, EECP doesn't involve any of the risks or recovery time associated with surgery! In fact, one study found that patients do just as well five years after EECP as those who have surgery (http://www.bravermancenters.com/abouteecp.html).

According to an article in the March 8, 2004 issue of *Time* magazine, the idea behind EECP *"is to decrease the demand on an ailing heart by helping it push blood through the body."* The article describes the procedure, as follows:

Patients lie down during the procedure, which lasts an hour and is performed once a day, five times a week, for seven weeks. (The cost is about $6,000, compared with as much as $60,000 for bypass surgery.) The pneumatic cuffs are timed to inflate in progression – starting with the section around the calves – when the heart reaches its resting phase between beats. As each cuff inflates, it squeezes blood out of the legs and back to the heart. "It feels like a deep muscle massage," says Dr. Debra Braverman, who administers EECP to patients in Philadelphia.

Intriguingly, recent studies suggest that the heart responds to this extra flow of blood by producing tiny blood vessels to better nourish the heart. That may be why the benefits of EECP may also be useful in other hard-to-treat conditions, like congestive heart failure.

EECP has been found to be particularly beneficial for people who have already had angioplasty, stints, or bypass surgery, but their heart disease symptoms have returned or persisted. It has also been suggested that EECP may benefit those with diabetes, diabetic neuropathy, peripheral vascular disease, coronary heart disease, coronary artery disease, hypertension, memory disorders, Parkinson's disease and kidney disease.

EECP is now performed at more than 600 locations throughout the US, (as well as around the world). Following are just a few of the facilities that perform EECP:

- The Mayo Clinic
- The Cleveland Clinic
- University of Pittsburgh
- Texas Heart Institute
- University of Virginia
- University of Pittsburgh
- Emory University
- The Miami Heart Institute
- Kaiser Permanente of Denver

- Christ Hospital and Medical Center
- University of California at San Diego
- Beth Israel Medical Center, New York City
- John Hopkins Medical Center
- University of California at San Francisco
- The Ochsner Foundation Hospital
- JFK Medical Center, Atlantis, FL
- University of New York at Stony Brook
- University of Florida at Gainseville

Other Considerations

Something considerably less expensive than EECP for resolving angina pain that you might also consider, is a natural whole food form of vitamin E by Standard Process™, called Cataplex-E™. Other high-potency vitamin E supplements are normally missing the important vitamin E_2 found in Cataplex-E™, which appears to be beneficial for those suffering from angina pain. That is very similar to another whole food product previously discussed, also from Standard Process™, called Cataplex-B™, which contains vitamin B_4 not found in most B-complex vitamins.

If you choose the EECP option, I would I would suggest doing that therapy first, followed by either oral or IV chelation. The objective would be to first start building a new network of arteries to supply the heart muscles more efficiently. Then, you could follow up with the chelation therapy to begin removing the plaque from the original arteries. It seems logical that you might possibly be able to provide an even greater supply of oxygen to the heart muscles than before you had the restriction.

It would be beneficial if you could also supplement with as much as 200 mg of CoQ_{10}, along with both Cardio-plus™ and Cataplex-B™. I believe this would be a winning combination that could very possibly allow you to go from an invalid to an athlete, as well as avoiding a great deal of unnecessary pain and suffering. The heart has tremendous restorative capability, and with the many natural resources at our disposal, seldom should anyone be required to resort to bypass or heart transplant surgery.

CHAPTER TWENTY-EIGHT
CANCER THERAPIES – NATURAL Vs. TRADITIONAL

The Problem with Current Cancer Therapies (Profit Potential)

I recently saw a special on TV talking about the high cost of healthcare. One woman for example was forced to sell her home, as she was temporarily without insurance coverage when her teenage son was diagnosed with cancer. In just three months her medical expenses had already exceeded $75,000, and he was just getting started. Keep in mind that there are many other natural options available. Seriously consider those that are not toxic, and normally much less expensive, but unfortunately as usual will not be covered by your insurance. In my opinion, that is an out and out crime, and the author Kenny Ausubel did an excellent job of bringing that issue to light in his book *When Healing Becomes a Crime* (2001).

In his book, Ausubel explains how a man in the 1940's and 1950's named Harry Hoxsey, was effectively curing tens of thousands of people in the last stage of cancer that doctors had sent home to die. He was using an herbal formula called the Hoxsey formula. It was the very same formula his father, a veterinarian, had successfully used to cure horses of cancer for years. Harry stressed that his most difficult cases were those who had received radiation and chemotherapy treatment, due to the associated anemia and immune suppression. The AMA, FDA, and even the American Cancer Society did everything within their power to suppress the information. After years of court battles and persecution, Harry finally gave up the battle. His nurse eventually moved across the border and started and ran a cancer clinic in Mexico for years, successfully saving many lives.

Even today, oncologists are still employing the very same toxic therapies that were utilized over thirty years ago when president Nixon declared the war on cancer. The current use of radiation and chemotherapy seem as archaic as the blood letting and mercury employed when medicine was still in the dark ages. Although billions of dollars were spent on research, the focus was always on drugs, and natural therapies were basically never considered. Unfortunately, healing is often still a crime today. That is especially true if an M.D. might attempt to implement a natural therapy (no matter how effective), as the AMA would likely threaten to revoke his license to practice medicine. That is obviously a serious threat, as it could easily end his career. Anyone who claims to have a cure for cancer often runs into some kind of trouble, especially if they chose to advertise the fact as Harry Hoxsey did.

Mangosteen's Anti-Tumor Effects and Cancer Prevention Potential

Mangosteen contains powerful phytoceuticals called xanthones. One xanthone, Garcinone E, was tested against six chemotherapy agents (5 Flouraurcil, cisplatin, vincristine, methotrexate, mitoxantrone and taxol®) to compare its ability to kill cancer cells in laboratory preparations. The cell lines came from lung, stomach and primary liver cancer. Garcinone E was found to be more effective than all the drugs tested except Taxol®.

Additionally, it is an established fact that antioxidants (like xanthones) act as modulators of gene expression. This means that they act at the level of the cell's DNA to prevent both mutation and the activation of oncogenes (cancer genes). Once again, no medicines commonly prescribed have the ability to perform these protective functions. The question to be asked is, why wouldn't we use the mangosteen for these benefits? (A Doctor's Challenge, Dr. J Frederic Templeman, M.D., 2003, pp. 42-43).

First, I might explain that *the Insider* (Vol. II, Number 1, 2005), which I am about to quote from, is something I subscribed to, (and unfortunately is no longer available). It was a monthly publication, along with a companion CD, which kept subscribers informed of the latest research by Dr. Templeman and Dr. Morton, regarding new discoveries on the benefits of mangosteen. Following are the results of one of Professor Matsumoto's studies:

In the Journal of Natural Products last year, a group of Japanese researchers from Gifu Pharmaceutical University, led by Prof. Matsumoto, wrote of their results studying 6 xanthones from the mangosteen for their effects against several cell lines of human leukemia. This was an in vitro (in a laboratory using cell cultures and not animals) study. They found that all 6 xanthones had the power to inhibit the growth of cancer cells at all the concentrations tested (p. 6).

On the companion CD, Dr. Templeman indicated that after reading some of the research published by professor Matsumoto, he decided to consult with him. Unfortunately, the pharmaceutical company, Merck, got to him first. They not only hired him, but had also placed him on a non-disclosure (basically a gag order). They would prefer to hide the information from the public, while searching desperately for a drug that might duplicate the benefits of the xanthones in mangosteen, (God's creation), which man can't possibly duplicate.

Without a doubt, if Merck (or any other drug company) could develop a symptom-free drug, with the cancer-fighting potential of mangosteen, it would definitely cost a fortune. An article published on October 1, 2006 in the *New York Times*, shows just how corrupt and out of control our healthcare system has become. It's titled "Hope, at $4,200 A Dose," (incidentally, that's not a misprint!) We're actually talking about a modified version of the old chemotherapy drug Taxol™, as follows:

Charging $4,200 a dose for a new version of an old cancer drug has helped make Dr. Patrick Soon-Shiong a billionaire.

The drug, Abraxane, does not help patients live longer than the older treatment, though it does shrink tumors in more patients, according to clinical trials.

In clinical trials, Abraxane's overall side-effect profile was similar to that of paclitaxel [Taxol], which was approved as a chemotherapy treatment in 1992 and is still widely used. Both Abraxane and Taxol can kill white blood cells, leaving patients open to infection, as well as damage nerves in the hands and feet. **Taxol causes more damage to white blood cells, while Abraxane causes more nerve damage.**

Drug industry experts say **Abraxane's price reflects the fact that makers of cancer drugs can charge high prices for new medicines even if they are only marginally better than their older counterparts.**

Drug companies have sharply increased prices for new cancer drugs in the last decade. Since 1998, for example, Celgene, a biotechnology company based in Summit, N.J., has raised the price of Thalomid, a drug for a cancer called multiple myeloma, to more than $35,000 a year from $4,000.

Since 2000, when Bristol-Myers Squibb's patent on Taxol expired, the drug has been available both as **nonbranded generic paclitaxel and as branded Taxol, at a cost of about $150 a dose for the generic and $1,000 for the branded version,** *which is now sold mostly outside the United States.*

In the largest clinical trial comparing Abraxane and Taxol, covering 454 patients, the two drugs produced similar side effects – although Taxol caused more patients to have low white blood cell counts.

After two years, roughly 75 percent of patients in the study had died, whether they received Abraxane or Taxol
(http://www.nytimes.com/2006/10/01/business/yourmoney/01drug.html?ex=1162616400&en=e24bc8ad6de10258&ei=5070).

This is a prime example of the major price gouging going on, leading to the dramatic increase in the cost of our over-inflated healthcare system, reflected in the constantly increasing insurance rates.

Now let's take a moment and evaluate what we just learned. One doctor has become extremely wealthy by promoting the use of a slightly modified version of Taxol (which now sells for only $150 a dose for the generic version). Although the new drug, Abraxane, now sells for an outrageous price of $4,200 a dose! If my math is correct, "that's 280 times as much!" Not only that, but even if they both cost the very same amount, and I was considering chemotherapy, "which I definitely wouldn't," I would likely still opt for the Taxol. Why, you might ask? Simply because it still wouldn't extend your life any more than Taxol would, but in my opinion, poses a "much greater risk" than Taxol regarding its side effects, if you do manage to survive.

Although Taxol causes more damage to the white blood cells, "Abraxane actually causes more nerve damage!" A far greater concern in my opinion, as it is much easier to restore white blood cells, than to restore nerve damage, (which is often irreversible). Not only that, but 75% will still die after taking either drug. So if there is any real benefit for the patient, it's definitely not obvious to me.

One little known fact (although one that oncologists are fully aware of), is: a great deal of their income actually comes from the sale of chemotherapy drugs, (something I recently discovered myself). They buy them wholesale, and then sell them for retail to their patients. So, the more the medication costs, and the larger the dosage the patient receives, the greater the profit potential for the oncologist. That's why, in my opinion, most oncologists tend to totally ignore the much safer insulin potentiation therapy (we will be discussing next), which utilizes only minute doses of the chemo drug, as it basically targets only the cancer itself. As a result, there is not nearly the amount of side effects, or collateral damage inflicted to the healthy cells (normally associated with traditional chemotherapy). Unfortunately, as it's much less profitable for oncologists, (as are natural therapies), neither are normally discussed as options with their patients. Isn't medicine fascinating? It's quite amazing just how naïve, and totally unaware most people really are, regarding this serious flaw in our healthcare system, sometimes referred to as our sick care system. A system that has continually placed profit potential above lives, a very serious flaw in our healthcare system that can't be over stressed, and absolutely must be addressed, as millions of lives are at stake! Only by focusing on prevention, can we possibly expect to begin experiencing true vibrant health, as well as having a cost-effective healthcare system.

One Cancer Therapy With Potential – Insulin Potentiation Therapy

Something you should be aware of is a therapy that uses a very low dose of chemo, along with insulin for delivery. The therapy is referred to as Insulin Potentiation Therapy (IPT). No surgery or radiation is required, and the toxic side effects of high levels of the standard chemotherapy can be avoided. So why have you likely not heard of IPT before? Chemo drugs are not only very toxic, but also very expensive. Using only minute doses of an expensive drug is obviously not very profitable, and the companies producing chemo drugs would prefer doctors use large amounts, rather than the small amounts employed with IPT, for obvious reasons. The procedure appears to be more successful, and much less invasive, thus standard chemotherapy and radiation could be avoided.

It's interesting that IPT has not only been used to treat cancer, but also several other diseases including arthritis, cardiovascular, and respiratory diseases. As a result, the therapy might bring about multiple benefits. If you are interested in finding a doctor who practices IPT, that information is also available on the Internet at http://getipt.com/location.htm. As of this writing, February 24, 2005, there are doctors in 26 states who practice IPT, and in the state of California there are currently seven, and the number continues to grow.

Employing Protolytic Enzymes To Attack The Cancer

One example is a therapy employed by a dentist named Dr. William D. Kelley, D.D.S., M.S., who used a combination of detoxification, juice fasting and diet. The basis of his therapy though was based on implementing a protolytic (protein digesting) enzyme. In my opinion, the best protolytic enzyme currently on the market is called Vitalzyme™. This particular form of enzyme actually digests the layer of protein the cancer creates in order to hide from the immune system. The remainder of his program was removing toxins, and strengthening the immune system. He encountered a great deal of opposition, basically attacking his credibility, as he was "just a dentist", (as if it really made any difference). It's the results, and not the title, that should be the real issue.

Dr. Kelley was actually successful in curing all 33 cases of supposedly incurable pancreatic cancer that he treated. You certainly can't find a better success rate. This might not be the best option following radiation and chemotherapy, unless the compromised immune system can first be restored. The immune system must be strong enough to destroy the exposed cancer. For more information on his therapy, or to find an alternative practitioner familiar with Dr. Kelley's work, call the Cancer Coalition for Alternative Therapies, Inc. in Canada at (709) 726-7060, or visit http://www.whale.to/a/kelley1.html.

A Recent Discovery With A Good Track Record – Poly-MVA

One recent natural discovery that appears to hold a great deal of promise is called Poly-MVA. A few months ago I met a cancer survivor in a naturopathic conference in Seattle, with an incredible story. He was a 69-year-old minister named Ken Walker, who by all counts should not have been alive. In the book *Fire in the Genes – Poly-MVA – The Cancer Answer?*, Michael L Culbert, Sc.D. tells his story. Following are some excerpts:

It all began on March 19, 2001, and at the age of 67 my wife Deana and I were devastated by the news that I had only a short time to live. I was diagnosed as being in the latter stages of a rare form of bone marrow cancer, multiple myeloma.

Then, by May 2001, I was in really bad shape. My oncologist told me the cancer was "ravaging my bone marrow."

I now had bone lesions in my head (holes in my skull), three broken ribs, cancer in my spine and, was unable to get up from a chair without help. I was trying to sleep sitting upright in a motorized recliner, taking both pain and sleeping pills. I was told I only had about three months to live.

Finally, by Nov. 27, 2001, all of my cancer markers have fallen to just slightly above normal. My oncologist told me that if I were coming in for a first visit, they would not suspect cancer (pp. 33-34).

In Dr. Culbert's book you will find not only Ken Walker's story, but also several other amazing success stories. You will find true stories of those given a death sentence by their doctor, due to supposedly incurable cancer that eventually was discovered actually curable. You will also learn more about what Poly-MVA actually is, and how it was developed. One thing unique about Poly-MVA is its ability to cross the blood-brain barrier, something chemotherapy is apparently incapable of. You can also find many success stories of survivors at http://www.polymvasurvivors.com. Incidentally, Ken told me personally that he hadn't felt as good in years. You will discover that most, including Ken, also incorporated other adjunctive therapies in order to help insure their success. That is something I would also highly recommend. The more ammunition you utilize, the more successful the battle will likely be. Cancer is a formidable foe that we must take seriously.

Just remember, the objective should be to not only destroy the enemy within, but also discourage him (the cancer) from ever returning. Also, keep in mind that you can't continue doing the same things and somehow expect to get different results. Although you were likely unaware of the fact, you apparently were doing something wrong that resulted in DNA damage, and eventually the development of cancer.

The things that can resolve cancer in a natural way will restore your immune system (contrary to the toxic effect of radiation and chemotherapy), as well as improving your overall health in general. This will not only help prevent the occurrence of cancer in the future, but also help you avoid other diseases as well. Cancer, and disease in general, begins with unhealthy cells, which normally results from an accumulation of toxins, along with a deficiency of important nutrients. And as we learned, prescription medications contribute to both unhealthy conditions. Drugs are toxic chemicals, the liver must attempt to deal with, and they also deplete many important vitamins and minerals. That is a perfect combination for creating an unhealthy environment in your body (as is radiation and chemotherapy). Remember, those who live long, healthy, productive lives, are not the ones taking medications, but normally those living in remote areas, who have never heard of them. Unfortunately, too many of us **(myself excluded)** tend to depend upon them, assuming their survival is somehow dependent upon their medications. Although, nothing could be further from the truth.

Surviving Traditional Cancer Therapies
(Standard Procedure Following Traditional Chemotherapy)

First, we might just take a moment, and evaluate the approach traditional medicine would normally take, in an attempt to repair the damage they just inflicted on the poor cancer patient. Of course incorporating nutrients are not an approved procedure, or covered by insurance, thus they are normally not an option to be considered.

After evaluating the typical drug approach, of using medications such as Procrit™ with its many potentially serious side effects, I believe you will find our natural approach much more refreshing. It also makes considerably more sense, as I believe you will soon discover. Working with our body in a natural way, rather than forcing various functions in an unnatural way, seems much more logical. As our body is organic in nature, all our therapies should be also. One thing we must never forget is: God doesn't make mistakes, and He obviously wouldn't have designed our body with flaws that we would somehow be required to resort to drugs to resolve. Our body is amazingly complex and super efficient. Only after studying quantum medicine, and looking at the body from the molecular perspective, did I begin to appreciate just how minute and extremely complex each individual cell really is. Cells actually communicate with each other, as do our organs, as well as the master controller our brain. It's quite obvious that God is, and always will be, far more intelligent than man.

Anyone who watches the national evening news has to have heard of Procrit™, the solution to anemia following chemotherapy. The chemo survivors seem to suddenly go from barely enough energy to drag through the day, to a sudden burst of energy and enthusiasm. Don't believe the commercial? Neither do I. Then what's the real story? First, you must ask for your doctor's for permission, and then if he approves, you will have to begin receiving **injections of Procrit™.** Obviously not a lot of fun, although neither was the radiation and chemotherapy. I can't help but wonder, what would be the most painful and depressing, the cancer or the therapy, especially when the therapy has such a poor track record?

As we evaluate the rest of the story (Paul Harvey's famous approach), we will soon find a whole different story. A rather disturbing story I might add. We find the objective is to treat anemia by stimulating red blood cell production. What's amazing is **the mineral iron, along with the vitamin B$_{12}$ and folic acid normally used to treat anemia, are all three actually depleted by Procrit™** (quite amazing I would say)! A deficiency of both B$_{12}$ and folic acid can also lead to an increase in the level of the cardiovascular risk factor homocysteine, which is another serious concern.

Two other cardiovascular risk factors listed as common side effects were: high blood pressure, and blood clots at the site of injection. When considering Procrit™, you are also supposed to tell your doctor if you have any one of five different cardiovascular risk factors, including **high blood pressure**, (the most common side effect). Even **stroke** was listed as a rare side effect (possibly due to the risk of migration of the clot from the site of injection to the brain). The question is: **Could we possibly be going from cancer to cardiovascular disease, along with gaining weight (just one more side effect)?** This would likely lead to the typical combination of a blood pressure medication and a diuretic. Two of the most popular classes of blood pressure medications appear to be the calcium channel blockers, and beta-blockers. The calcium channel blockers are known to cause the shrinkage of brain neurons, which along with a deficiency of both B$_{12}$ and folic acid would greatly increase the potential risk of developing Alzheimer's disease also. Then the beta-blockers pose a couple risks, as they can easily lead to an oxygen deficiency. That is especially a concern during exercise or any physical activity, as an oxygen deficiency can lead to loss of brain cells. The oxygen deficiency, along with the suppressed immune system, would then considerably increase the risk of cancer, and the anemia would just compound the problem. But unfortunately, there's even more to the story. We also find that **"stimulated tumor growth" is also a possible severe side effect associated with Procrit™** (WOW!). And finally, we have the typical extensive list of potential side effects resulting from taking a drug that is in this case, supposed to help rebuild red blood cells that were destroyed by the chemotherapy. Some additional particularly troubling side effects listed are:

1. **Dizziness**
2. **Blurred vision**
3. **Convulsions or Seizures**
4. **Fainting**
5. **Sudden loss of coordination**
6. **Sudden and severe inability to speak**
7. **Difficulty breathing**
8. **Closing of your throat**
9. **Double vision**
10. **Partial or complete loss of vision in one eye**
11. **Sudden vision changes**

What might happen if you suddenly experienced one or more of the above symptoms while driving in traffic? Quite possibly a sudden seemingly unexplainable accident, potentially leading to death or injury. As usual, after close evaluation, the potential risks associated with medications normally outweigh any possible benefits.

For Those Who Already Had Radiation or Chemotherapy
(A Natural Approach For Repairing The Damage)

Many herbalists and natural practitioners throughout history were often able to cure cancer patients who had been given a death sentence by their doctor. These were those patients that were basically sent home to get their affairs order, assuming their days were numbered. The most difficult patients of all to save were those who had undergone radiation and chemotherapy, and for very good reason, due to the terrible destruction inflicted on the immune system and the body in general.

The question still remains: What can we now possibly do to help restore the health of those who survived the therapy, in order to help prevent the future threat of cancer? Considering the terrible side effects, and obvious damage associated with radiation and chemotherapy, there some critical issues to consider. Damage control should be our first priority.

Goji specifically has been found to help neutralize the side effects of chemotherapy and radiation, and is considered the top nutritional support for cancer patients. Studies have shown that goji also helps significantly prolong remission rates in those who drink it, compared with those who do not.

As our best defense against cancer is our immune system, which has been greatly compromised from the toxic therapy, rebuilding our immune system will now be our primary focus.

Naturally Restoring the Immune System

1. **Goji, mangosteen, and noni**. All three of these amazing fruits (juices) naturally enhance, strengthen and support the immune system. In addition, the antioxidants and other nutrients in these juices *"may have the ability to restore and repair vital DNA, preventing cancerous genetic mutations that might otherwise overwhelm the immune system."* Research suggests two to four ounces of high-quality juice daily (*Breakthroughs In Health*, August 2006, Vol. 1, Issue 1, p. 8).

2. **Astragalus** is one little known, but excellent herbal resource. In an article in the July 2001 issue of *Dr. Jonathan V Wright's Nutrition & Healing* newsletter, Kerry Bone, FNIMH, FNHAA, states that Astragalus is *"More than just an immune booster. It has been shown to actually **increase the number of immune cells (white blood cells) in the body!**"* The article continues:

> *In one clinical trial, 115 patients with low white blood cell counts were given between 10 and 30 grams of Astragalus per day for eight weeks. At the end of that time period, the patients' white blood cell counts were measured again. The numbers had increased significantly.*

> *It is this action of Astragalus that makes it particularly useful for chronic states of immune system debilitation like chronic fatigue syndrome or **following chemotherapy or radiation therapy*** (p. 5)

3. **Vitamin C** is a good antioxidant, as well as an immune system booster. I would recommend taking at least 5 grams (5,000 mg) daily, in divided doses. The best form is ester-C with bioflavonoids. It is alkaline rather than acidic as ascorbic acid is. It is also more efficiently utilized by the body.

4. **Water.** I recommend drinking ten 8-ounce glasses of water, along with one teaspoon of Celtic sea salt daily. Just make sure the water is free of both chlorine and fluoride, as they are thyroid and enzyme suppressors. This will help provide an alternate source of energy for the brain, reducing the need for glucose. Adequate water intake is also important for the effective removal of toxins, thus reducing an acidic environment, which increases oxygen efficiency in the body.

5. **Avoid Sugar.** Not only does cancer thrive on sugar, but sugar is also a known immune suppressant (obviously something that must be avoided). As eliminating sugar is something many people

find rather difficult, you may want to refer to the chapter on Sugar, earlier in this book, in the section titled "Breaking the Sugar Habit" for some helpful hints.

Rebuilding The Red Blood Cells

That brings us to the other problem of reduced red blood cells. As usual, we have a much better solution than the drug Procrit™ that most doctors normally resort to. We will begin by adding, (rather than depleting), the nutrients necessary for building red blood cells.

The First Consideration – Adequate Thyroid Function

A thyroid deficiency can be associated with, and contribute to many different conditions. Adequate thyroid function actually plays a critical role in many functions throughout the body (including building red blood cells). For that very reason, it is unbelievable that most doctors continue to overlook this major issue.

Very few doctors are aware of the connection between the thyroid function and anemia. The problem is the low body temperature, or hypothyroid condition, normally resulting in cold hands and feet, leads to cold bones. The end result is, a reduction in the production of red blood cells by the bones in the extremities that are the coldest. One major contributor to suppressed thyroid function is stress. And common contributors to stress, and thus thyroid suppression, are major surgery or a serious disease such as cancer. If your metabolism is suppressed, that should be the first issue to address. You will find a considerable amount of information on this issue, in the Hypothyroidism chapter of this book. Wearing warm clothing and stockings, especially in the winter, can also be helpful in increasing the production of red blood cells. Just remember: The warmer the body, the warmer the bones, which helps build red blood cells.

Now we will be looking at a few supplements beneficial for building red blood cells in order to help resolve the anemia.

1. **Liver** just happens to contain everything normally necessary for producing red blood cells. I personally use a product from *Universal Nutrition*, called Uni-Liver™. It contains 18 amino acids, several vitamins and minerals, and natural heme iron. You can contact the company at (800) USA-0101. When building red blood cells, I would recommend taking four 30-grain (1940 mg) tablets with each meal.

2. **Blackstrap Molasses.** To assure an adequate supply of iron, I would also recommend taking a tablespoon of molasses twice a day. By taking iron in the natural form, you do not risk getting an overdose. This could be a potential risk factor if an inorganic form of iron was used, as the body can accumulate toxic levels of iron when too much of the wrong form is used.

3. **Vitamin C** potentiates the absorption of iron, and is also important for many other functions in the body. I would recommend from 2,000 mg to 5,000 mg of Ester-C with bioflavonoids in divided doses. Take along with the blackstrap molasses in order to assist in the absorption of iron.

4. **Copper and Zinc.** Taking 2 mg daily of copper, and 30 mg of zinc daily would be helpful in building red blood cells. Although zinc is needed to balance the copper, they would be best taken separately, as zinc tends to cancel the copper when taken together.

5. **B-vitamins.** You will need a good vitamin B-complex in order to provide adequate levels of folic acid, vitamin B_6 and B_{12}, (necessary for preventing elevated homocysteine), along with the other B-vitamins. To assure the most efficient absorption, the coenzyme form of B-complex capsules might be the best form. The coenzyme form is especially beneficial for those whose liver might have been compromised, from the use of drugs, or a toxic substance such as chemo. The coenzyme B-vitamins are already in the form utilized by the body, and the normal conversion by the liver is thus unnecessary. The one formula I use is produced by Country Life, and contains 50 mg or more of all the B vitamins, plus

some additional cofactors. There are also B-100 formulas available, or you can take a B-50 formula twice daily, if you prefer. The B-50 indicates that the formula contains 50 mg of each B-vitamin.

6. **Taking extra B$_6$ and B$_{12}$** would also be helpful. As we age especially, we will normally benefit from additional B$_6$ and B$_{12}$. An extra 100 mg of B$_6$ should be adequate. And two 1,000 mcg (1 mg), twice daily of B$_{12}$ would normally be sufficient. I would recommend using the sublingual lozenges (absorbed under the tongue) for better absorption. For those who do no absorb oral vitamin B$_{12}$ very well, the injections would likely be the best option. Either you or your doctor can do the injections of 2 cc of vitamin B$_{12}$ serum once a week. Your doctor can provide the injectable B$_{12}$ and needles. It is relatively inexpensive, especially if you choose to do them yourself.

7. **Alfalfa** is an excellent herb with multiple benefits. It contains many beneficial minerals, in a balanced and easily absorbable form. Alfalfa has the distinct advantage of having a tenacious root system that can penetrate nearly 130 feet into the earth. Alfalfa thus has access to minerals that other plants don't. It is sometimes referred to as the king of herbs. And best of all, it is readily accessible, and very inexpensive. Alfalfa is alkaline and thus also beneficial for preserving oxygen in the body. It is useful for arthritis, liver disorders, and high blood pressure, but is of special benefit for our concerns: Cancer and anemia. So we definitely want to add alfalfa to our list of resources. I would recommend 2,000 mg, twice daily, although more should be perfectly safe. Cattle and horses thrive on alfalfa.

8. **Vitamin E.** Last, we come to vitamin E, which has been proven to be beneficial in preventing blood clots, and is an excellent antioxidant for fats. In our case, vitamin E also helps prolong the life of the red blood cells. I would recommend 800 IU of vitamin E in the form of D-alpha-tocopherol daily. It would be best if taken at a different time than the molasses, to prevent reducing iron absorption. Be sure to use the natural form of E, (**there should not be an "L"** following the D, as that is the artificial form).

9. **One final consideration – Your Attitude.** Your state of mind and your will to live have a tremendous influence on your overall success of surviving cancer. Just assume that you now have multiple resources (without all the toxic side effects). Once you do, you now have the potential to not only destroy the enemy within, but also improve your overall health in the process. My theory is, you must gang up on the cancer with all your resources (basically show him that you are in charge). Just consider it a challenge, and a battle you are destined to win. Set some future goals (things you always intended to do) so you have something to live for. It's amazing the powerful influence this can have on strengthening your immune system (your very best defense against cancer). My guess is that many people are dreading dealing with the terribly toxic radiation and chemotherapy, (and rightfully so). Using the natural approach, you can look forward to feeling better, not worse.

A prime example is reflected in one study conducted at Kings Hospital in London. All the women who were found to have had breast cancer from a biopsy, were interviewed three months following their diagnosis of cancer. In those who expressed feelings of hopelessness, four out of five had died by the five-year follow up period. In contrast, only two of the twenty who had a positive fighting spirit actually died. Four in five, versus two in twenty (quite amazing statistics)! Imagine the potential you have for beating cancer, and thus having a future to look forward to. A positive attitude and a fighting spirit might very well be one of your most valuable assets.

Good luck, and start rebuilding those red blood cells in order to finally get your energy level back. And remember, more red blood cells mean more cancer-fighting oxygen to every single cell. When it comes to cancer, gaining and then maintaining the upper hand is the key to success (so hold the sugar please).

CHAPTER TWENTY-NINE
ACID REFLUX "DISEASE" –
Also Known As GERD (Gastro-Esophageal Reflux Disease)

Hydrochloric (HCL) acid is produced in our stomach during the initial stage of protein digestion, and performs at least two important functions, (and thus **should not be suppressed**). One function is the digestion of proteins, and the other is killing virus and bacteria, which can't survive in the highly acidic environment.

In an article in *The Insider* (Vol. 1, No. 8, December 2004), Dr. J. Frederic Templeman, M.D. gives an excellent description of GERD, as follows:

Hydrochloric acid is the potent acid that the body produces in the early phases of digestion, which occur in the stomach. It has a pH of 1.5 and is strong enough to corrode metal. It is the first agent used in beginning the digestion of protein.

As the term reflux suggests, GERD refers to the return of acidic stomach contents back into the lower esophagus or the swallowing tube that connects the mouth to the stomach. Such acidic contents will literally burn the tissues of the esophagus, producing the heartburn we feel. This damage, if repeated often, will cause scarring of the esophagus. Failure to stop the damage can lead to esophageal cancer.

Obesity is increasing rapidly in our society. Obesity results in the deposition of mesenteric or belly fat that pushes down on abdominal organs and causes excessive intra-abdominal pressure. This excessive pressure pushes upon the stomach and forces the acidic gastric contents up into the esophagus. This occurs more easily at night when the person is recumbent and the advantage of gravity is lost (p. 3).

The Effects of Sugar on Digestion

Sugars in all forms (i.e. commercial sugars, syrups, sweet **fruits**, honey, etc.) have an inhibiting affect upon the secretion of gastric juice and upon the motility of the stomach. Sugars undergo **no** digestion in the mouth and stomach. They are digested in the intestine. If ingested alone, they do not remain in the stomach for any length of time, as they are rapidly sent into the intestine. However, when sugars are eaten with other foods, either proteins or starches, they are detained in the stomach, waiting the digestion of the other foods, resulting in fermentation. **So as you can see, it is best to avoid eating sugars and proteins at the same meal.**

Fruits should be eaten at least ½ hour before or 2½ hours following a meal, but not at the same time, as they take longer to digest if ingested during or immediately following a meal. The sugar (fructose) from fruits eaten after a meal will end up in a full stomach, most often containing fats, and the fructose will mix with them. This will prevent the fruit's sugar from being used as a source of energy, and will instead be stored as fat.

Quite possibly, another way sugar negatively affects digestion, is its depletion of the very nutrients necessary for the production of hydrochloric acid and a healthy digestive tract. We will now look at another common contributor to the problem.

Your Prescription Medication Is A Contributing Factor To Your "Acid Reflux Disease"

While reviewing a list of the top 200 most prescribed drugs, of the 180 prescription medications that were tested for nutrient depletion, **every single one depletes nutrients that can contribute to acid reflux disease!** Considering there are actually at least 21 nutrients involved in digestion or the production of hydrochloric acid, there is a good chance that your medications could be depleting more than one nutrient, just compounding the problem. And as usual, these nutrients are often depleted by the very medication prescribed to heal the condition.

Following are nutrients important for the production of hydrochloric acid and healthy digestion, in addition to the drugs or conditions that deplete them:

1. **Vitamin B$_1$ (thiamine)** – Assists in the production of hydrochloric acid, and a healthy digestive tract. Deficiency can produce gastrointestinal disturbances. A high-carbohydrate diet and smoking increases the need for this vitamin.
   Vitamin B$_1$ is depleted by sulfa drugs, SSRI antidepressants, smoking, estrogen and oral contraceptives, diuretics, caffeine, **sugar,** antiseizure medication (i.e. barbiturates, phenytoin), antiarrhythmic agents (i.e. digoxin), antibiotics, **antacids,** alcohol, cooking, food processing methods, physical and mental stress.

2. **Vitamin B$_2$ (riboflavin)** – Assists in the metabolism of carbohydrates, fats, and proteins. Necessary for the metabolism of tryptophan (an amino acid), which is converted into niacin in the body (necessary for the production of hydrochloric acid). Deficiency can produce poor digestion. Strenuous exercise increases the need for this vitamin.
   Vitamin B$_2$ is depleted by sulfa drugs, steroids and corticosteroids, muscle relaxants, mineral oil and laxatives, estrogen and oral contraceptives, diuretics, diabetes medication, antidepressants (SSRI and tricyclics), antiseizure medication (i.e. barbiturates, phenytoin), antibiotics, alcohol, **antacids, sugar,** ultraviolet light, physical and mental stress.

3. **Vitamin B$_3$ (niacin)** – Assists in the production of hydrochloric acid, and is involved in the normal secretion of bile and stomach fluids. Also assists in the metabolism of carbohydrates, fats, and proteins. Deficiency can produce indigestion.
   Vitamin B$_3$ is depleted by sulfa drugs, SSRI antidepressants, steroids and corticosteroids, sleeping pills, estrogen (and oral contraceptives), caffeine, antibiotics, alcohol, **sugar,** and physical and mental stress.

4. **Vitamin B$_5$ (pantothenic acid)** – Needed for normal functioning of the gastrointestinal tract. Also assists in the metabolism of carbohydrates, fats, and proteins.
   Vitamin B$_5$ is depleted by sulfa drugs, sleeping pills, estrogen (and oral contraceptives), caffeine, alcohol, **sugar,** cooking, and physical and mental stress.

5. **Vitamin B$_6$ (pyridoxine)** – Necessary for the production of hydrochloric acid, and maintains the body's pH balance. Also assists in the metabolism of carbohydrates, fats, and proteins. Smoking and a diet high in protein increase the need for this vitamin.
   Vitamin B$_6$ is depleted by vasodilators (i.e. nitroglycerin), sulfa drugs, steroids and corticosteroids, smoking, sleeping pills, estrogen (and oral contraceptives), diuretics, diabetic medication, caffeine, asthma medications, antidepressants and MAO inhibitors, antibiotics, alcohol, **sugar,** heat (canning & roasting), and physical and mental stresses.

6. **Vitamin B$_{12}$** – Needed for proper digestion, food absorption, and a healthy gastrointestinal tract. Also assists in the metabolism of carbohydrates, fats, and proteins. Deficiency can produce digestive disorders. Smoking and a diet high in protein increase the need for this vitamin.
   Vitamin B$_{12}$ is depleted by sulfa drugs, SSRI antidepressants, sleeping pills, smoking, **proton pump inhibitors (i.e. Nexium™),** muscle relaxants, mineral oil and laxatives, **histamine H$_2$**

blockers (i.e. Tagamet™, Pepcid™, Zantac™), estrogen and oral contraceptives, diuretics, diabetic medication, calcium deficiency, caffeine, all cholesterol-lowering drugs, including statins and bile acid sequestrants (i.e. Questran™, Colestid™), antiseizure medication (i.e. barbiturates, phenytoin), amphetamines and diet pills, antibiotics, and alcohol. Certain anti-gout medications, anticoagulant drugs, potassium supplements, medications for high blood pressure and Parkinson's disease, and excess cholesterol also interfere with absorption of this vitamin.

7. **Biotin** – Assists in the metabolism of carbohydrates, fats, and proteins. Also assists in the utilization of the other B vitamins.

   Biotin is depleted by sulfa drugs, estrogen and oral contraceptives, caffeine, antiseizure medication (i.e. barbiturates, phenytoin), antibiotics, alcohol, and saccharin. Fats and oils that have been subjected to heat or exposed to air, and raw egg whites inhibit biotin absorption.

8. **Choline** – Assists in fat and cholesterol metabolism. Deficiency can produce an inability to digest fats and gastric ulcers.

   Choline is depleted by sulfa drugs, lithium, estrogen and oral contraceptives, caffeine, **sugar,** and alcohol.

9. **Folic acid** – Promotes a healthy digestive and intestinal trace and protects the body from intestinal parasites (candida). Also assists inositol in the metabolism of carbohydrates, fats, and proteins. Deficiency can produce digestive disturbances. Smoking increases the need for this vitamin.

   Folic acid is depleted by sulfa drugs, SSRI antidepressants, steroids and corticosteroids, smoking, NSAIDs (i.e. ibuprofen), mineral oil and laxatives, **Histamine H$_2$ blockers (i.e. Tagamet™, Pepcid™, Zantac™),** estrogen (and oral contraceptives), diabetic medication (especially Metformin), diuretics, decongestants (i.e. pseudoephedrine), caffeine, all cholesterol-lowering drugs, including statins and bile acid sequestrants (i.e. Questran™, Colestid™), aspirin, antiseizure medication (i.e. barbiturates), antibiotics, **antacids,** alcohol, food processing, heat and boiling, and physical and mental stress.

10. **Inositol** – Assists choline in the metabolism of carbohydrates, fats, and proteins.

    Inositol is depleted by depleted by sulfa drugs, lithium, food processing, estrogen (and oral contraceptives), caffeine, antiseizure medication, antibiotics, and alcohol.

11. **PABA (Para-Aminobenzoic Acid)** – Assists the body in assimilation of protein and vitamin B$_5$ (which is important for digestion). PABA is one of the basic constituents of folic acid (also important for digestion), and can be converted into folic acid by intestinal bacteria. Assists in the maintenance of healthy intestinal bacteria, thus preventing candida. Deficiency can produce gastrointestinal disorders.

    PABA is depleted by sulfa drugs, estrogen and oral contraceptives, and alcohol.

12. **Vitamin C (Ascorbic Acid)** – **Needed for more than 300 metabolic functions in the body.** Necessary for the metabolism of folic acid (which is important for digestion). Deficiency can produce poor digestion. There is an increased need for vitamin C in smokers, diabetics, the elderly, people under stress, and allergy sufferers.

    Vitamin C is depleted by steroids and corticosteroids, smoking, NSAIDs (i.e. ibuprofen), muscle relaxants, estrogen and oral contraceptives, diuretics, diabetic medication, antihistamines, asthma medications, aspirin, anticoagulants, antidepressants (most), antiseizure medication (i.e. barbiturates, phenytoin), antibiotics, analgesics, amphetamines and diet pills, alcohol, caffeine, cooking (heat), high fever, physical and mental stress.

13. **Bioflavonoids (sometimes referred to as vitamin P, often combined with vitamin C supplements)** – Stimulates the production of bile, thus assisting in digestion.

    Bioflavonoids are depleted by boiling, cooking, heat, light, and smoking.

14. **Coenzyme Q$_{10}$ (CoQ$_{10}$)** – Beneficial in treating peptic ulcers, obesity, candida, and protects the stomach lining.

CoQ$_{10}$ is depleted by diuretics, vasodilators (i.e. nitroglycerin), diabetic medication, all cholesterol-lowering drugs, including statins and bile acid sequestrants (i.e. Questran™, Colestid™), antipsychotic class of drugs called phenothiazines, Antihypertensive (blood pressure lowering) drugs (including beta-blockers and calcium channel blockers), antihistamines, antidepressants (especially tricyclics), and antiarrhythmics (i.e. digoxin).

15. **Calcium** – Assists in the breakdown of fats, and increases the body's resistance to parasites and bacteria. A diet high in protein and/or saturated fat, soft drinks, excess salt, and/or white flour increases the need for calcium.

    Calcium is depleted by sulfa drugs, steroids and corticosteroids, SSRI antidepressants, NSAIDs (i.e. ibuprofen), mineral oil (laxatives), **Histamine H$_2$ blockers (i.e. Tagamet™, Pepcid™, Zantac™),** high fluoride intake (Prozac™), estrogen (and oral contraceptives), diuretics, caffeine, all cholesterol-lowering drugs, including statins and bile acid sequestrants (i.e. Questran™, Colestid™), aspirin, antiseizure medication (i.e. barbiturates), antifungals, antibiotics, antiarrhythmic agents (i.e. digoxin), **antacids**, alcohol, high protein diet, **high sugar diet,** high saturated fat diet, soft drinks, excess salt or white flour, excess sweating, smoking, and emotional and physical stress.

16. **Iron** – Assists in the production of carnitine (an amino acid), which is necessary for the metabolism of fatty acids. **There must be sufficient hydrochloric (HCL) acid in the stomach in order for the body to absorb iron.** Deficiency can produce digestive disturbances and obesity. A diet high in phosphorus or bran increases the need for iron.

    Iron is depleted by NSAIDs (i.e. ibuprofen), mineral oil and laxatives, narcotics, **histamine H$_2$ blockers (i.e. Tagamet™, Pepcid™, Zantac™),** choline magnesium trisalicylate (an anti-inflammatory), all cholesterol-lowering drugs, including statins and bile acid sequestrants (i.e. Questran™, Colestid™), Carisoprodol™ (pain reliever), caffeine (especially the tannic acid in coffee and tea), aspirin, antibiotics, **antacids,** high phosphorus diet (bran), excess sweating, heavy bleeding (i.e. menstruating women, bleeding ulcers), candida yeast infection, phosphate food additives and EDTA (a food preservative). Excessive dairy products and eggs also inhibit the absorption of iron.

17. **Magnesium** – Necessary for the metabolism of carbohydrates, proteins, and fats. Relieves indigestion and assists in maintaining the body's proper pH balance. Deficiency can produce gastrointestinal disorders and indigestion. **More than 300 enzymes are activated by magnesium, and low magnesium levels make nearly every disease worse.** A diet high in fat, refined flour, and/or soft water increases the need for magnesium. There is an increased need for magnesium in diabetics.

    Magnesium is depleted by steroids and corticosteroids, SSRI antidepressants, NSAIDs (i.e. ibuprofen), Immunosuppressants, high levels of zinc, estrogen and oral contraceptives, diuretics, diabetic medication, all cholesterol-lowering drugs, including statins and bile acid sequestrants (i.e. Questran™, Colestid™), antiseizure medication (i.e. barbiturates, phenytoin), antifungal medication, antibiotics, antiarrhythmic agents (i.e. digoxin), **antacids,** alcohol, antihypertensive (blood pressure lowering) drugs (including ACE inhibitors, beta-blockers and calcium channel blockers), large amounts of fats, **sugar**, refined flour, fluoride, soft water consumption, and physical and emotional stress. Large amounts of fats, cod liver oil, calcium, iron and protein also decrease the absorption of magnesium, as do the fat-soluble vitamins (A, D, E, and K) and foods high in oxalic acid (i.e. almonds, chard, cocoa, rhubarb, spinach, and tea).

18. **Manganese** – Necessary for the metabolism of proteins and fats, and assists in the proper digestion and utilization of food. Heavy consumption of meat or dairy products increases the need for manganese.

    Manganese is depleted by steroids and corticosteroids, SSRI antidepressants, diuretics, caffeine, alcohol, and **sugar.**

19. **Zinc** – Necessary for the metabolism of protein, fats, and carbohydrates.

Zinc is depleted by depleted by steroids and corticosteroids, SSRI antidepressants, HIV medication, **Histamine H$_2$ blockers (i.e. Tagamet™, Pepcid™, Zantac™),** estrogen (and oral contraceptives), diuretics, caffeine, all cholesterol-lowering drugs, including statins and bile acid sequestrants (i.e. Questran™, Colestid™), antibiotics, aspirin, antiseizure medication (i.e. barbiturates, phenytoin), **antacids and ulcer medication,** alcohol, ACE inhibitors and other blood pressure lowering drugs (including beta-blockers), diarrhea, perspiration, kidney disease, cirrhosis of the liver, food processing, physical and mental stress, a diet high in fiber, and the consumption of hard water. Zinc is also depleted by diarrhea, perspiration, kidney disease, cirrhosis of the liver, and diabetes.

20. *Bifidobacterium Bifidum* – The predominant healthy strain of bacteria (intestinal flora) in the large intestine. Assists in the syntheses of the B vitamins and vitamin K by creating healthy intestinal flora. Improves digestion and bowel function, which prevents digestive disorders. Deficiency can produce digestive disorders, gas and bloating, candida yeast infection.
    Bifidobacterium Bifidum **is depleted by** all antibiotics (especially steroids and corticosteroids), estrogen and oral contraceptives, and sulfa drugs.

21. *Lactobacillus Acidophilus* – The predominant healthy strain of bacteria (intestinal flora) in the small intestines. Produces a natural antibiotic against more than 20 types of harmful bacteria in the gastrointestinal tract, as well as enhancing several aspects of the immune system. Produces enzymes that assist in digesting fats, proteins, and dairy products. Promotes healthy digestion, enhances the absorption of nutrients, and metabolizes cholesterol. Deficiency can produce gas, bloating, intestinal and systemic toxicity, candida yeast infection.
    Lactobacillus Acidophilus **is depleted by** all antibiotics (especially steroids and corticosteroids), estrogen and oral contraceptives, and sulfa drugs.

The Potential For Mineral Malabsorption

Minerals need an acidic base to be broken down and assimilated, and if your stomach does not produce sufficient stomach acid (hydrochloric acid) to help the absorption of these nutrients, you can become deficient in important minerals. As our level of hydrochloric acid normally lowers as we age, this should be taken into account.

In addition, it is important to note that people with type "A" blood not only have an abnormally low level of hydrochloric acid (which is why they have difficulty digesting meats, and are more inclined to get bacteria and virus infections), but they are also missing the intrinsic factor in the intestine necessary for effective assimilation of vitamin B$_{12}$. This is a prime example of an instance where the coenzyme form of the B vitamins would prove beneficial. Another instance would be if you were a vegetarian, especially on the strict vegetarian (vegan) diet, as the foods we normally find vitamin B$_{12}$ in, would be missing from your diet. The vegan diet also lacks an adequate level of salt. Vegetarians will feel better, and have more energy, if they take one teaspoon of Celtic sea salt daily.

And incidentally, the sodium chloride in Celtic sea salt aids in the production of hydrochloric acid necessary for the digestion of proteins (and the absorption of minerals). Hydrochloric acid and pepsin have also proven to be quite helpful, and can be taken in capsule form if necessary.

A Possible Connection Between GERD (Acid Reflux Disease) And CoQ$_{10}$ Depletion (Often Caused by Statin Drug Use)

Although poor eating habits, improper food combining, and insufficient hydrochloric acid and pepsin (common in the elderly) could contribute to the problem, I believe there might also be a connection to statin drugs, due to their muscle weakening from the CoQ$_{10}$ depletion. It involves the circular muscle between the lower esophagus and the stomach, called the sphincter. A major function of the stomach is to churn and mix the digestive enzymes with food. The content of the stomach is very acidic, for one of two reasons. Either from a deficiency of the hydrochloric acid necessary for the digesting proteins, or from undigested food remaining in the stomach for an extended period of time (from improper food combining). Either one would result in a very acidic condition in the stomach. When the undigested food remains in the stomach for an extended period of time, it causes the contents to ferment and become acidic.

It appears that statin drugs are not selective, but basically influence and weaken muscles in general (all muscle tissue depend upon CoQ_{10} for energy). In my opinion, the weakening of the sphincter muscle could allow the acid reflux of the contents in the stomach to pass up through the opening into the lower esophagus. Dr. Templeman mentioned one more concern, regarding another influence on this important muscle. He indicated that when eating a meal high in fat, the sphincter muscle tends to relax, additionally increasing the risk of acid reflux.

Although the stomach lining was created to withstand the acid, the esophagus was not. The result is the painful burning and potential damage to the esophagus, so a new disease *"acid reflux"* was born. Unfortunately, the drugs prescribed to treat the condition just create additional problems. For one thing, they suppress part of the normal digestion, thus reducing the absorption of some very important nutrients. This is just one more way drugs contribute to the reduction of available vitamins, minerals, and amino acids, necessary for health.

A Closer Look At Two Popular Stomach Acid Reducers - Zantac™ and Prilosec™

Not only do acid-suppressing medications reduce our ability to efficiently digest and assimilate important proteins, and protect us against pathogens, but as usual they also deplete some critical nutrients, and can create many very troubling side effects as well.

We will now take a quick look at the importance of the nutrients depleted by these two medications, (incidentally, both deplete the exact same nutrients), as follows:

1. **Vitamin A**
   - Enhances immune system.
   - Assists in new cell growth.
   - Helps to protect cells against cancer, and the degenerative effects of aging, alcohol consumption, and smoking.
   - Important for healthy skin, hair, bones, and teeth.
2. **Vitamin B$_{12}$**
   - Assists folic acid in the formation of red blood cells, thus preventing anemia and contributing to the utilization of iron.
   - **Needed for proper digestion, food absorption, and a healthy gastrointestinal tract.**
   - **Assists in the metabolism of carbohydrates, fats, and proteins.**
   - Assists in memory, concentration and learning.
   - Maintains a healthy nervous system and prevents nerve damage.
   - Assists in cell formation, and promotes normal cell growth.
   - **Deficiency can produce digestive disorders.**
3. **Folic Acid**
   - Assists in the formation of blood cells and tissue functions, thus maintaining normal patterns of growth.
   - **Promotes a healthy digestive and intestinal tract, and protects the body from intestinal parasites (candida).**
   - Maintains the nervous system. Beneficial for depression and anxiety.

- Regulates homocysteine.
- **Assists in the metabolism of carbohydrates, fats and proteins.**
- Prevents and treats folic acid anemia.
- **Deficiency can produce digestive disturbances.**

4. **Vitamin D**
   - Reduces cholesterol and prevents atherosclerosis.
   - Assists in the regulation of the heartbeat. Prevents muscle weakness.
   - Enhances immune system.
   - Assists in building strong bones and teeth. Deficiency can produce softening of bones and teeth in adults.
   - Assists in the prevention and treatment of osteoarthritis, osteoporosis and hypocalcemia.
   - Necessary for healthy thyroid function.
   - Assists in normal blood clotting.
   - Necessary for the absorption and utilization of calcium and phosphorus.
   - Assists in the prevention and treatment of breast and colon cancer.

5. **Vitamin E**
   - Thus far, vitamin E has been shown to protect against approximately eighty diseases.
   - Improves circulation, strengthens capillary walls, and relaxes leg cramps.
   - Maintains healthy nerves and muscles.
   - Assists in the prevention of cancer and cardiovascular disease. Low levels of vitamin D has been linked to both bowel cancer and breast cancer.
   - Reduces blood pressure and assists in normal blood clotting.
   - Assists in the prevention of anemia and cataracts.
   - Prevents heart attacks and cell damage.

6. **Vitamin K**
   - Necessary for normal blood clotting and prevents internal bleeding.
   - Necessary for bone formation and repair.
   - Prevents osteoporosis.
   - Enhances immune system and helps prevent cancers that target the inner linings of the organs.
   - Assists in converting glucose to glycogen for storage in the liver, thus promoting healthy liver function.
   - Deficiency interferes with insulin release and glucose regulation in ways similar to diabetes.

7. **Calcium**
   - Necessary for maintenance of a regular heartbeat and the transmission of nerve impulses.
   - Necessary for the formation of strong bones, teeth and healthy gums.
   - Prevents bone loss associated with osteoporosis
   - Lowers cholesterol and prevents cardiovascular disease.
   - Necessary for muscular growth and the prevention of muscle cramps.
   - Lowers blood pressure and assists with blood clotting.
   - Assists in the prevention of cancer.
   - Assists in the breakdown of fats, thus utilizing it for energy.
   - Assists in the neuromuscular activity and the entire nervous system.
   - **Increases the body's resistance to parasites and bacteria.**

8. **Copper**
   - Necessary for the utilization of vitamin C, thus assisting in the healing process and enhancing the immune system.
   - Assists in the formation of red blood cells and hemoglobin.

- Stimulates the absorption of iron in the body.
- Necessary for healthy nerves and joints. Reduces the degeneration of the nervous system.
- Assists in the formation of collagen, one of the fundamental proteins for bones, skin and connective tissue.

9. Iron
   - **There must be sufficient hydrochloric acid (HCL) in the stomach in order for the body to absorb iron.**
   - Responsible for the conversion of blood sugar to energy.
   - Necessary for a healthy immune system.
   - Responsible for the transportation of oxygen within blood and muscle, and the oxygenation of red blood cells, by the production of hemoglobin and myoglobin.
   - Assists in the production of carnitine (an amino acid), which is necessary for the metabolism of fatty acids.
   - **Deficiency can produce digestive disturbances,** obesity, and a decreased immune system

10. Magnesium
    - **More than 300 enzymes are activated by magnesium. Low magnesium levels make nearly every disease worse.**
    - Responsible for the production and transfer of energy.
    - **Necessary for the metabolism of carbohydrates, proteins, and fats.**
    - Necessary for healthy nervous and muscular tissues, and nerve transmission and impulses, needed to maintain normal heart rhythm and muscular contraction.
    - Reduces cholesterol, reduces blood pressure, and assists in maintaining the body's proper pH balance.
    - Reduces stress, assists in the prevention and treatment of depression
    - Protects the arterial linings from the effects of stress caused by sudden blood pressure changes.
    - Assists in the formation of healthy bones and teeth.
    - Assists in the prevention of cardiovascular disease, osteoporosis, and certain forms of cancer.
    - Increases the rate of survival following a heart attack.
    - **Relieves indigestion.**
    - **Deficiency can produce gastrointestinal disorders and indigestion.**

11. Phosphorus
    - Necessary for blood clotting.
    - Necessary for bone and tooth formation.
    - Necessary for cell growth and cell reproduction.
    - Necessary for contraction of the heart muscle and normal hearth rhythm.
    - Necessary for kidney function.
    - Assists the body in utilization of vitamins and the conversion of food to energy.

12. Zinc
    - Important in prostate gland function and the growth of the reproductive organs.
    - Reduces cholesterol deposits.
    - Promotes mental awareness.
    - **Necessary for the metabolism of protein, fats, and carbohydrates.**
    - Promotes a healthy immune system and the healing of wounds.
    - Zinc is a constituent of insulin.
    - Necessary for bone formation.
    - Protects the liver from chemical damage.

All you have to do is look at the importance of each of the twelve nutrients depleted, and you will begin to realize their potential for contributing to many serious conditions. Some I can immediately recognize at a glance are: osteoporosis, elevated homocysteine, calcification of the arteries, dementia, depression, hypertension, anemia, irregular heartbeat, fatigue, and infections. You may also notice that **of the twelve nutrients depleted, SIX (half!) are necessary for the digestion of carbohydrates, proteins, and fats, or the resistance to parasites and bacteria (candida).**

Now let's take a look at some very troubling potential side effects noted:

Zantac™ / generic name = Ranitidine HCL

* Headache	* **Agitation**	* **Anemia**
* **Changes in liver function**	* **Depression**	* **Difficulty sleeping**
* Dizziness	* Hallucinations	* Heart Block
* Hypersensitivity reactions	* **Hepatitis**	* **Inflamed blood vessels**
* **Inflammation of the pancreas**	* Joint pain	* Irregular heartbeat
* Involuntary movements	* Muscle pain	* **Rapid heartbeat**
* **Reduced white blood cells**	* **Weight gain**	* Swollen face and throat
* **Reversible mental confusion**	*Severe allergic reactions	

Additional Concerns:
   * **Confusion and dizziness may be especially likely to occur in elderly patients,** who are usually more sensitive than younger adults to the effects of H$_2$ blockers.
   * If you have kidney disease, liver disease, or diabetes, this drug should be used with caution.
   * Be sure to tell your doctor if you already have a weakened immune system (difficulty fighting infection). **The decrease in stomach acid caused by H$_2$ blockers may increase the possibility of a certain type of infection.**

Prilosec™ / generic name = Omeprazole

* **Aggression**	* **Anemia**	* **Anxiety**
* **Breast development in males**	* Apathy	* **Blood in urine**
* **Changes in liver function**	* **Confusion**	* **Depression**
* **Difficulty sleeping**	* Dizziness	* Fatigue / weakness
* **Fluid retention and swelling**	* **Hepatitis**	* Fluttery heartbeat
* Frequent urination	* **Irritable colon**	* **High blood pressure**
* **General feeling of illness**	* **Low blood sugar**	* Joint and leg pain
* Muscle cramps and pain	* Nervousness	* Pain in testicles
* **Rapid heartbeat**	* Sleepiness	* Stomach tumors
* Taste distortion	* Throat pain	* Urinary tract infection
* **Upper respiratory infection**	* **Tremors**	* Weight gain

Additional Concerns:
   * **Long-term use of this drug can cause severe stomach inflammation.**

Doctors often prescribe proton pump inhibitors such as these, in order to prevent Acid Reflux "Disease" (or GERD). All these drugs do is reduce the production of hydrochloric acid (HCL), thus reducing the ability to efficiently digest proteins. By resorting to medications such as Zantac™ or Prilosec™, we are also depleting important nutrients that the body needs for many critical functions, thus the reason for the many side effects. The problem would be even worse for someone with type "A: blood, who is already experiencing a deficiency of HCL. The same would also apply to seniors, as our level of HCL acid normally decreases as we age.

According to the January 8, 2001 issue of *Business Week*, **Prilosec™ was the top selling prescription drug in the world at that time, earning its maker, Astra Zeneca, $6 billion per year!** However, studies revealed in the *New England Journal of Medicine* (March 29, 2001; 344:967-973), found that **Prilosec™ and Prevacid™ are ineffective for many,** noting the following:

> *A recent online survey of over 4200 patients taking Prilosec or Prevacid found:*
> - *35% to 41% of the respondents continue to experience daily heartburn symptoms.*
> - *As many as 60% of the respondents reported experiencing symptoms three or more times per week.*
> - *75% of PPI patients also take nonprescription medications, such as Pepcid, Maalox and Tums.*

The Importance of Food Combining

In the November 1992 issue of *Health Alert* (November 1992), Dr. Bruce West, D.C. explains that **improper combinations of foods** (like meat with potatoes, or peanut butter with jelly – i.e. **fats with carbohydrates**) make it extremely difficult for your system to digest the meal. When you choose to combine your foods in this manner, the following problems can occur:

1. Digestion is drastically reduced.
2. The entire digestive process will require much more energy than is normally required, resulting in severe fatigue.
3. Because your digestive system is being compromised, your food ends up being only partially digested. This causes your body to receive just a small portion of the nutrients, leaving you with chronic nutritional deficiency, which will only worsen over time.
4. Much of your food may end up never being digested at all.
5. Over time, chronic nutritional deficiencies will take their toll. The heart and other organs are usually the first to feel the effects.
6. With poor digestion, there is constant indigestion, as well as no energy.

When foods are not eaten in compatible combinations, it can take up to eight hours to digest, causing the food to be stored in the warm environment of our stomach for an extended period of time. This often results in fermentation, causing alcohol to be produced in the digestive tract. This is the same ethanol alcohol that is found in liquor, which is absorbed immediately through the stomach wall into the bloodstream, promoting liver damage, leaky gut syndrome, slowing metabolism, and often resulting in weight gain.

Another potential problem with improper food combining is a resultant yeast infection called Candida, which thrives on sugar (causing extreme sugar cravings), and is also very effective in fermenting, and converting sugar into ethanol alcohol, and its toxic metabolite acetaldehyde. In fact, people who had consumed an excessive amount of sugar, and also had the Candida infection, have actually been arrested for high alcohol levels, even though they had never drank alcohol. Incidentally, Candida is a common cause of sugar cravings and obesity that is often overlooked.

According to Dr. Bruce West, D.C., there are five principles to food combining:
1. Do not combine fruit with any other food.
2. Do not combine a protein with a starch.
3. Do not combine bread with a protein.
4. Eat fresh whole foods and drink only pure water with your meal.
5. After your dinner, do not eat anything else until morning.

Dr. West claims you should try this for one week, in order to experience a drastic difference in the way you feel, and lose weight in the process.

The Beneficial Effects of Nature's Miracles (mangosteen, noni and goji)

➤ **Mangosteen** has acid-lowering, anti-inflammatory, and antioxidant effects, with no side effects. Following is Dr. Templeman's explanation of how this works:

The mangosteen possesses histamine-blocking capabilities. Histamine is a cellular messenger that you will recognize as being involved in the symptoms of allergic diseases. Some medications block histamine release or block histamine molecules that have been released from attaching to their receptors. Such blockade prevents histamine from causing its intended and often deleterious effects. In the case of allergies, the type of histamine molecule that is blocked is called histamine 1. In the case of the stomach, the histamine 2 molecule is blocked. Histamine 2 stimulates the production of acid by the specialized (parietal) cells of the stomach. Medications which block histamine 2 and reduce acid secretion are Zantac™, "Tagamet™" and similar drugs now sold over the counter. As with all drugs, they have many side effects. The mangosteen effectively blocks both H_1 and H_2 receptors in laboratory experiments. Clinically, the mangosteen is apparently capable of reducing the allergic response and reducing stomach acid (The Insider, Vol. 1, No. 8, December 2004, p. 4).

For prevention and treatment of digestive disease of the upper gastrointestinal tract, Dr. Templeman's recommendation (and mine) is to try either one or two ounces of mangosteen before each meal. The mangosteen's potent antioxidants help repair and protect the lower esophagus. Its acid-suppression effects reduce the acidity of stomach contents when reflux does occur, and its anti-inflammatory effects reduce the changes that lead to cancer.

Dr. Templeman's conclusion, as usual: ***"Why would anyone ever use a drug when a food could do the same thing? My experience with the mangosteen reveals greater efficacy in treating GERD than the prescription medications used to do the same thing."*** Prescribing medications was something he had done for 20 years, prior to learning about mangosteen.

Incidentally, I knew a man who started taking two ounces of mangosteen (XanGo™) three times daily, in order to help stabilize his blood sugar, reduce his sugar cravings, and help phase out his medications in general. I eventually learned that he was also taking Zantac™, (as was his wife), for Acid Reflux "Disease". His wife began taking the Mangosteen along with her husband, and soon they both began experiencing relief, and no longer needed Zantac™. Although part of his improvement was the result of taking mangosteen, additional benefit was likely the result of eliminating his medications. To make a long story short, they both soon discovered their Acid Reflux "Disease" was gone, and neither needed to continue taking the Zantac™ they had been taking for years. That is an important issue considering the extensive list of both potential side effects, and depleted nutrients associated with Zantac™. Mangosteen provides many benefits, and one more is its ability to kill pathogens such as viruses, bacteria, fungus, and parasites.

➤ **Noni** is a "digestive bitter", naturally rich in enzymes that promote healthy digestion, stimulating the activity of the entire digestive process, increasing necessary secretion and bile flow. Noni has been used to assist with indigestion and stomach ulcers, and has antibacterial properties that can protect against digestive damage.

➤ **Goji** improves digestion, and has long been used in the treatment of atrophic gastritis, a weakening of digestion caused by reduced activity of stomach cells. It contains fiber that is easily digested and assimilated.

Other Natural Solutions For "Acid Reflux Disease"

1. Water and Celtic sea salt. Dr. Batmanghelidj recommends drinking a glass of water along with a pinch of Celtic Sea Salt approximately ½ hour before each meal, as this will greatly assist in the breakdown and digestion of the food. It also promotes a balanced pH level in your body, thus reducing acidity.

2. Digestive enzymes. During the main meal, especially if it consists mostly of cooked foods, a complete digestive enzyme should be beneficial. Taking a complete digestive enzyme, which includes amylase for digesting carbohydrates, protease for digesting proteins, and lipase for digesting fats, will assist in digestion and reduce the load on the pancreas.

3. Hydrochloric acid (HCL) and pepsin have also proven to be quite helpful for those deficient, and may be taken in capsule form with your meal, if necessary.

4. Vinegar stimulates the production of bicarbonate, which reduces the acidity in the stomach. According to Dr. Julian Whitaker, by drinking one glass of warm water with a teaspoon each of raw honey and organic apple cider vinegar each morning, one of his patients was able to stop taking Zantac™ (which he had been taking for years).

5. Avoid drinking excessive liquid with a meal, as it will have a tendency to dilute the digestive enzymes.

6. Avoid acid-stimulating substances. It can also be helpful to eliminate acid-stimulating substances, such as caffeine, alcohol, and spicy or fatty foods.

7. Avoid overcooking your food. Cooking or canning foods removes the natural enzymes, which would normally aid in the digestion. The more the food is cooked, the more difficult it is to digest and metabolize.

8. MSM (Methyl sulfonyl methane) is a special type of dietary sulfur produced from DMSO. Sulfur is used by the liver to manufacture bile and is important for digestion, as well as crucial to our overall health. MSM levels normally decline as we age, which is likely one reason so many of the elderly suffer from "acid reflux disease."

According to Robert Herschler, a pioneer MSM researcher, unless people eat their fish and meat raw, and their vegetables unwashed and uncooked, (which is highly unlikely), people **will be** sulfur-deficient.

MSM can be found in the powder form, or in 500 mg or 1,000 mg capsules. I personally take two to four 1,000 mg capsules daily, although more is perfectly OK. As MSM tends to be bitter, rather than using the powder form, I prefer the capsules.

CHAPTER THIRTY
NATURALLY RESOLVING PAIN

What Do We Know About Pain?

I believe we can all agree that unrelenting pain can be a real pain, as well as terribly distracting. There are varying degrees of pain, as well as acute (short-term) versus chronic (long-term) pain. We can experience pain in just about any area of the body where we have nerves. There are different causes of pain, although inflammation or an oxygen deficiency (such as angina pain), seem to be the most common. The question remains: What lead to the inflammation, or the restriction of oxygen? Although the degree of pain often varies from slightly uncomfortable, to outright excruciating and thus intolerable, we normally experience pain for a very good reason. We can't periodically take a look inside our body or joints, thus we have an early warning system, as well as a constant reminder, and we call it pain. If we never experienced any kind of pain or discomfort, we would be totally unaware that a problem exists!

Traditional medicine just focuses on suppressing the symptom (our body's way of communication), which as usual is not properly addressing the underlying cause of pain to begin with. Unless we do, continued suppression (never-ending medication) would be necessary. Then as we will soon learn, the source of your pain could very well be your medications (one very common side effect). Your pain medication itself could in turn lead to another condition, such as depression or possibly hypertension (or whatever), and seldom is the source ever identified. This is a very common problem associated with medications, and the primary reason that very few are on only one medication, at least for any length of time. Quite often, just suppressing the symptom (pain) without addressing the underlying cause of pain, can eventually lead to a worsening of the condition. Thus, our objective will be to identify the underlying condition, and do our utmost to fix, rather than ignore it. We will now look at an all too common source of many people's mysterious and seemingly unexplainable pain.

Your Prescription Medications Are A Contributor to Pain

According to a list of the top 200 most prescribed drugs, <u>**every single prescription medication,**</u> **listed some form of pain as a potential side effect!** One blood pressure medication (an ACE inhibitor) actually listed 12 different kinds of pain!

A few of the types of pain listed include:

* Chest pain	* Back (or lower back) pain	* Joint pain
* Bone pain	* Muscle pain (or cramps)	* Foot pain
* Shoulder pain	* Leg (or calf) pain	* Hand pain
* Arm pain	* Painful urination	* Breast pain
* Nerve pain	* Pain around cheek bones	* Eye pain
* Kidney pain	* Ear pain (or earache)	* Neck pain
* Dental pain	* Painful erection	* Headache
* Sore throat	* Mouth pain (or ulcers in mouth)	* Bladder pain
* Painful menstruation	* Stabbing pain in extremities	* Side pain
* Painful glands	* Pain at place of injection	

* Abdominal pain (includes stomach pain, gastrointestinal pain)

Then, on that same list, although 20 medications have not yet been evaluated to determine nutrient depletion, **of the 180 prescribed medications that were tested, 142 medications (nearly 79%) actually depleted nutrients which, when deficient, can result in pain.** As usual, drugs are obviously not the answer for truly resolving any health issue, but are all too often contributors to the underlying problem as well.

The depletion (or a deficiency) of the following nutrients can result in pain. Also listed are the drugs, or class of drugs, substances, and conditions (i.e. stress) that can contribute to their depletion:

1. **Vitamin B$_6$ (Pyridoxine)** – depleted by vasodilators (i.e. nitroglycerin), sulfa drugs, steroids and corticosteroids, smoking, sleeping pills, estrogen (and oral contraceptives), diuretics, diabetic medication, caffeine, asthma medications, antidepressants and MAO inhibitors, antibiotics, alcohol, **sugar,** heat (canning & roasting), and physical and mental stress.
   NOTE: ALL diuretics block the absorption of vitamin B$_6$.

2. **Biotin** – depleted by sulfa drugs, estrogen (and oral contraceptives), caffeine, antiseizure medication (i.e. barbiturates, phenytoin), antibiotics, alcohol, food processing, and saccharin.

3. **Calcium** – depleted by sulfa drugs, steroids and corticosteroids, SSRI antidepressants, NSAIDs (i.e. ibuprofen), mineral oil (laxatives), Histamine H$_2$ blockers (i.e. Tagamet™, Pepcid™, Zantac™), high fluoride intake (Prozac™), estrogen (and oral contraceptives), diuretics, caffeine, **all cholesterol-lowering drugs, including statins and bile acid sequestrants (i.e. Questran™, Colestid™),** antiseizure medication (i.e. barbiturates), antifungals, antibiotics, antiarrhythmic agents (i.e. digoxin), aspirin, antacids, alcohol, high protein diet, **high sugar diet,** high saturated fat diet, soft drinks, excess salt or white flour, excess sweating, smoking, and emotional and physical stress.

4. **Magnesium** – depleted by steroids and corticosteroids, SSRI antidepressants, NSAIDs (i.e. ibuprofen), Immunosuppressants, high levels of zinc, estrogen and oral contraceptives, diuretics, diabetic medication, **all cholesterol-lowering drugs, including statins and bile acid sequestrants (i.e. Questran™, Colestid™),** antiseizure medication (i.e. barbiturates, phenytoin), antifungal medication, antibiotics, antiarrhythmic agents (i.e. digoxin), antacids, alcohol, antihypertensive (blood pressure lowering) drugs (including ACE inhibitors, beta-blockers and calcium channel blockers), large amounts of fats, **sugar,** refined flour, fluoride, soft water consumption, and physical and emotional stress.

5. **Phosphorus** – depleted by ACE inhibitors, beta-blockers and other Antihypertensive (blood pressure lowering) drugs, antacids, antiarrhythmic agents (i.e. digoxin), **all cholesterol-lowering drugs, including statins and bile acid sequestrants (i.e. Questran™, Colestid™),** diuretics, mineral oil (laxatives), excess iron or magnesium, a diet high in processed cooked foods and junk food.

Nature's Miracles Relieve Years of Chronic Pain Caused By A Prior Injury

Most pain is the result of inflammation, which can become chronic and last for many years, or even a lifetime. As quoted from *Health Journal* (2004, Volume 44, Number 2), we will now learn what some doctors discovered regarding the miraculous influence the mangosteen (a very effective anti-inflammatory) had, in relieving their own pain, as well as that of their patients.

First, we will learn what a prominent surgeon named Armondo V. DeGuzman, M.D. discovered, regarding the resolution of pain following a very serious biking accident, as follows:

In 1989 I was in a very serious accident while bicycle racing. I had several facial injuries and fractures, and I fractured my cervical spine and lower back. It is a miracle I'm not a quadriplegic today. I started having problems with severe, traumatic arthritis and compression syndrome in my back. It had become so painful that I needed to take Celebrex and Vioxx for the pain. I also had to take some narcotics at night because the pain was so severe I couldn't sleep.

I was going to have surgery on my back to decompress it, but I decided to hold off. Then a friend of mine called me and told me about the launch of a mangosteen juice. I began using three ounces twice a day. After the first week, I didn't have to take the narcotics at night. After another week, I didn't have to use any medications because I was completely pain free (p. 2).

We will now see what Dr. Kenneth J Finsand, a board certified chiropractic physician and author of the book *Mangosteen: Healing Secrets Revealed* (2003) has personally experienced, resolving twenty years of pain following a major back injury while surfing in Hawaii, in his own words:

In 1981, while surfing in Hawaii, I sustained a back injury. At the time, I was thrown to the bottom of the surf with such force that it bent my entire body backward, breaking my back in four areas. Over the last 20 years through chiropractic care, I have been able to lead a fairly normal life. However, the pain has increased because spurring has advanced and degeneration has occurred in certain areas of the spine.

Then I learned about mangosteen juice. I was given an ounce of the juice, and that was the beginning of a major change in my health, my life and my career. I have implemented this product in my clinic and recommended its use to my patients with incredible results. Never have I encountered a natural fruit so powerful that it could do the job of so many other herbs. Because of the amazing results I have had with mangosteen, I am now drug free and virtually pain free for the first time in 21 years (p. 4).

Following is an account of Dr. Gil Alvarado, N.D., L.Ac., who has practiced medicine for over 30 years, regarding his experience with a patient who had suffered with arthritic pain for 25 years. Dr. Alvarado states that:

One person with whom I worked had been suffering with arthritic pain for at least 25 years. She had consulted every type of health practitioner she could find, both conventional and alternative, and still the pain and stiffness stayed with her every day. I suggested she drink a mangosteen beverage daily, and after 2.5 months she called to tell me that because of mangosteen her 25 years of constant pain had completely disappeared (p. 3).

We now come to a very successful and talented doctor, Dr. Sam Walters, N.M.D., who has treated more than 55,000 patients over the past 30 years. He also experienced a major back injury, although from a parachute injury. As told in his book *Tame The Flame* (2004), he explains his experience as follows:

In 1988, during a parachuting accident, I had sustained some pretty intense injuries to my spine that resulted in chronic arthritis. Despite all I knew, I had never been able to rid myself of this pain. After drinking mangosteen juice for about a month, my arthritic pain disappeared. I couldn't believe it! We're talking almost two decades of pain gone (p. 8).

Dr. Walters also describes a quite amazing experience he had with a patient who had been confined to a wheelchair for over six years, as follows:

One patient had been in a wheelchair for five to six years. He had several pages of medical problems and complains. At the top of his list were pain, fatigue, and a lack of energy. I had him drink large quantities of mangosteen juice as his entire treatment. He is no longer in the wheelchair, and he is actively enjoying life (p. 9).

As you can see, the mangosteen is a quite amazing fruit, with outstanding anti-inflammatory qualities, necessary for resolving pain. That is a particular concern if you consider the dangers associated with the COX-2 inhibitors such as Vioxx, Celebrex, and Bextra. There are absolutely no pain medications I am aware of that come without risks. It's comforting to know we have a completely safe juice that appears to be very effective in resolving even chronic long-term pain.

Goji is another amazing fruit with outstanding anti-inflammatory qualities. One study in China found that *"ingesting goji resulted in a 40 percent increase of the extremely important anti-inflammatory enzyme"* (*Breakthroughs In Health*, August 2006, Vol. 1, Issue 1, p. 16).

Noni is also quite an effective anti-inflammatory, and one of its major benefits is relieving most types of pain. Dr. Bryan Bloss, M.D., faculty at the University of Louisville Hospital and Orthopedic Surgeon from Indiana, tells his own personal experiences with noni in the Genesis Today™ Master Training Manual, as follows:

Before I used Noni in my practice, I tried it myself and had a lot of personal success with it. I used to be unable to sleep on my stomach because of back pain. Noni not only took care of that, but it relieved the pain in my left shoulder. Noni has also increased my energy level. My opponents on the tennis court have noticed that my reaction time is much faster.

Since the, I have used Noni on about 70 of my patients. Fifteen of my patients with chronic back pain found that noni significantly relieved their pain. Eight other patients had knee pain from Osteoarthritis, until noni made them almost pain free. Several of my patients with Type II diabetes (adult onset, non-insulin dependent_ lowered their blood sugar after taking noni. One diabetic with chronic back pain found that for the first time in 15 years, he could bend over and pick up balls on the tennis court. He could also golf again without always being laid up afterward.

Fibromyalgia Pain

Many women suffer from the very painful and debilitating condition known as fibromyalgia. It appears that elevated estrogen contributes to the build-up of fibrin in the contractile (muscle) tissue, causing ischemia (pain from a deficiency of oxygen) in the muscles, due to any obstruction. The pain can also be exacerbated by cholesterol lowering medications, which can contribute to muscle pain for even a healthy individual (one common side effect, due to CoQ_{10} depletion). Beta-blockers, often prescribed for hypertension, could also contribute to the problem (especially during exercise), as they suppress the heart rate, reducing the oxygen supply the muscles, as well as depleting CoQ_{10}.

Another consideration is, according to a study of thyroid function, 63% of a group of fibromyalgia patients suffered from some degree of hypothyroidism (*Life Extension Disease Prevention and Treatment Protocols – Expanded 2nd edition*, 1998, p. 112). Elevated estrogen not only stimulates the production of fibrin, but is also a thyroid suppressant.

According to Dr. James Balch, M.D. (*Prescription for Nutritional Healing, 3rd edition*, 2000), *"Chronic pain sufferers, especially those with fibromyalgia, tend to be deficient in magnesium"* (p. 377).

Depression and fatigue are often associated with the condition (likely due to the chronic pain). Unfortunately, modern medicine normally just suggests prescriptions such as painkillers, sleeping pills, antidepressants, muscle relaxants, and a variety of anti-inflammatories. Fortunately, we have some natural options to help relieve the effects of fibromyalgia, without the potential side effects associated with dangerous prescription drugs.

1. Follow the recommendations in this book for solving a hypothyroid condition.

2. Then, **natural progesterone** cream should be used to control the estrogen. When taken in supplement form, it would be metabolized by the liver, and thus not effective. As a result, it is best to use the cream instead, as the delivery must be transdermal (through the skin) to be effective, and is slowly absorbed and released internally.

3. And finally, I would recommend taking 3 capsules of the protolytic (protein digesting) enzyme Vitalzyme™, three times daily, to begin breaking down and removing the fibrin. It selectively digests only abnormal proteins, such as the fibrin. Sometimes pain caused by ischemia (an oxygen deficiency) can only be completely eliminated by removing any restriction of oxygen flow to the muscles.

4. Following are a few nutrients that have been found to be beneficial in reducing pain. Just experiment and find what works the best for you:

- **Mangosteen** is one of the best anti-inflammatories I am aware of. Mangosteen is also a good mood elevator and energizer, and it should also help with pain and depression.
- **Goji juice** is also a potent anti-inflammatory, and may help soothe fibromyalgia symptoms. It also helps with depression and, as reported in several medical study groups, *"nearly all patients taking goji reported better quality of sleep – a crucial factor in managing fibromyalgia"* (*Breakthroughs In Health*, August 2006, Vol. 1, p. 17).
- **Noni** is another anti-inflammatory, as well as a mood elevator, and in clinical trials noni was shown to have an analgesic effect.
- **SAMe** (a derivative of the essential amino acid methionine) has proven beneficial in treatment of disorders of the joints and connective tissue, including arthritis and fibromyalgia.
- **Folic acid** is a natural analgesic or painkiller. It is one of the B vitamins normally found in a vitamin B-complex containing all the B vitamins.
- **Copper** is necessary for healthy nerves and joints, and has an anti-inflammatory affect for some forms of arthritis.
- **Magnesium** is necessary for healthy nervous and muscular tissues, and is a natural tranquilizer. It is beneficial in the treatment and prevention of depression. A deficiency can produce muscle cramps, as well as weakness and fatigue.
- **Bromelain** is an enzyme found in pineapple, and is good for reducing pain and inflammation, as well as improving joint mobility. It is normally taken in tablet form. Incidentally, it is one ingredient included in the protolytic enzyme formula called Vitalzyme™, which we just discussed.
- **Curcumin, found in the spice Turmeric**, is good for inflammatory conditions, as well as improving circulation.
- **MSM** contains sulfur, and has been proven to be extremely effective for killing pain, especially tissue and joint pain.
- While **Willow bark** contains many beneficial phytochemicals, and contains compounds from which aspirin was derived. It is beneficial for both joint and nerve pain, and is also an anti-inflammatory.
- **Cats Claw, Feverfew, Ginger, and *Capsicum annum* (cayenne pepper),** are all herbs that have been found to be beneficial in relieving pain.

Although I'm sure there are others, this should give you plenty to choose from. As usual, the above all have multiple benefits. Along with the SAMe and the EFAs such as flax seed oil, this should resolve most cases of depression, which could be important, as the majority suffering with Fibromyalgia are also experiencing depression. SAMe can also prevent the elevation of the major cardiovascular risk homocysteine, by methylation converting it into the very beneficial amino acid methionine. Although in this case we are focusing on pain, combined they also provide dozens of other benefits (the distinct advantage associated with all nutrients).

Arthritis – From Joint Deterioration

As you now know, most pain medications actually contribute to joint deterioration, and should thus be avoided. And as you also have learned, most pain is normally caused by inflammation.

Once the inflammation has been eliminated, not only is the pain resolved, but a more efficient flow of nutrients to the joints can also be an additional benefit. Inflammation impedes the circulation, and thus the very first issue that should be addressed, allowing the nutrients to be delivered and the toxins to be removed efficiently.

With the inflammation issue out of the way, our focus will now be providing nutrients for rebuilding the cartilage, and strengthening the tendons and ligaments. There are several formulas available. The one I personally use is in a liquid form. It is produced by the Rockland Corporation and called "Liquid Life™ Joint Care". It comes in a 32-ounce bottle and the serving size is one ounce, which contains:

- 200 mg of vitamin C
- 1,000 mg of Glucosamine HCl
- 800 mg of Condroitin Sulfate
- 500 mg of MSM
- 50 mg of collagen (liquid protein)
- 10 mg of aloe vera (200:1 concentrate)

The mineral manganese (not magnesium) is also beneficial for rebuilding cartilage. I take one 5 mg tablet daily.

A sufficient supply of water (8 to 10 eight-ounce glasses daily), along with one teaspoon of Celtic sea salt daily, is also important. If the joints are not properly hydrated, the cartilage dries and begins flaking, contributing to degeneration. When properly hydrated, cartilage acts as a cushion as intended.

The Wrong Diet Can Be A Rather Painful Experience

Several years ago, after the Atkins Diet was first announced, my wife decided to try the diet in an attempt to lose a few pounds. Rather than the necessity of preparing different foods for me, I decided to try the diet with her. As a diet concentrating on eating mostly fats and proteins is obviously very acidic, it eventually caught up with me while on vacation in Maui. Although I was used to hiking several miles non-stop on some steep mountain trails at home, I suddenly ran into a problem while hiking only two miles (on the level) in Maui. After hiking only about a mile, my joints suddenly began to hurt and felt very unstable. I wasn't sure if I would be able to make the mile back to our condo.

At first, it didn't seem to make a bit of sense. I wondered what could possibly have such a negative influence on the stability of my joints in such a short span of time? It was then that I recalled a lecture by a doctor several years prior, addressing a particular problem associated with excessive acidity in the body. He mentioned that when the body becomes too acidic, it causes a leaching (removal) of the synovial fluid from the joint. I learned first hand, the tremendous influence an acidic diet can have on the joints. An acidic condition is actually unhealthy in other ways also, such as contributing to an overall oxygen deficiency in the body. Anyone who has adhered to a similar high protein/high fat diet, could easily be experiencing the very same problem, and not have a clue why, (thus, the reason for this discussion). In my forthcoming book on Weight Loss, I will provide what I consider a much healthier, more alkaline diet that anyone can easily follow, along with some other important recommendations that should even work for those who have been the most resistant to weight loss.

As many in the nation are currently attempting to lose weight, and are under the impression this might be an appropriate diet, they might want to reconsider. Just remember to avoid simple sugar in all forms, as well as starchy foods, and instead get your complex carbohydrates from fruits and vegetables that are alkaline, which provide many healthy nutrients as well. Also remember that both coffee and soft drinks are very acidic, as well as dehydrating. It's interesting that although common table salt is acidic, Celtic sea salt is instead alkaline, and thus beneficial for your joints.

In my case, I was basically dealing with two different problems: (1) Joint instability from the loss of synovial fluid and, (2) Pain as the result of the acidic condition in the joints. The synovial fluid helps nourish and lubricate the joints, as well as providing stability. Then, from his *Special Report on Pain: Arthritis Pain and Back Pain*, Dr. F. Batmanghelidj, M.D. helps explain the part that both salt and water play in the acid removal process as follows:

> *Salt helps to extract the acidity from the inside of the cartilage cells and pass it into the water that carries the acid away from the cells. This is a constant process. For the acid extraction process to be effective, two elements are vital: water and salt. Adequate salt supply is essential for the prevention of arthritis pain, be it in the joints of the limbs or the spine. It is the added salt level in the blood's serum that increases the serum's water content for more abundant flow through the cartilage* (p. 4).

Not only does an acidic condition contribute to pain, but also according to Dr. James Balch, ***"If the blood is too acidic, the cartilage in the joints may dissolve. The joints loose their normal smooth sliding motion, bones rub together, and the joints become inflamed, causing pain"*** (*Prescription for Nutritional Healing*, 3*rd* edition, 2000, p. 193). So as we can see, getting the acid out of the joints could not only help prevent the pain, but also reduce the destruction of cartilage. And water also has the added benefit of hydrating the cartilage, thus preventing another cause of cartilage deterioration.

After identifying the problem, I immediately began eating a much more alkaline diet. I also began drinking more water, along with Celtic sea salt to help remove the acids. In addition, I took alfalfa tablets, algae, chlorella, and MSM, to assist in both alkalizing and detoxification. It took approximately three weeks (to reverse the process), before my joints again became stable and pain-free, as they had always been in the past.

You can purchase a roll of test paper to help monitor your pH (acid/alkaline), and track your progress if you choose. On the back of the dispenser is a chart with colors identifying your pH level. One common tape is called Phydron™. It can evaluate a pH ranging from 5.5 (yellow, very acidic) to 8.0 (blue, very alkaline), and in between (varying shades of green). The healthy saliva range falls somewhere between 7.0 and 7.4. Although **most people are too acidic**, too alkaline is not considered healthy either. It was found that people with cancer typically have a pH of 4.5 to 5.0 (very acidic). Your body is similar to a swimming pool, as they both have a healthy pH range, where they function the most efficiently.

Dehydration – A Common Contributor to Back Pain

I consider Dr. Batmanghelidj to be a foremost authority regarding the many influences of dehydration throughout the body. His most comprehensive book is *Your Body's Many Cries For Water* (1992/1998), and a book I would highly recommend. Dr. Batmanghelidj did an excellent job of describing the structure and function of the spine, in his *Special Report on Pain: Arthritis Pain and Back Pain*. Most importantly, he explained exactly how dehydration causes both pain and dehydration of the spinal column. Now in his own words, we will see what he has to say on the subject as follows:

> *Low back pain has two components. One component is muscle spasm, which is the simple cause of back pain in 80 percent of people that suffer this infliction. The second component is disc degeneration. This puts added strain on the tendons and ligaments in the spinal column. Both of these components, that cause the same back pain, are initiated by the onset of chronic dehydration.*

All joint surfaces are padded with cartilage that covers and separates the joints' bone structures. This firm layer of cartilage, which is attached to the ends of the bones in all joints, contains a vast quantity of water that gives the cartilage its lubricative and smooth gliding properties. A water-lubricated cartilage has the ability to glide over the opposing cartilage surface, and makes it possible for the joint to go through its normal motions without pain or clicking noises. Thus, prolonged local drought, that leaves the cartilage short of water, will produce a more-than-normal amount of friction and shearing stress at the cartilage contact points within the joint.

A healthy joint is fully hydrated.

When cartilage is dehydrated, its gliding ability is decreased. The cartilage cells sense their dehydration, and give out alarm signals of pain, because they would soon die and peel off from their contact surfaces if used in their dehydrated state. The way this pain is produced is truly simple. The environment of cartilage is alkaline. In dehydration it becomes acid. This acidity sensitizes the nerve endings, and they register this drastic environmental change by producing pain.

Seventy-five percent of the weight of your upper body mass is supported by the hydraulic properties of the discs that absorb and hold water in their central cores. In a dehydrated state, when the body mass constantly squeezes out the water content of the discs during movement and bending, not enough of the lost water can be replaced. The dehydrated discs with their shrunken cores gradually become less supportive of the weight of the body. In dehydration, the discs lose their wedge quality and the spinal joints become less firm.

The discs, when fully hydrated, act as wedges between each of the 24 vertebrae, at the same time that they are effective shock absorbers.

When discs are effective wedges, the muscles at the back of the spine do not have to overwork to keep the body upright. In their dehydrated state, the discs become poor wedges, and the muscles of the back have to work proportionately harder to hold the body upright. The overworked muscles gradually become fatigued and begin to suffer spasm. It is this spasm of the back muscles that in 80 out of 100 cases of back pain is the culprit. The muscles that develop spasm also have an increased toxic waste content that cannot be washed away because of local dehydration – thus causing more pain (pp. 3-8).

That certainly helps explain why so many in the nation are experiencing back pain, if you consider the average person's beverage of choice is not water. Dr. Bruce West, N.D. discovered that 95% of his patients complaining of back pain were just dehydrated.

Our Final Step – Lubricating Those Stiff Creaky Joints

We now come to our final step regarding healthy pain-free fully functioning joints. Anytime we have any kind of friction from two opposing surfaces (especially weight-bearing), adequate lubrication is of primary importance. Although proper hydration of the cartilage is an important issue, there is actually more we can do to assure our success. We also need to keep all those joints adequately lubricated, for optimum performance, (our primary objective).

When it comes to our blood, the lower the viscosity (the thinner), the better for efficient circulation and delivery of nutrients and oxygen. Although the opposite is true regarding the lubricant in our joints, called synovial fluid. We will be looking at natural ways to not only assure an adequate supply, but also proper viscosity, in order to provide the best possible protection and assure joint efficiency. I might add that I not only have absolutely no joint pain, but my joints also appear to be even stronger, and more stable than they were years ago when in my youth. Who says our bodies or joints necessarily have to deteriorate as we age? Speaking from experience, I assure you it's not really necessary, although it is totally impossible if you are willing to settle for a lifetime of damaging medications to suppress your body's cries for help. If you begin forming an alliance with your body, you will be amazed at what it can accomplish, when provided the adequate resources.

We are about to discover one very effective solution to this particular issue that I learned about from a book published more than a decade ago, but the original discovery dates back 150 years, from a medical book actually published in 1855! It's inexcusable in my opinion, that a discovery of this magnitude (as with many other important findings) was ignored and not implemented in medicine just because it was too cost effective, and thus not profitable. My objective is to bring these findings out of obscurity, so we can again take advantage of the many exceptional resources deliberately suppressed, often for decades. It appears this discovery is possibly one of the most outstanding findings of all, even in regards to long-term arthritis.

My resource for this information is one of hundreds of books in my library, titled *Sam Biser's Course of Curing Hopeless Health Conditions*, published in 1993. The author, Sam Biser, also published a newsletter for several years, titled *The Last Chance Health Report*, which is just one of several that I have subscribed to over the years. I was always searching for answers, and will likely continue to do so the remainder of my life. In his book, Sam Biser interviewed a layman named Dale Alexander, who became interested in arthritis back in the late 1920's when his mother was stricken with arthritis. After watching her suffer for ten long years, and seeing the gradual deterioration from the debilitating disease, he began a quest searching for an answer. He spent many years looking at all the latest medical findings, as well as researching old folk remedies. By chance, one day he came across an old medical book published back in 1855, authored by a medical doctor named L. J. DeJongh, who made an amazing discovery. He discovered something that worked with his patients for arthritis, far better than anything he had ever heard of, or tried in the past.

You are likely wondering what this outstanding discovery might possibly be, and understandably so. Alexander stated that *"I came upon one old-time folk remedy that was to prove to be the lost 'key' to solving the problems of arthritis"* (p. 449). Would you believe it was just plain old cod liver oil, something I rather detested as a child. Fortunately, it can be found today in a variety of flavors, as well as in soft gel capsules. If you recall, I recommended both cod liver oil and flax seed oil as good sources of essential fatty acids (EFAs). Well in our case, the type of delivery is a critical issue, and although the soft gel capsules work fine when dealing with other issues, it won't work very well for lubricating the joints.

All nutrients have multiple benefits throughout the body and brain. The very reason nature's pharmacy should be our only resource if we truly respect our body, and if optimal health is our primary objective. Exactly how, and sometimes even when we take some substances, will determine how the body might possibly use them. As you begin establishing a closer relationship with your body, that will eventually become second nature, and will as a result be reflected in your overall health. We will be taking a look at Sam Biser's interview of Dale Alexander, who incidentally wrote the number one best selling non-fiction book in England, titled *Arthritis and Common Sense*. As the interview was rather lengthy, for the sake of brevity we will just extract some of the most pertinent information.

We will be addressing the primary issue of most effectively getting the very important lubricating oil into all those joints covered with cartilage. But first let's look at a report that Dale Alexander found in Dr. Pemberton's book titled *The Medical Management of Arthritis*. The report showed that **there was a tremendous variation in the viscosity of the synovial fluid in a non-arthritic person, versus that of those suffering with arthritis.** Would you believe <u>a normal person's synovial fluid is over 15 times as thick</u>? That's a tremendous variation, and most importantly, we will soon discover how we can quite easily influence the viscosity of our joints (and as usual, it's not with drugs).

Under the chapter on Acid Reflux Disease (GERD), we learned the importance of proper food combining for efficient digestion and assimilation of foods. Then, in regards to diabetes, we find the combination of foods eaten during a meal will determine the release rate of glucose into the bloodstream. Now we will learn what the negative influence of combining some of the wrong liquids with a meal might have on efficiently assimilating cod liver oil (as well as where it will be deposited).

We will be evaluating two primary issues, and in Mr. Alexander's own words, he will be discussing:

*...**foods and habits that inhibit or destroy the oil in your joints**, and **foods and habits that enhance or increase the quality of synovial fluid in the joints**. Let's start with the oil-inhibiting foods and habits.*

The first oil-inhibiting habit is drinking our oil-free liquids like water, tea or coffee with your meal.

When you drink liquids with meals, very little oil gets to the joints. Let me explain, because it's very important.

Remember the old adage that oil and water don't mix. Well, it's also true in matters of diet. I'll explain.

When you eat a meal, the food is broken down into minute oily particles and mixed with the stomach juices. The heat in the stomach changes any fats in the food into tiny oily globules. Now – if you've drank no liquids – here's what happens.

The tiny oily globules (about half of them) are collected by something called the cisterna chyle. This is a passageway leading out of the stomach and emptying eventually into the bloodstream. The oily globules travel along this passageway, get to the bloodstream and are transported to the joints. The remaining oils will travel on and eventually enter the portal vein and go to the liver.

However – if you've drank an oil-free beverage with your meal, the picture changes. The beverage causes the oil globules to rupture into one large pool. Now, only about 20% of them can enter the cisterna chyle, bypass the liver, and go directly to the joints. The other 80% go on to the portal vein. They end up in the liver, which uses them for energy and other metabolic purposes – not as lubricants.

If you want your dietary oils to act as lubricants, you've got to get them to bypass your liver. The way to accomplish this is to avoid all mealtime beverages, except milk or soups. These two beverages cause no problems because they already contain tiny particles of oil. Hence they don't disturb the globules in the stomach.

So, to sum up, avoid oil-free beverages at mealtime. You will actually triple the amount of oils available for joint lubrication. This isn't an idle speculation of mine. It's been proven by no less an authority than Dr. Abraham White of Yale University.

I'm not against drinking water – but you have to do it at the right time, which is ten minutes before a meal or three hours afterward.

One more thing: You have to drink your liquids at the right temperature. Don't drink iced liquids with meals. The cold liquids will congeal (harden) the oils in your food, making it almost impossible for them to bypass the liver.

Next to water (drank at the wrong time), the most harmful dietary mistake is drinking acid liquids.

When you drink citrus juices, the citrus acid they contain cuts the oil out of your system. Lemon kills off the lubricating oils we need most.

Other fruit juices are equally bad. The reason for this is that they are all acidic. When you drink them, the acidity goes into your system without being neutralized by your saliva. So avoid fruit juices, including apple juice and pineapple juice.

Besides citrus juices, there are a number of acid foods which are also bad for arthritis.

Vinegar is one. It contains acetic acid. Another is soda pop. It contains phosphoric acid, an acid strong enough to dissolve a tooth in two weeks. Imagine what it can do to the linings of your joints.

Regular non-herbal tea should be dropped. *It contains another acid, tannic acid. This is what the tanning industry uses to remove the oil from hides. It does the same thing to joints.* ***When I visited England, a land of tea drinkers, I saw more cases of deformed arthritis than anywhere else in the world.***

Finally, ***eliminate all white sugar and products made with it. Sugar attacks the oils in your joints, leaving them subject to scarring*** (*Sam Biser's Course of Curing Hopeless Health Conditions, 1993, pp. 449-451*).

According to Alexander, you will experience the very best results if the cod liver oil is taken on an empty stomach. The best time is one hour before breakfast, or four hours after the last meal of the day. Apparently if you do, it should go directly through your arteries to your joints. He also discovered that if the cod liver oil is consumed with warm (not hot) whole milk, the entire mixture is more easily assimilated, and will reach the arthritic joints in greater supply. According to Alexander, both butter and egg yolks are also good sources of oil, and that soft-boiled eggs are best. He also noted that coffee can turn the egg yolk into a rubbery material, which taxes the gall bladder, heart, and arteries.

We will finally evaluate what kind of results you might expect, as well as an approximate time frame. According to Alexander:

Generally speaking, after taking cod liver oil, your fingers and your arms will lose their stiffness and swelling first. Arthritis of the back and spine will require the longest time before any change is noticed.

Don't be discouraged. You may think nothing is happening when all of a sudden, the improvement will come from nowhere. Just know that you are no different from anyone else. ***The program will work for you if you stick to it*** (*Sam Biser's Course of Curing Hopeless Health Conditions, 1993, p. 457*).

He also noted, that ***"Usually it takes from 3 to 6 months or more to get results. But sometimes it happens in only two weeks"*** (p. 452).

Keep in mind that your results will obviously depend on how strictly you adhere to the program. It's encouraging that Alexander discovered from years of experience that ***"It doesn't' matter what kind of arthritis you have, they all respond to cod liver oil.*** *The reason for this is that all arthritis – regardless of the symptoms – has the same basic cause: poorly lubricated joints. It's just that each person reacts differently"* (p. 444).

Alexander was looking for the very best oil, and in his own words, he states that:

I have spent years testing every kind of oil and I discovered that cod liver oil is one of the best lubricants of the joints.

Cod liver oil is the best all-around oil, not only for arthritics, but for everyone. Besides being such an excellent lubricant, it has other benefits. For one, it contains plenty of vitamins A and D. You need vitamin A for eyes and skin moisture.

You need vitamin D to make strong bones and joints. ***You also need vitamin D to make natural cortisone, which is manufactured by your adrenal glands. Without cortisone in our bodies, we'd all have arthritis. Cortisone's purpose is to increase the stickiness of the joint oil. Without it, joint oils thin out and leak into surrounding*** *tissues.* Cod liver oil helps you make your own cortisone, which is far better than any synthetic product.

Cod liver oil also contains iodine and some fifty other different nutrients. It's the best single food an arthritic could use (*Sam Biser's Course of Curing Hopeless Health Conditions, 1993, p. 453*).

Unfortunately, millions of Americans have been taking potentially dangerous arthritis medications for years. Some of the worst offenders were Vioxx™, Celebrex™, and Bextra™, as well as being the most widely prescribed. This is one more example where doctors normally prescribe very risky medications, when much safer and more effective natural options are available. As long as traditional medicine insists on excluding anything but drugs or surgery, the problem will continue to worsen.

In summary, we learned that:
- Medications are major contributors to pain.
- Inflammation is the most common cause of pain.
- Insufficient oxygen also contributes to pain.
- Dehydration can contribute to pain.
- Acid in the joints sensitizes the nerves causing pain.

We also learned (from my experience), that an acidic diet can lead to leaching (removal) of the synovial fluid from the joint capsule. Thus the combination of excess acid in the joint, as well as a deficiency of synovial fluid, can lead to both pain and joint instability.

As usual, we not only identified the various causes of pain, but also several viable solutions. We learned of ways we can remove acids from the joints and prevent the serious dehydration of cartilage. We also found that several nutrients can help to restore worn or damaged cartilage. And finally was the discovery that cod liver oil will lubricate the joints and thus complete the process of restoring joint health, and eliminating pain. Truly resolving any disease or condition can only take place once all the contributing factors have been identified, which as you noticed we were able to do. Once that has been accomplished, a solution for each one must be found, which we did. Medications instead simply suppress symptoms such as pain, while allowing the condition to worsen, and often even contribute to the deterioration in the process, which is true regarding many arthritis medications.

We will now look at another reason for eliminating back pain, and a potential consequence if you don't.

A Good Reason To Resolve Back Pain – It May Alter Brain Chemistry

The following article was obtained through *The Chiropractic Health Research Information Service* (February 9, 2001):

Back pain doesn't just affect patients' backs – it also influences their brains, say scientists. *According to a recently published report in the journal Pain,* **chronic back pain (CBP) alters patients' brain chemistry.**

Researchers at SUNY Upstate Medical University in Syracuse, New York used magnetic resonance spectroscopy to measure the relative concentrations of several brain chemicals (N-acetyl aspartate, creatine, choline, glutamate, glutamine, gamma-aminobutyric acid, inositol, glucose and lactate) in 9 CBP sufferers and 11 pain-free volunteers. Measurements were conducted in six different brain regions. Patients with CBP also underwent evaluations for pain and anxiety.

Findings revealed that, "in chronic back pain, the interrelationship between chemicals within and across brain regions was abnormal, and there was a specific relationship between regional chemicals and perceptual measures of pain and anxiety. These findings provide direct evidence of abnormal brain chemistry in chronic back pain" (Pain, December 2000, 15;89:7-18)
(http://hub.elsevier.com/pii/S0304395900003407).

Consider Visiting A Chiropractor

If you are suffering with back pain and haven't been to a chiropractor lately, I would suggest finding a good chiropractor and at least get checked. If you just happen to have a subluxation (basically out of adjustment), just an adjustment or two could possibly solve your problem. If not, you will at least have eliminated that possibility. A pinched nerve can influence various organs, based on where the misalignment might be. It can even cause pain in the legs. Most chiropractors are normally inexpensive, so it might be a good investment. Years ago, my wife suffered with terrible intermittent headaches for months. Nothing showed up in any of the many tests the doctors made. They suggested she see an ophthalmologist and have her eyes tested. Between visits her vision even changed. I finally took her to a very experienced chiropractor. In a matter of minutes he located the problem and with just one adjustment, the headaches disappeared!

Possibly one of the most surprising discoveries I made was an unusual contributor to mysterious unexplainable pain, which few have likely heard of, but could potentially influence many. So, if all else fails, get ready for a surprise!

If All Else Fails, The Pain Could Be Caused By Your Brain
(Although not necessarily all in your head)

Following is something very interesting that I learned from Dr. Bruce West, D.C., which he in turn learned from Dr. John Sarno, M.D. (as noted by Dr. West, in the April 2005 issue of his *Health Alert* newsletter, Volume 22, Issue 4, pp. 4-6):

Thanks to careful evaluation over the years and research from men like John Sarno, M.D., we now know without a doubt that lots of chronic pain is caused by the brain.

*It is Dr. Sarno's contention that **most people with incurable pain are suffering from TMS (Tension Myositis Syndrome) – a condition whereby repressed anxiety, anger, and rage trigger muscle spasms and joint problems.** In human nature we all suffer from repressed anger and rage. This is a relatively natural condition caused by all kinds of damages heaped on us throughout childhood and adult life. **This repressed anger and rage is kept in the unconscious mind.** In other words, you do not know you have this anger inside of you because you are not conscious of it.*

*When this rage becomes overwhelming and begins to become **conscious,** your brain creates TMS to divert attention away from the anger and rage by using pain. It is as simple as that. And the cure can be equally simple for most people. **Once you have reached the stage where you know that your pain is chronic and incurable, you must accept that you are suffering from TMS.** Upon this acceptance, it is a simple matter of realizing that there is nothing wrong with your back and that your pain is nothing more than TMS. **The realization and acceptance along is enough to break the cycle and put an end to chronic pain.***

What to Do about TMS

Here are the ways to recognize and accept TMS – thereby finally overcoming chronic pain.

1) You must acknowledge that TMS and nothing else is the cause of your pain, numbness, tingling, weakness, etc.

2) To get well, you must put your past medical experiences behind you and concentrate on your program to get well. That means forgetting everything you have been told in the past by your doctors, including diagnoses and what you should and shouldn't do.

*3) **Concentrate on understanding that your brain is causing tension and slight oxygen deprivation to your muscles and joints. This can cause the most severe pain or symptoms imaginable.** The crushing pain of angina or a heart attack brought about by a deprivation of oxygen to the heart muscle is a perfect example. When you suffer from TMS, your back, neck, arms, shoulders, and legs are **normal** no matter what you have been told.*

4) The when and where of your pain is not important. Rather, the cure involves changing your brain's programming with proper thinking. The pain is actually caused by unconscious rage. This may have been generated in infancy or childhood. It stays with you your entire life, even if you have never been angry. Often, personality traits induce TMS. People who must please everyone often are filled with unconscious rage. If you are a type "A" personality, you may also be filled with unconscious rage. Your job, your spouse, your friends, or even your kids can contribute to unconscious rage.

*5) Remember that you (your brain) unconsciously fears that this rage may become conscious. Therefore, **you unknowingly produce pain to distract yourself from these intense emotions.** Now comes the best part – you don't have to solve or undo all these emotional problems and pains. You simply need to recognize them and accept that they are the cause of your chronic pain.*

6) Once you start on this enlightening voyage, you will quickly begin to recognize the phenomenon, toss all past medical diagnoses in the garbage heap, and as soon as you get better, resume all normal activities – even if warned against them.

*So, get started. Remember that all joint problems require common sense – and that means good nutrition to supply the nutrients needed by the body to regenerate joints. It may also require physical therapy. For problems that simply cannot be cured, you must recognize TMS. **I know that this phenomenon is true. And certainly Dr. Sarno does, since he has successfully resolved incurable pain in tens of thousands using this method.***

*For a simple and awakening voyage to becoming pain free, get a copy of Dr. John Sarno's book, **Healing Back Pain** (Warner Books). As soon as you get it and start reading it, send for his two videotapes. They come with a Study Guide that together, within a few weeks to months, will help you to finally become pain free.*

So as you can see, your pain can at times have multiple sources, as well as multiple solutions, for whatever the source your pain might possibly be.

CHAPTER THIRTY-ONE
SUMMARY

Some Basic Flaws In Our Current Health Care System

As a nation, we are currently experiencing a terrible insidious increasingly serious plague spreading throughout the nation.

For lack of a better description, I will refer to them as "Syndromes". A few of the most obvious, and easily recognizable, although curable, are:

A. Regarding your Doctor:
- "There's Nothing We Can Do Until It Becomes a Disease"
- "I Don't Have Time To Research All The Drug Interactions"
- "I Can't Afford to Spend that Much Time With My Patients"
- "I'm Only Following What I was Taught In Medical School"
- "I'm Just Following AMA Approved Procedures"
- "I Could Lose My License If I Tried That Unapproved Therapy"
- "I Only Know What My Pharmaceutical Rep Told Me"

B. Regarding the Pharmaceutical Industry:
- "Natural Supplements are Becoming a Serious Threat"
- "If They Find That Out, Our Drugs will Never Sell"
- "How Can We Best Buy Influence In the Government?"
- "What Authorities Can We Place in Strategic Positions?"
- "Is There Some Way We Can Justify Regulating Vitamin Safety?"
- "How Can We Discredit the Benefits of Natural Supplements?"
- "How Can We Best Influence a Positive Outcome Of This Study?"
- "How Long Can We Stall the Production of This Generic Drug?"
- "How Can We Create a New Disease to Develop Drugs For?"
- "How Can We Best Promote Our Drugs to the Public?"
- "How Can We Modify Our Study In Order to Get FDA Approval?"
- "How Can We Stop Canada from Undermining Our Drug Profits?"
- "How Can We Convince the Public that Canadian Drugs are Unsafe?"
- "How Can We Control The Public's Access to Vitamins?"
- "How Can We Promote Government Supported Drug Coverage?"
- "How Can We Control What's Covered By Patients' Insurance?"
- "How Long Can We Effectively Continue Our Deception?"
- "How Can We Reduce Our Legal Liability For Risky Drugs?"
- "This Drug is Too Profitable To Pull, So What Can We Do About It?"
- "We Can't Let People Know About the Risk Associated With This Drug"
- "Disease Prevention Is Not Profitable, and Shouldn't Be Promoted"
- "How Can We Best Keep the Public In The Dark About Drug Risks?"
- "What Doctors Might Be Willing to Make a Statement for a Price?"

Unfortunately, these are syndromes that have a tremendous influence on your overall health, and have for decades. In the majority of cases, these are not things you are doing yourself, but are the external influences by others that still directly influence your health (or lack thereof). The objective should be to first identify the syndromes, just like identifying the various underlying contributors to a disease. We then need to no longer allow them to treat us as immature adolescents, incapable of thinking for ourselves.

What is the answer to this terrible corruption of medicine, at our expense, and just for the sake of profit? One can't help but recognize that the driving force behind the obvious corruption in medicine begins and ends with the tremendous influence of the very profitable and thus powerful pharmaceutical industry. It all begins with their influence on your doctor's training in medical school, as well as his follow-up training later.

The Tremendous Lobbying Power of The Pharmaceutical Industry

Sexual performance drugs such as Viagra™ will soon be covered under Medicare's new prescription drug program. The new prescription coverage for Viagra™ was scheduled to begin January 2006, and **is expected to cost more than $500 billion over the next decade.**

According to Gary Karr, spokesman for the Centers for Medicare and Medicaid Services, which administers the health insurance program for older Americans, the law says if it is an FDA-approved drug and it is medically necessary, it must be covered. The key word here is "medically necessary," and I think anyone would be hard-pressed to prove that Viagra™ is in any way medically necessary. And expecting taxpayers to pay for Medicare coverage for sexual performance drugs for 76 million baby boomers would just assure the impending collapse of Medicare.

In fact, it was discovered that hundreds of convicted rapists and sex offenders had been receiving Medicaid reimbursements for Viagra™ for years. A spokesman for the Health and Human Services department claims that confusion over a federal directive is to blame. How in the world could anyone possibly overlook something so outright ridiculous? Providing Viagra™ for free is a perfect way to promote rape by stimulating increased sexual desire (one thing Viagra™ is promoted for). And worst of all, we the taxpayers are footing the bill.

One can't help but recognize the unbelievable lobbying power by the drug industry to successfully promote the approval of the recreational drug Viagra™ for improving sexual performance, and force the taxpayers to pick up the tab. This comes at a time when the solvency of both Medicare and Medicaid are at the greatest risk of any time in history. The greatest contributor to the problem is the cost of medications. Promoting the use of more drugs to the general public just adds to the problem. More people are being unnecessarily placed on medications that are often inappropriate, and based only on patients' requests. We must put a stop to that kind of obvious abuse that threatens the very financial structure of organizations that so many in the nation depend upon, and just for the sake of profit.

These very profitable drug companies have become more and more aggressive in promoting their terribly inflated medications, with no consideration for ethics, or the best interest of the many patients being placed at risk, or the solvency of Medicare and Medicaid.

Now that we have completed our research, and identified the underlying problems, we can begin focusing on the appropriate solutions, (implementing our drug-free therapies).

Based on the evidence, the current approach to medical care has proven to be fundamentally unsound, and obviously flawed. That fact is reflected in the statistics, which don't lie, but should instead bring the serious concern to our attention, and ignoring the facts won't make the problem somehow go away. As I have stated before, **we can't continue doing the same things, and somehow expect to get different results (an irrefutable fact).** So the obvious question is: What exactly must we do to rectify the problem? Based on the evidence provided herein, what would you suggest? I believe by now you are fully aware of my recommendation: **Just say no to all unnecessary drugs!** So now what's next? (Plenty!)

My Latest Release:
Antidepressants, Antipsychotics, and Stimulants – Dangerous Drugs on Trial

I recently discovered what I consider to be a serious concern, especially regarding our kids. There is currently a concerted effort by the pharmaceutical giants, to place as many of our children as possible on their extremely dangerous mind-altering stimulants, antidepressants, and antipsychotics. They are highly profitable drugs that were never tested on, or FDA-approved, for children! Not only that, but they are even attempting to circumvent parental consent!

Their aggressive campain is a federally mandated program, called TeenScreen. It is specifically targeting our kids, preschool and over. Worst of all, is the tremendous potential for serious damage from their use. They not only damage the brain, and lower IQs, but they are behind the dramatic increase in diseases such as cancer and diabetes, once considered as adult diseases. I provide ample scientific evidence in my book to back up all my claims.

There were two very telling studies conducted, by the major pharmaceuital provider Scripts, Inc., who has millions of customers. Incidentally, both studies involved 3.7 million children. In the first study, it was discovered that in only four years' time, twice as many children had also been placed on antidepressants (the result of the aggressive promotional campaign). Then in another study conducted two years later, on the exact same number of children, (from the same database), twice as many children had been placed on diabetes medications. The drugs that so many children are being placed on, are actually contributing to that very problem, (both SSRI antidepressants, and antipsychotics, contribute to diabetes).

Once you learn the facts, you will want to get your kids (or yourself) off, ASAP! Just don't stop suddenly. I explain why it's important to withdraw slowly, and exactly how, in order to avoid a serious reaction. This book is an absolute must-read for anyone with school-age children, or grandchildren, or even for any adults who are currently taking them, or considering doing so.

Future projects:

I hope to conduct a clinical study in the future, focusing on identifying the most efficient method of withdrawing from medications, while also resolving the different underlying conditions they were prescribed for. That is often surprisingly easy, as many medications are prescribed just to suppress the side effects associated with other medications a patient might have been placed on, (the typical domino effect). Although all drugs create side effects, some are often not even accomplishing what they were prescribed for to begin with.

I was surprised to find that although my findings (many published in this book) could quite easily save billions of dollars in Medicare and Medicaid healthcare expenses, none of the legislators I wrote proposals to, have seemed the least bit interested. I rather feel as though I have been basically fighting fires lately, with very little success. Hopefully, with a new administration, things might finally change.

Although the book on weight loss was intended to be my next, it keeps getting superseded, by what appear to be even greater concerns. As Alzheimer's is becoming an epidemic, and such a devastating disease, I decided to tackle that condition next. I soon discovered that by far the greatest contributors to both dementia and Alzheimer's are the medications the majority of seniors are being placed on. As more seniors are being placed on more medications, (due to the recent prescription drug "benefit" plan), more are also acquiring Alzheimer's, and often at a much earlier age as well. I will also be adressinsg other contributors, as well as how to prevent (and at times, even reverse) the condition.

Stay tuned by checking my Website at http://www.drtanton.com periodically, as I will be announcing my new books, along with a brief description of each.

CHAPTER THIRTY-TWO

REFERENCE GUIDE
VITAMINS – MINERALS – SUPPLEMENTS

In this chapter you will learn the many benefits of vitamins, minerals, and other supplements that are being depleted by your medications. It is not only important to learn of the many nutrients that medications deplete, but also the important contributions that each provide to your overall health. Only then can you more fully appreciate the seriousness of taking multiple medications known to contribute to their depletion. You will also better understand why taking supplements, along with eating a healthy diet, could likely eliminate the need for taking potentially dangerous medications in the first place.

Due to the extensive depletion of nutrients by medications, maintaining an adequate level of each nutrient, as well as a proper balance, is extremely difficult, (if not impossible). Microwave cooking is one major contributor to vitamin depletion. Sugar and stress are also notorious for the depletion of many nutrients. So, we actually have two primary areas of concern. First, is to assure that you are getting an adequate level of vitamins, minerals, amino acids, and phytonutrients (plant extracts), from your diet and supplements. And then, be sure to avoid anything that could possibly contribute to their depletion, such as medications, stress, sugar, or microwave cooking.

You should also be aware that there can be a considerable difference in the quality of supplements that you might purchase. Just don't expect to benefit much from any one-a-day type multivitamin/mineral supplement. Although they normally contain an extensive list of ingredients, they contain an insufficient amount of each one to be of any real value. There is obviously no way you could possibly expect to get a sufficient amount of supplements in one pill (or a bowl of cereal), as often advertised. Unfortunately, by producing poor quality vitamins, the manufacturers are just providing the public with a false sense of security.

Would you believe that some pharmaceutical companies actually produce vitamins? The problem is, their objective is definitely "not" to keep you healthy! Their real profit comes from the highly inflated medications that they patent, and then make huge profits on. When you are healthy, you won't likely be experiencing symptoms, or visiting your doctor, where all the prescriptions for medications originate. If you have been taking a once-a-day type vitamin or mineral, you need to find a better quality supplement. You can't possibly expect to realize any real benefit from one or two pills, which normally contain "minute amounts" of an extensive list of vitamins and minerals. They won't begin to compensate for the extensive depletion of nutrients caused by your medications, (if you are taking any). Sewer systems often contain thousands of vitamin pills. Most are still intact, and thus not even absorbed!

As you will soon discover, many vitamins and minerals are actually codependent, and thus synergistic (or more beneficial when others are also present). You will also discover that every single vitamin or mineral has a surprising number of benefits. Going through the entire list, will help you better appreciate the importance of maintaining an adequate level of each one.

Vitamin A (Retinol and Carotene)

- **Vitamin A is depleted by:**

  o **Alcohol**
  o **Antacids**
  o **Antibiotics**
  o **Antiseizure medication (i.e. barbiturates, phenytoin)**
  o **All cholesterol-lowering drugs, including statins and bile acid sequestrants (i.e. Questran™, Colestid™)**
  o **Aspirin**
  o **Caffeine**
  o **Estrogen (and oral contraceptives)**
  o **Laxatives (mineral oil)**
  o **NSAIDs (i.e. ibuprofen)**
  o **Steroids and corticosteroids**

- Vitamin A is fat-soluble. It needs fats and minerals to be adequately absorbed into the body.

- Prevents night blindness and other eye problems.

- Important for healthy skin, hair, bones, and teeth.

- Vitamin A is an antioxidant, which helps to protect cells against cancer, and the degenerative effects of aging, alcohol consumption, and smoking.

- Enhances the immune system and assists in new cell growth.

- Protein cannot be utilized by the body without vitamin A.

- An emulsified form of vitamin A puts less stress on the liver.

- Most beneficial when taken with niacin, vitamin C, vitamin D, vitamin E, vitamin B_5, and zinc.

- Deficiency can produce: night blindness, chronic infections, dry hair/skin, insomnia, fatigue.

- Insufficient vitamin A can cause a deterioration of the pituitary gland's basophil cells where the thyroid-stimulating hormone is synthesized, limiting the amount of iodine that the thyroid gland can absorb, and reducing the amount of thyroid hormone it produces.

- CAUTION: Do not take more than 100,000 IUs daily, as it can be toxic to the liver.

Vitamin B₁ (Thiamine)

- **Vitamin B₁ is depleted by:**

  o **Alcohol**
  o **Antacids**
  o **Antibiotics**
  o **Antiarrhythmic agents (i.e. digoxin)**
  o **Antiseizure medication (i.e. barbiturates, phenytoin)**
  o **Caffeine**
  o **Diuretics**
  o **Estrogen (and oral contraceptives)**
  o **Smoking**
  o **SSRI antidepressants**
  o **Sulfa drugs**

- **Vitamin B₁ is also depleted by sugar, cooking (heat), food processing methods, and physical and mental stress.**

- Assists in blood formation and enhances circulation.

- Assists in the production of hydrochloric acid, which is necessary for proper digestion and a healthy digestive tract.

- Reduces stress and anxiety.

- Enhances energy and learning capacity.

- Important for healthy nervous system functioning.

- Needed for proper muscle tone of the intestines, heart, and stomach.

- Vitamin B₁ is an antioxidant, which helps to protect cells against cancer, and the degenerative effects of aging, alcohol consumption, and smoking.

- A high-carbohydrate diet increases the need for vitamin B₁.

- Most beneficial when taken with vitamin B₁₂ and vitamin C.

- Deficiencies can produce: beriberi (a rare nervous condition), constipation and other gastrointestinal disturbances, edema (swelling), fatigue, poor coordination, forgetfulness, weak and sore muscles, numbness of the hands and feet, heart changes, irritability or nervousness, general weakness, severe weight loss.

Vitamin B$_2$ (Riboflavin)

- **Vitamin B$_2$ is depleted by:**

  o **Alcohol**
  o **Antacids**
  o **Antibiotics**
  o **Antiseizure medication (i.e. barbiturates, phenytoin)**
  o **Antidepressants (SSRI and tricyclics)**
  o **Diabetic medication**
  o **Diuretics**
  o **Estrogen (and oral contraceptives)**
  o **Mineral oil (laxatives)**
  o **Muscle relaxants**
  o **Steroids and corticosteroids**
  o **Sulfa drugs**

- **Vitamin B$_2$ is also depleted by sugar, ultraviolet light, and physical and mental stress.**

- **Strenuous exercise increases the need for vitamin B$_2$.**

- Vitamin B$_2$ is water-soluble. The body cannot store it. It is lost easily and needs replaced daily.

- Necessary for red blood cell formation and normal cell growth.

- Assists in the metabolism of carbohydrates, fats, and proteins, thus enhancing energy.

- Enhances vision. Reduces eye fatigue.

- Promotes healthy skin, nails and hair.

- Assists in converting protein to energy.

- Necessary for the metabolism of tryptophan (an amino acid), which is converted into niacin in the body.

- Strongly influences how well the thyroid gland synthesizes its hormones.

- Best taken with vitamin A, vitamin B$_1$ and vitamin B$_3$.

- Deficiency can produce: cracks and sores at the corners of the mouth, inflammation of the mouth and tongue, skin lesions and dermatitis, dizziness, hair loss, insomnia, light sensitivity, poor digestion, slowed mental response, fatigue, hypertension (high blood pressure), anxiety.

Vitamin B₃ (Niacin, Nicotinic Acid, Niacinamide)

- **Vitamin B₃ is depleted by:**

  - **Alcohol**
  - **Antibiotics**
  - **Caffeine**
  - **Estrogen (and oral contraceptives)**
  - **Sleeping pills**
  - **Steroids and corticosteroids**
  - **SSRI antidepressants**
  - **Sulfa drugs**

- **Vitamin B₃ is also depleted by sugar, and physical and mental stress.**

- Vitamin B₃ is water-soluble. The body cannot store it. It is easily lost and needs replaced daily.

- Needed for proper circulation and healthy skin.

- Enhances memory and prevents senility.

- Reduces blood pressure and lowers cholesterol.

- Assists in normal functioning of the nervous system.

- Essential to the good health of all glands, especially the thyroid.

- Assists in the metabolism of carbohydrates, fats, and proteins, thus enhancing energy.

- Assists in the production of hydrochloric acid, which is necessary for proper digestion. It is involved in the normal secretion of bile and stomach fluids.

- Most beneficial when taken with vitamin B₁, vitamin B₂, vitamin B₆ and tryptophan.

- Deficiencies can produce: depression, dementia, canker sores, dizziness, fatigue, headaches, indigestion, insomnia, loss of appetite, low blood sugar, muscular weakness.

- CAUTION: Excess niacin may elevate blood sugar levels.

- CAUTION: Do not take more than 500 mg daily, as it may cause liver damage.

Vitamin B₅ (Pantothenic Acid)

- **Vitamin B₅ is depleted by:**

  o **Alcohol**
  o **Caffeine**
  o **Estrogen (and oral contraceptives)**
  o **Sleeping pills**
  o **Sulfa drugs**

- **Vitamin B₅ is also depleted by sugar, heat (canning & roasting), and physical and mental stress.**

- Vitamin B₅ is water-soluble. The body cannot store it. It is easily lost and needs replaced daily.

- Assists in the production of the adrenal hormones and needed for proper functioning of the adrenal glands.

- Assists in the formation of antibodies.

- Assists in vitamin utilization.

- Assists in converting fats, carbohydrates, and proteins into energy.

- Is required by all cells in the body and is concentrated in the organs.

- Assists in the production of neurotransmitters, thus assisting in reducing stress, anxiety, and depression.

- Needed for normal functioning of the gastrointestinal tract.

- Prevents certain forms of anemia.

- Most beneficial when taken with folic acid and biotin.

- Deficiency can produce: fatigue, headache, nausea and tingling in the hands, and hypoglycemia.

Vitamin B$_6$ (Pyridoxine)

- **Vitamin B$_6$ is depleted by:**

  o **Alcohol**
  o **Antibiotics**
  o **Antidepressants and MAO inhibitors**
  o **Asthma medications**
  o **Caffeine**
  o **Diabetic medication**
  o **Diuretics**
  o **Estrogen (and oral contraceptives)**
  o **Sleeping pills**
  o **Smoking**
  o **Steroids and corticosteroids**
  o **Sulfa drugs**
  o **Vasodilators (i.e. nitroglycerin)**

- **Vitamin B$_6$ is also depleted by sugar, heat (canning & roasting), and physical and mental stress.**

- **Diuretics and cortisone drugs block the absorption of this vitamin.**

- **Intake should be increased with diets high in protein.**

- Vitamin B$_6$ is water-soluble. The body cannot store it. It is easily lost and needs replaced daily.

- Involved in more bodily functions than almost any other single nutrient. It affects both physical and mental health.

- Necessary for the production of hydrochloric acid, which is needed for proper digestion.

- Assists in the metabolism of carbohydrates, fats, and proteins, thus enhancing energy.

- Acts as a diuretic, yet maintains sodium and potassium balance (pH).

- Promotes red blood cell formation.

- Required by the nervous system (stress resistance) and needed for normal brain function.

- Assists in the absorption of vitamin B$_{12}$.

- Enhances the immune system and antibody production.

- Maintains teeth and facial bones, thus preventing dental decay.

- Assists in the prevention of arteriosclerosis.

- Inhibits the formation of homocysteine, thus reducing cholesterol deposition surrounding the heart.

- Acts as an antihistamine, assisting in the treatment of allergies and asthma.

- Most beneficial when taken with vitamin C, biotin, vitamin B_3, vitamin B_5, and magnesium.

- Deficiency can produce: anemia, headaches, acne, sores or inflammation of the tongue and lips, convulsions, arthritis, depression, dizziness, fatigue, hypertension (high blood pressure), learning difficulties or memory loss, hair loss, impaired wound healing, numbness or tingling sensations.

- A thyroid gland deficient in vitamin B_6 (pyridoxine) has difficulty converting iodine into thyroid hormone.

- A deficiency of vitamin B_6 contributes to the *"plateau phenomenon"* – a period of time during dieting when weight loss is at a stand still.

- Carpel tunnel syndrome has also been linked to a vitamin B_6 deficiency.

- CAUTION: Prolonged use of high doses of vitamin B_6 (over 1,000 milligrams per day) can be toxic, and may result in nerve damage and loss of coordination.

Vitamin B₁₂ (Cobalamin, Cyanocobalamin)

- **Vitamin B₁₂ is depleted by:**

  o **Alcohol**
  o **Amphetamines and diet pills**
  o **Antibiotics**
  o **Antiseizure medication (i.e. barbiturates, phenytoin)**
  o **All cholesterol-lowering drugs, including statins and bile acid sequestrants (i.e. Questran™, Colestid™)**
  o **Caffeine**
  o **Calcium deficiency**
  o **Diabetic medication**
  o **Diuretics**
  o **Estrogen (and oral contraceptives)**
  o **Histamine H₂ blockers (i.e. Tagamet™, Pepcid™, Zantac™)**
  o **Mineral oil (laxatives)**
  o **Muscle relaxants**
  o **Proton pump inhibitors (i.e. Nexium™)**
  o **Sleeping pills**
  o **Smoking**
  o **SSRI antidepressants**
  o **Sulfa drugs**

- **Certain anti-gout medications, anticoagulant drugs, potassium supplements, medications for high blood pressure and Parkinson's disease, excess cholesterol, and a low thyroid interfere with B₁₂ absorption.**

- **Intake should be increased with diets high in protein.**

- Vitamin B₁₂ is water-soluble. The body cannot store it. It is easily lost and needs replaced daily.

- Assists folic acid in the formation of red blood cells, thus preventing anemia and contributing to the utilization of iron.

- Needed for proper digestion, food absorption, and a healthy gastrointestinal tract.

- Assists in the metabolism of carbohydrates, fats, and proteins, thus promoting high energy levels.

- Assists in cell formation, prevents nerve damage, and promotes normal cell growth.

- Assists in memory, concentration and learning.

- Maintains a healthy nervous system.

- Prevents insomnia by enhancing sleep patterns and REM sleep.

- Vitamin B₁₂ is not easily absorbed and must be combined with calcium for proper absorption.

- In addition to calcium, it is most beneficial when taken with folic acid, vitamin A, vitamin B_1, vitamin B_3, vitamin B_5, vitamin B_6, and biotin.

- Deficiency can be caused by malabsorption, most commonly in elderly people and in those with digestive disorders. Taking sublingual (under the tongue) tablets allows for easier absorption. The most effective delivery of B_{12}, for those who have difficulty absorbing it, is weekly injections.

- Deficiency can produce: anemia, chronic fatigue, weight gain, constipation, digestive disorders, dizziness, fatigue, enlargement of the liver, memory loss, depression, moodiness or nervousness, palpitations or labored breathing, bone loss, degeneration of nerves.

- Deficiency can result in a significant reduction in the conversion of T4 to T3 thyroid hormones.

Biotin (Vitamin H)

- **Biotin is depleted by:**

  o **Alcohol**
  o **Antibiotics**
  o **Antiseizure medication (i.e. barbiturates, phenytoin)**
  o **Caffeine**
  o **Estrogen (and oral contraceptives)**
  o **Sulfa drugs**

- **Biotin is also depleted by food processing and saccharin**

- **Fats and oils that have been subjected to heat or exposed to air, and raw egg whites inhibit biotin absorption.**

- Biotin is water-soluble. The body cannot store it. It is easily lost and needs replaced daily.

- Is actually a member of the B vitamin family.

- Assists in the utilization of the other B vitamins.

- Assists in cell growth.

- Maintains healthy skin.

- Prevents baldness and hair from turning gray.

- Assists in the metabolism of carbohydrates, fats, and proteins, thus enhancing energy.

- Promotes healthy sweat glands, nerve tissue, and bone marrow.

- Relieves muscle pain.

- Most beneficial when taken with vitamin A, vitamin B_2, vitamin B_3, and vitamin B_6.

- Deficiency can produce: anemia, depression, hair loss, high blood sugar, inflammation of the mucous membranes, insomnia, loss of appetite, muscular pain, nausea, and soreness of the tongue.

Choline

- **Choline is depleted by:**

  o **Alcohol**
  o **Caffeine**
  o **Estrogen (and oral contraceptives)**
  o **Lithium**
  o **Sulfa drugs**

- **Choline is also depleted by sugar and food processing.**

- Choline is water-soluble. The body cannot store it. It is easily lost and needs replaced daily.

- Is a cofactor of the B vitamin family.

- Necessary for proper transmission of nerve impulses from the brain through the central nervous system.

- Assists in gallbladder regulation.

- Assists in kidney and liver function.

- Assists in hormone production.

- Assists in fat and cholesterol metabolism, thus reducing fat in the liver.

- Prevents and treats arteriosclerosis. Important for cardiovascular health.

- Most beneficial when taken with vitamin A, B-complex, inositol, and folic acid.

- Deficiency can produce: impaired brain and memory function, fatty buildup in the liver, inability to digest fats (and weight gain), high blood pressure, gastric ulcers, cardiac symptoms.

Folic Acid (Folacin, Folate, vitamin B₉)

- **Folate is depleted by:**

  o **Alcohol**
  o **Antacids**
  o **Antibiotics**
  o **Antiseizure medication (i.e. barbiturates, phenytoin)**
  o **Aspirin**
  o **All cholesterol-lowering drugs, including statins and bile acid sequestrants (i.e. Questran™, Colestid™)**
  o **Caffeine**
  o **Decongestants (i.e. pseudoephedrine)**
  o **Diabetic medication (especially Metformin)**
  o **Diuretics**
  o **Estrogen (and oral contraceptives)**
  o **Histamine H₂ blockers (i.e. Tagamet™, Pepcid™, Zantac™)**
  o **Mineral oil (laxatives)**
  o **NSAIDs (i.e. ibuprofen)**
  o **Smoking**
  o **Steroids and corticosteroids**
  o **SSRI antidepressants**
  o **Sulfa drugs**

- **Folate is easily lost in boiling, sunlight, heat, food processing, and physical and mental stress.**

- Folate is water-soluble. The body cannot store it. It is easily lost and needs replaced daily.

- Is a cofactor of the B vitamin family, sometimes referred to as vitamin B₉.

- Promotes a healthy digestive/intestinal tract and protects the body from intestinal parasites (candida).

- Is considered a brain food, and is needed for energy production.

- Assists in the formation of blood cells and tissue functions.

- Maintains normal patterns of growth.

- Assists in treating depression and anxiety, and maintains the nervous system.

- Regulates homocysteine levels.

- Prevents and treats folic acid anemia.

- A natural analgesic or painkiller.

- Assists inositol in the metabolism of carbohydrates, fats, and proteins.

- Deficiency may lead to high levels of homocysteine contributing to heart disease.

- Deficiency can produce: a red and sore tongue, anemia, digestive disturbances, fatigue, graying hair, insomnia, labored breathing, memory problems, paranoia, weakness.

Inositol

- **Inositol is depleted by:**

  o **Alcohol**
  o **Antibiotics**
  o **Antiseizure medication**
  o **Caffeine**
  o **Estrogen (and oral contraceptives)**
  o **Food processing**
  o **Lithium**
  o **Sulfa drugs**

- Inositol is water-soluble. The body cannot store it. It is easily lost and needs replaced daily.

- Is a cofactor of the B vitamin family.

- Vital for hair growth. Prevents balding.

- Reduces cholesterol levels and prevents hardening of the arteries.

- Assists choline in the metabolism of carbohydrates, fats, and proteins, thus enhancing energy. Assists in fat removal from the liver.

- High doses assist in the treatment of depression and anxiety, as it helps regulate mood swings.

- Most beneficial when taken with choline, B-complex and vitamin B_{12}.

- Deficiency can produce: arteriosclerosis, constipation, hair loss, skin eruptions, high blood cholesterol, irritability and mood swings.

PABA (Para-Aminobenzoic Acid)

- **PABA is depleted by:**

  o **Alcohol**
  o **Estrogen (and oral contraceptives)**
  o **Food processing**
  o **Sulfa drugs**

- PABA is water-soluble. The body cannot store it. It is easily lost and needs replaced daily.

- Is a cofactor of the B vitamin family.

- Assists the body in assimilation of protein and pantothenic acid (vitamin B_5).

- Is one of the basic constituents of folate and can be converted into folate (folic acid) by intestinal bacteria.

- Assists in the maintenance of healthy intestinal bacteria, thus preventing candida.

- Assists in the formation of red blood cells.

- Necessary for normal skin and hair growth.

- High doses can restore gray hair to its natural color.

- PABA is an antioxidant. Prevents wrinkles. Protects against effects of secondhand smoke, ozone and other air pollutants.

- Protects against sunburn (through absorption of ultraviolet radiation), and thus skin cancer. Reduces the pain of burns.

- Reduces inflammation due to arthritis.

- Enhances flexibility.

- Deficiency can produce: depression or irritability, fatigue, gastrointestinal disorders, graying of the hair, nervousness, and patchy areas of white skin.

Vitamin C (Ascorbic Acid)

- **Vitamin C is depleted by:**

  o **Alcohol**
  o **Amphetamines and diet pills**
  o **Analgesics**
  o **Antibiotics**
  o **Anticoagulants**
  o **Antiseizure medication (i.e. barbiturates, phenytoin)**
  o **Antidepressants (most)**
  o **Aspirin**
  o **Asthma medications**
  o **Antihistamines**
  o **Caffeine**
  o **Diabetic medication**
  o **Diuretics**
  o **Estrogen (and oral contraceptives)**
  o **Muscle relaxants**
  o **NSAIDs (i.e. ibuprofen)**
  o **Steroids and corticosteroids**

- **Vitamin C is also depleted by cooking (heat), light, high fever, physical and mental stress, and is seriously depleted by smoking.**

- **There is an increased need for vitamin C in smokers, diabetics, the elderly, people under stress, and allergy sufferers.**

- Vitamin C is water-soluble. The body cannot store it. It is easily lost and needs replaced daily.

- Reduces cholesterol and prevents atherosclerosis.

- Lowers blood pressure and strengthens blood vessels.

- Necessary for the growth and repair of body tissue cells, bones, gums and teeth.

- Vitamin C is an antioxidant needed for more than 300 metabolic functions in the body. When combined with toxic substances (i.e. heavy metals, pollution), vitamin C can render them harmless, allowing them to be eliminated from the body.

- Enhances adrenal gland function.

- Enhances the immune system, thus promoting the healing of wounds and burns, preventing infection, and fighting bacterial infection.

- Assists in the prevention and treatment of cancer.

- Assists in the production of anti-stress hormones.

- Necessary for the metabolism of folic acid, tyrosine, and phenylalanine.

- Protects against abnormal blood clotting and bruising.

- High doses of vitamin C can reduce the symptoms of asthma.

- Enhances the absorption of iron by 30%.

- Assists the body with oxygen use.

- Most beneficial when taken with vitamin A, vitamin B_6, pantothenic acid (vitamin B_5), and zinc.

- For maximum benefits, supplemental vitamin C should be taken in 2 or 3 doses daily, as it is quickly absorbed and lost through urine.

- Deficiency can produce: soft and bleeding gums, tooth loss, easy bruising, tissue swelling (edema), prolonged wound healing, extreme weakness and fatigue, increased susceptibility to infection (especially colds and bronchial infections), poor digestion.

NOTE: The form of vitamin C that I prefer is called Ester-C, with bioflavonoids. Although ascorbic acid is acidic, Ester-C is instead alkaline, which helps maintain a healthier pH balance. This is especially important when taking high doses of vitamin C. Ester-C is also assimilated more efficiently and retained longer in the tissues than ascorbic acid.

Vitamin D (Calciferol)

- **Vitamin D is depleted by:**

  o **Alcohol**
  o **Analgesics**
  o **Antacids**
  o **Antiarrhythmics (i.e. digoxin)**
  o **Antidepressants**
  o **Antibiotics**
  o **Antiseizure medication (i.e. barbiturates, phenytoin)**
  o **Aspirin**
  o **Asthma medications**
  o **All cholesterol-lowering drugs, including statins and bile acid sequestrants (i.e. Questran™, Colestid™)**
  o **Diabetic medication**
  o **Diuretics**
  o **Estrogen (and oral contraceptives)**
  o **Histamine H$_2$ blockers (i.e. Tagamet™, Pepcid™, Zantac™)**
  o **Mineral oil (laxatives)**
  o **Muscle relaxants**
  o **Smoking**
  o **Steroids and corticosteroids**

- **Vitamin D is also depleted by cooking (heat), light, high fever, and physical and mental stress.**

- **Thiazide diuretics such as chlorothiazide (Diuril™) and hydrochlorothiazide (Esidrix™, HydroDIURIL™, Oretic™) alter the body's calcium-to-vitamin D ratio.**

- Vitamin D is fat-soluble. It needs fats and minerals to be adequately absorbed into the body.

- Prevents muscle weakness.

- Reduces cholesterol and prevents atherosclerosis.

- Assists in the regulation of the heartbeat.

- Enhances immune system.

- Assists in building strong bones and teeth.

- Necessary for healthy thyroid function.

- Assists in normal blood clotting.

- Assists in the prevention and treatment of breast and colon cancer.

- Assists in the prevention and treatment of osteoarthritis, osteoporosis and hypocalcaemia.

- Assists in the treatment of conjunctivitis.

- Necessary for the absorption and utilization of calcium and phosphorus.

- There are several forms of vitamin D:

  o Vitamin D_2 (ergocalciferol) – derived from food sources. This form requires conversion by the liver and kidneys before it becomes fully active.

  o Vitamin D_3 (cholecalciferol) – synthesized in the skin in response to exposure to the sun's ultraviolet rays.

  o Vitamin D_5 – a synthetic form of vitamin D

- Vitamin D_3 is considered the natural form of vitamin D and is the most active.

- Most beneficial when taken with vitamin A, vitamin C, calcium, and phosphorus.

- Deficiency can produce: skeletal malformations, softening of bones and teeth in adults, retarded growth in children, loss of appetite and weight loss, a burning sensation in the mouth and throat, diarrhea, insomnia, visual problems, and insulin resistance.

- Intestinal disorders and liver and gallbladder malfunctions interfere with the absorption of vitamin D.

- Intake of vitamin D should be increased during the winter and reduced exposure to sunlight, or in areas where the level of smog is high.

- CAUTION: Doses over 5000 IU daily can be toxic. Doses over 1,000 IU daily can cause a decrease in bone mass.

Vitamin E (Tocopherol)

- **Vitamin E is depleted by:**

  o **Alcohol**
  o **Antibiotics**
  o **Aspirin**
  o **Estrogen (oral contraceptives)**
  o **Mineral oil (laxatives)**
  o **Orlistat™ (fat-blocking weight loss agent)**
  o **All cholesterol-lowering drugs, including statins and bile acid sequestrants (i.e. Questran™, Colestid™)**
  o **NSAIDs (i.e. ibuprofen)**

- **Vitamin E is also depleted by heat, frying, oxygen, freezing temperatures, air pollution, inorganic iron, and chlorine.**

- Vitamin E is fat-soluble. It needs fats and minerals to be adequately absorbed into the body.

- Thus far, vitamin E has been shown to protect against approximately eighty diseases.

- Reduces blood glucose levels and improves insulin sensitivity.

- Improves circulation, strengthens capillary walls, and relaxes leg cramps.

- Maintains healthy nerves and muscles, while improving athletic performance (enhances energy).

- Promotes healthy skin and hair.

- Reduces blood pressure and assists in normal blood clotting.

- Assists in the prevention of cancer and cardiovascular disease.

- Assists in the prevention of cataracts.

- Assists in the prevention of anemia.

- Necessary for tissue repair and reduces scarring from some wounds, when taken internally or externally.

- Prevents heart attacks. Some studies have shown that daily use of vitamin E is more protective than aspirin for prevention of heart attacks, with no harmful side effects.

- Vitamin E is an antipolutant for the lungs. Long-term use of vitamin E has been shown to reduce prostate cancer risk in smokers (*National Cancer Institute*, 1998).

- Vitamin E is an antioxidant, which prevents cell damage, retards aging and prevents age spots.

- Enhances sperm production in some men.

- **There are 8 naturally occurring fat-soluble nutrients in vitamin E, called tocopherols: alpha, beta, gamma, delta, epsilon, zeta, eta and theta.**

  o **Alpha has the highest biological activity.**

  o **The D-alpha tocopherol form is the most potent (twice the benefit of the synthetic form).**

  o **The DL-alpha tocopherol form is synthetic.**

- Assists in the utilization of vitamin A.

- The body needs zinc in order to maintain the proper level of vitamin E in the body.

- Most beneficial when taken with vitamin C, vitamin B_{12}, manganese, and selenium.

- Do not take vitamin E with iron supplements, as *in*organic forms of iron (i.e. ferrous sulfate) destroy vitamin E. However, *organic* iron (i.e. ferrous gluconate or ferrous fumarate) leaves vitamin E intact.

- Deficiency can produce: fatigue, blood clotting, red blood cell destruction resulting in anemia, coronary thrombosis, infertility (in both men and women), menstrual problems, spontaneous abortion (miscarriage), uterine degeneration, neuromuscular impairment, neurological dysfunction, and oxygen-starved cells making them susceptible to cancer.

Vitamin K (Menadione)

- **Vitamin K is depleted by:**

  o **Alcohol**
  o **Antibiotics**
  o **Aspirin**
  o **Antiseizure medication (i.e. barbiturates, phenytoin)**
  o **All cholesterol-lowering drugs, including statins and bile acid sequestrants (i.e. Questran™, Colestid™)**
  o **Blood thinners (i.e. Coumadin™)**
  o **Mineral oil (laxatives)**
  o **Rancid fat**
  o **Sulfa drugs**
  o **X-ray therapy.**

- **All antibiotics and anticoagulants not only deplete vitamin K, but they also interfere with the absorption of vitamin K.**

- Vitamin K is fat-soluble. It needs fats and minerals to be adequately absorbed into the body.

- Vitamin K is needed for the production of prothrombin, which is necessary for blood clotting.

- Controls the rate of blood clotting and prevents internal bleeding.

- Necessary for bone formation and repair.

- Assists in converting glucose to glycogen for storage in the liver, thus promoting healthy liver function.

- Enhances immune system and helps prevent cancers that target the inner linings of the organs.

- There are 3 forms of vitamin K:

  o Vitamin K_1 (phylloquinone or phytonactone) – derived from plants.
  o Vitamin K_2 – from a family of substances called menaquinones, which are made by intestinal bacteria. The majority of the body's supply of vitamin K is synthesized by the "friendly" bacteria normally present in the intestines.
  o Vitamin K_3 – a synthetic form of vitamin K.

- Necessary for the synthesis of osteocalcin, the protein in bone tissue on which calcium crystallizes (thus preventing osteoporosis).

- Deficiency can produce: abnormal and/or internal bleeding disorders, osteoporosis. Deficiency also interferes with insulin release and glucose regulation in ways similar to diabetes (*Life Extension* magazine, March 2004, p. 67).

Bioflavonoids

- **Bioflavonoids are depleted by boiling, cooking, heat, light and smoking.**

- Although bioflavonoids are not vitamins in the strictest sense, they are sometimes referred to as **vitamin P**.

- Bioflavonoids have an antibacterial effect.

- Promote circulation.

- Stimulate bile production, thus assisting in digestion

- Lower cholesterol levels.

- The human body cannot produce bioflavonoids, therefore supplementation is essential.

- Bioflavonoids are essential for the absorption of vitamin C, and the two should be taken together.

Coenzyme Q$_{10}$ (CoQ$_{10}$)

- **CoQ$_{10}$ is depleted by:**

  o **Antiarrhythmics (i.e. digoxin)**
  o **Antidepressants (especially the tricyclics)**
  o **Antihistamines**
  o **Antihypertensive (blood pressure lowering) drugs (including beta-blockers and calcium channel blockers)**
  o **Antipsychotic class of drugs called phenothiazines**
  o **All cholesterol-lowering drugs, including statins and bile acid sequestrants (i.e. Questran™, Colestid™)**
  o **Diabetic medication**
  o **Diuretics**
  o **Vasodilators (i.e. nitroglycerin)**

- CoQ$_{10}$ is fat-soluble. It needs fats and minerals to be adequately absorbed into the body.

- CoQ$_{10}$ is a vitamin-like substance that resembles the actions of vitamin E, and is one of the most important nutrients in the human body.

- Is a natural antihistamine, thus beneficial for those who suffer from allergies, asthma or respiratory disease.

- Is an even more powerful antioxidant.

- Plays a critical role in energy production.

- Enhances the immune system.

- Lowers blood pressure.

- Assists in circulation and increases tissue oxygenation.

- Beneficial in treating anomalies of mental function (i.e. schizophrenia and Alzheimer's disease).

- Beneficial in treating obesity.

- Beneficial in treating candida.

- Beneficial in treating peptic ulcers, and protects the stomach lining.

- Beneficial in treating periodontal disease.

- Beneficial in treating multiple sclerosis

- Beneficial in treating diabetes.

- Beneficial in preventing and treating cardiovascular disease and congestive heart failure.

- Reduces the side effects of cancer chemotherapy.

- NOTE: The level of CoQ$_{10}$ naturally declines with age. It is believed that as many as 75 percent of people over fifty may be deficient in coenzyme Q$_{10}$.

- Deficiency can produce: congestive heart failure, high blood pressure, angina, mitral valve prolapse, stroke, cardiac arrhythmias, cardiomyopathy, fatigue, decreased immune system.

- Deficiency has been linked to diabetes, muscular dystrophy, and periodontal disease.

NOTE: As CoQ$_{10}$ is:

1. Critical for so many bodily functions, as well as our energy levels.
2. A nutrient so many are deficient in.
3. Very difficult for the body to produce (a 17-step process requiring several vitamins and minerals).
4. One of the most expensive supplements.

Any medication that can directly deplete CoQ$_{10}$ should be avoided if at all possible. That also applies to any medication that depletes the vitamins and minerals the body requires for producing this very valuable nutrient. Although the cholesterol-lowering drugs appear to be the worst offenders, many other medications do also. Even drugs that don't directly deplete CoQ$_{10}$, normally deplete nutrients necessary for its production.

According to *The Drug-Induced Nutrient Depletion Handbook, 2nd Edition* (2001, Hawkins, Krinsky, LaValle, & Pelton, p. 320), the vitamins B$_2$, B$_3$, B$_5$, B$_6$, B$_{12}$, folic acid, vitamin C, *"and numerous other trace elements* [minerals]*"* are required for producing CoQ10. Most medications are responsible for depleting at least one, (normally more than one) of the above nutrients.

Calcium

- **Calcium is depleted by:**

  o **Alcohol**
  o **Antacids**
  o **Antiarrhythmic agents (i.e. digoxin)**
  o **Antibiotics**
  o **Antifungals**
  o **Antiseizure medication (i.e. barbiturates, phenytoin)**
  o **All cholesterol-lowering drugs, including statins and bile acid sequestrants (i.e. Questran™, Colestid™)**
  o **Aspirin**
  o **Caffeine**
  o **Diuretics**
  o **Estrogen (and oral contraceptives)**
  o **High fluoride intake (Prozac™)**
  o **Histamine H$_2$ blockers (i.e. Tagamet™, Pepcid™, Zantac™)**
  o **Mineral oil (laxatives)**
  o **NSAIDs (i.e. ibuprofen)**
  o **SSRI antidepressants**
  o **Steroids and corticosteroids**
  o **Sulfa drugs**

- **Calcium is also depleted by a diet high in protein, saturated fat and/or sugar, soft drinks, excess salt, and/or white flour, excessive sweating, smoking, emotional and physical stress.**

- Calcium is a water-soluble essential mineral that must be replaced daily. Minerals depend on each other for balance, thus if one is out of balance all mineral levels are affected. If not corrected, this can start a chain reaction of imbalances that leads to illness.

- Necessary for maintenance of a regular heartbeat and in the transmission of nerve impulses.

- Necessary for the formation of strong bones and teeth and healthy gums.

- Lowers cholesterol and prevents cardiovascular disease.

- Necessary for muscular growth and the prevention of muscle cramps.

- Assists in the prevention of cancer.

- Lowers blood pressure and assists with blood clotting.

- Prevents bone loss associated with osteoporosis.

- Assists in the breakdown of fats, thus utilizing it for energy.

- Assists in neuromuscular activity and the entire nervous system.

- Increases the body's resistance to parasites and bacteria.

- Too much calcium can interfere with the absorption of zinc, and excess zinc can interfere with calcium absorption.

- Do not take calcium with iron, as they bind together preventing the optimal absorption of both minerals. Take separately.

- Most beneficial when taken with vitamin A, vitamin C, vitamin D, and phosphorus.

- A proper balance of magnesium, calcium and phosphorus should be maintained at all times. If there is an excess of one of these minerals, it will have adverse effects on the entire body.

- Most effective when taken in smaller doses throughout the day, rather than one single big dose. Best when taken before bedtime, as food can sometimes interfere with absorption.

- Deficiency can be caused by lack of vitamin D (or sunshine) and intestinal inflammatory conditions.

- Deficiency can produce: aching joints, brittle nails, eczema, elevated blood cholesterol, hypertension (high blood pressure), heart palpitations, muscle cramps, insomnia, nervousness or depression, rheumatoid arthritis, tooth decay, hyperactivity, numbness in arms and/or legs.

- Deficiency allows lead to be absorbed by the body and deposited in the teeth and bones.

- Deficiency has been linked to colorectal cancer.

Chromium

- **Chromium is depleted by:**

    o **Diabetic medication**
    o **Excess iron**
    o **Processed foods (i.e. junk food)**
    o **Refined carbohydrates**
    o **Sugar**

- Chromium is a water-soluble essential trace mineral, which means only minute amounts are required. The body cannot store it, thus it must be replaced daily. Minerals depend on each other for balance, thus if one is out of balance all mineral levels are affected. If not corrected, this can start a chain reaction of imbalances that leads to illness.

- NOTE: Trace minerals should be taken with an acidic food or drink, preferably in the evening, for optimal utilization and absorption.

- Necessary for maintaining stable blood sugar levels through proper insulin utilization.

- Promotes the loss of fat and an increase in lean muscle tissue.

- Prevents osteoporosis.

- Lowers cholesterol.

- Necessary for energy.

- Assists in the treatment of diabetes and hypoglycemia.

- Deficiency can produce: anxiety, fatigue, glucose intolerance (especially in diabetics), increased risk of arteriosclerosis. Deficiency symptoms parallel those of diabetes.

- Diabetes and coronary heart disease have been linked to low chromium concentrations in human tissue.

- NOTE: Chromium levels naturally decrease with age.

Copper

- **Copper is depleted by:**

  o **Antacids**
  o **Antiviral HIV medication**
  o **Bile acid sequestrants (i.e. Questran™, Colestid™)**
  o **Ethambutol™ (tuberculosis treatment)**
  o **Excess zinc**
  o **Histamine H₂ blockers (i.e. Tagamet™, Pepcid™, Zantac™)**
  o **Penicillamine™ (chelating agent for copper removal)**
  o **High amounts of fructose (fruit sugar)**

- Copper is a water-soluble trace mineral, which means only minute amounts are required. The body cannot store it, thus it must be replaced daily. Minerals depend on each other for balance, thus if one is out of balance all mineral levels are affected. If not corrected, this can start a chain reaction of imbalances that leads to illness.

- NOTE: Trace minerals should be taken with an acidic food or drink, preferably in the evening, for optimal utilization and absorption.

- Assists in the formation of collagen, one of the fundamental proteins for bones, skin and connective tissue.

- Necessary for the utilization of vitamin C, thus assisting in the healing process.

- Assists in energy production and enhances energy.

- Assists in the formation of red blood cells and hemoglobin.

- Stimulates the absorption of iron in the body.

- It is involved in hair and skin coloring and taste sensitivity.

- Necessary for healthy nerves and joints. Has an anti-inflammatory affect for some forms of arthritis.

- Reduces the degeneration of the nervous system.

- Copper deficiency is directly related to the levels of zinc in the body. Excess zinc decreases copper absorption.

- Deficiency can produce: anemia, baldness, diarrhea, fatigue, impaired respiratory function, skin sores, inflammation, thickening of the heart muscle, increased blood fat levels, weakening of cells resulting in aneurysm or stroke.

- Copper deficiency is significantly worsened by high amounts of fructose (fruit sugar).

Iron

- **Iron is depleted by:**

  - o **Antacids**
  - o **Antibiotics**
  - o **Aspirin**
  - o **All cholesterol-lowering drugs, including statins and bile acid sequestrants (i.e. Questran™, Colestid™)**
  - o **Caffeine (especially the tannic acid in coffee and tea)**
  - o **Carisoprodol™ (pain reliever)**
  - o **Choline magnesium trisalicylate (an anti-inflammatory)**
  - o **Histamine H$_2$ blockers (i.e. Tagamet™, Pepcid™, Zantac™)**
  - o **Mineral oil (laxatives)**
  - o **Narcotics**
  - o **NSAIDs (i.e. ibuprofen)**

- **Iron is also depleted by strenuous exercise, heavy perspiration, a diet high in phosphorus, heavy bleeding (i.e. menstruating women, bleeding ulcers), candida yeast infection, bran, phosphate food additives and EDTA (disodium ethylene diamine tetra acetate – a food preservative).**

- **Alcohol, excessive dairy products and eggs inhibit iron absorption.**

- Iron is a water-soluble trace mineral, which means only minute amounts are required. Minerals depend on each other for balance, thus if one is out of balance all mineral levels are affected. If not corrected, this can start a chain reaction of imbalances that leads to illness.

- NOTE: Trace minerals should be taken with an acidic food or drink, preferably in the evening, for optimal utilization and absorption.

- Responsible for transporting oxygen within blood and muscle, and the oxygenation of red blood cells, by the production of hemoglobin and myoglobin.

- Responsible for the conversion of blood sugar to energy.

- Necessary for a healthy immune system.

- Assists in the production of carnitine (an amino acid), which is necessary for the metabolism of fatty acids.

- There must be sufficient hydrochloric acid (HCL) in the stomach in order for the body to absorb iron.

- Copper, manganese, molybdenum, vitamin A, and the B-complex vitamins are also needed for complete iron absorption.

- Taking vitamin C can increase iron absorption by as much as 30%.

- Deficiency can produce: anemia, decreased immune system, headache, fatigue and general weakness, impaired concentration, brittle hair or hair loss, fragile bones, digestive disturbances, dizziness, obesity, nervousness or depression, nails that are spoon-shaped or that have ridges running lengthwise.

- Deficiency has been reported to impair the body's ability to make its own thyroid hormones.

- CAUTION: High levels of iron have been linked to heart disease and cancer.

Magnesium

- **Magnesium is depleted by:**

  o **ACE inhibitors or Beta-blockers and other blood pressure lowering drugs**
  o **Alcohol**
  o **Antacids**
  o **Antiarrhythmic agents (i.e. digoxin)**
  o **Antibiotics**
  o **Antifungal medication**
  o **Antiseizure medication (i.e. barbiturates, phenytoin)**
  o **All cholesterol-lowering drugs, including statins and bile acid sequestrants (i.e. Questran™, Colestid™)**
  o **Diabetic medication**
  o **Diuretics**
  o **Estrogen (and oral contraceptives)**
  o **High levels of zinc**
  o **Immunosuppressants**
  o **NSAIDs (i.e. ibuprofen)**
  o **SSRI antidepressants**
  o **Steroids and corticosteroids**

- **Magnesium is also depleted by large amounts of fats, sugar, refined flour, fluoride (Prozac™), food processing, soft water consumption, emotional and physical stress, and diabetes.**

- **Large amounts of fats, cod liver oil, calcium, iron, and protein also decrease the absorption of magnesium, as do fat-soluble vitamins (A, D, E, and K) and foods high in oxalic acid (i.e. almonds, chard, cocoa, rhubarb, spinach, and tea).**

- Magnesium is a water-soluble essential mineral. Minerals depend on each other for balance, thus if one is out of balance all mineral levels are affected. If not corrected, this can start a chain reaction of imbalances that leads to illness.

- More than 300 enzymes are activated by magnesium.

- Low magnesium levels make nearly every disease worse.

- Responsible for the production and transfer of energy, thus reducing fatigue.

- Necessary for the metabolism of carbohydrates, proteins, and fats.

- Necessary for healthy nervous and muscular tissues, and nerve transmission and impulses.

- Necessary to maintain normal heart rhythm and muscular contraction.

- Magnesium is a natural tranquilizer, known as the anti-stress mineral.

- Protects the arterial linings from the effects of stress caused by sudden blood pressure changes.

- Assists in the prevention and treatment of depression and PMS.

- Relieves indigestion.

- Necessary for the prevention of calcification of soft tissue.

- A proper balance of magnesium, calcium and phosphorus should be maintained at all times. If there is an excess of one of these minerals, it will have adverse effects on the entire body.

- Assists in maintaining the body's proper pH balance.

- Assists in the prevention of cardiovascular disease, osteoporosis, and certain forms of cancer.

- Increases the rate of survival following a heart attack.

- Naturally reduces cholesterol and blood pressure.

- Along with vitamin B_6, magnesium helps reduce and dissolve calcium phosphate kidney stones.

- Assists in the formation of healthy bones and teeth. Helps bind calcium to tooth enamel, thus creating an effective barrier to tooth decay.

- Most beneficial when taken with vitamin B_6, vitamin C, calcium, and phosphorus.

- Deficiency can produce: muscle cramps, weakness and fatigue, insomnia, loss of appetite, gastrointestinal disorders and indigestion, kidney stones, osteoporosis, nervousness and anxiety, confusion, irritability, depression, seizures, asthma, chronic fatigue, rapid heart beat, high blood pressure, cardiac arrhythmia (fatal), sudden cardiac arrest, and is often synonymous with diabetes. Low levels of magnesium have been linked to asthma.

Manganese

- **Manganese is depleted by:**

  o **Alcohol**
  o **Caffeine**
  o **Diuretics**
  o **SSRI antidepressants**
  o **Steroids and corticosteroids**

- **Manganese is also depleted by excess sugar and heavy consumption of meat or dairy products.**

- Manganese is a water-soluble trace mineral, which means only minute amounts are required. Minerals depend on each other for balance, thus if one is out of balance all mineral levels are affected. If not corrected, this can start a chain reaction of imbalances that leads to illness.

- NOTE: Trace minerals should be taken with an acidic food or drink, preferably in the evening, for optimal utilization and absorption.

- Necessary for the use of biotin, vitamin B_1, vitamin C and vitamin E in the body. Manganese works well with the entire B-complex vitamins to give an overall feeling of well-being.

- Assists in reproduction, and the formation of mother's milk.

- Assists vitamin K in the regulation of blood clotting.

- Necessary in the syntheses of thyroxine, the principal hormone of the thyroid gland.

- Relieves fatigue, improves memory, and assists in energy production.

- Promotes a healthy nervous system and relieves nervous irritability.

- Promotes a healthy immune system.

- Assists with blood sugar regulation.

- Necessary for the metabolism of proteins and fats.

- Assists in the proper digestion and utilization of food.

- Necessary for normal bone growth, the formation of cartilage and synovial (lubricating) fluid of the joints.

- Deficiency can produce: confusion, convulsions, eye problems, hearing problems, heart disorders, high cholesterol levels, high blood pressure, irritability, memory loss, skeletal abnormalities (loss of muscle coordination, muscle contractions, sprains, strains, and weak ligaments), profuse perspiration, rapid pulse, tremors, breast ailments, abnormalities in insulin secretion, impaired glucose metabolism and pancreatic damage.

- Low levels of manganese are often found in people with epilepsy, hypoglycemia, schizophrenia, and osteoporosis.

Phosphorus

- **Phosphorus is depleted by:**

  o **ACE inhibitors or Beta-blockers and other blood pressure reducing drugs**
  o **Antacids**
  o **Antiarrhythmic agents (i.e. digoxin)**
  o **All cholesterol-lowering drugs, including statins and bile acid sequestrants (i.e. Questran™, Colestid™)**
  o **Diuretics**
  o **Mineral oil (laxatives)**

- **Phosphorus is also depleted by excess iron or magnesium, a diet high in processed cooked foods and junk food.**

- Phosphorus is a water-soluble trace mineral, which means only minute amounts are required. Minerals depend on each other for balance, thus if one is out of balance all mineral levels are affected. If not corrected, this can start a chain reaction of imbalances that leads to illness.

- NOTE: Trace minerals should be taken with an acidic food or drink, preferably in the evening, for optimal utilization and absorption.

- Necessary for blood clotting.

- Necessary for bone and tooth formation.

- Necessary for cell growth and cell reproduction. Is part of DNA and RNA.

- Necessary for contraction of the heart muscle and normal heart rhythm.

- Necessary for kidney function.

- Assists the body in utilization of vitamins and the conversion of food to energy.

- A proper balance of magnesium, calcium and phosphorus should be maintained at all times. If there is an excess of one of these minerals, it will have adverse effects on the entire body.

- Deficiency can produce: anxiety or irritability, bone pain, fatigue or weakness, irregular breathing, numbness, weight changes.

Potassium

- **Potassium is depleted by:**

  o **ACE inhibitors and other blood pressure lowering drugs**
  o **Acetazolamide™ (a carbonic anhydrase inhibitor)**
  o **Alcohol**
  o **Amphetamines and diet pills**
  o **Antibiotics**
  o **Antifungal medication**
  o **Aspirin**
  o **Asthma medication**
  o **Antiarrhythmic agents (i.e. digoxin)**
  o **Beta-blockers**
  o **Caffeine**
  o **Diuretics**
  o **Immunosuppressants**
  o **Laxatives**
  o **Muscle relaxants**
  o **NSAIDs (i.e. ibuprofen)**
  o **Parkinson's disease medication**
  o **Smoking**
  o **Sodium bicarbonate (Alka Seltzer™)**
  o **Steroids and corticosteroids**

- **Potassium is also depleted by sugar, refined foods, large amounts of licorice, and physical and mental stress**

- Potassium is a water-soluble essential mineral. Minerals depend on each other for balance, thus if one is out of balance all mineral levels are affected. If not corrected, this can start a chain reaction of imbalances that leads to illness.

- Assists sodium to neutralize acids and restore alkaline salts to the bloodstream, thus controlling the body's water balance (pH),

- Necessary for a healthy nervous system and the transmission of nerve impulses.

- Assists in regular heart rhythm and proper muscle contraction.

- Maintains blood pressure and prevents stroke.

- Assists magnesium in kidney stone prevention.

- Depletion can produce: hypertension (high blood pressure), abnormally dry skin, cognitive impairment, constipation, depression, diarrhea, salt retention and edema (swelling), nervousness, irrational behavior, insatiable thirst, fluctuations in heartbeat, glucose intolerance, high cholesterol levels, insomnia, muscular fatigue and weakness, drowsiness, nausea and vomiting, headaches, respiratory distress.

<u>Selenium</u>

- **Selenium is depleted by:**

    o **Alcohol**
    o **Caffeine**
    o **Excess zinc or copper**
    o **SSRI antidepressants**
    o **Steroids and corticosteroids**

- **Selenium is also depleted by food processing, high fat foods, infection, injury, blood loss, aging, and physical and mental stress.**

- Selenium is a water-soluble trace mineral, which means only minute amounts are required. Minerals depend on each other for balance, thus if one is out of balance all mineral levels are affected. If not corrected, this can start a chain reaction of imbalances that leads to illness.

- NOTE: Trace minerals should be taken with an acidic food or drink, preferably in the evening, for optimal utilization and absorption.

- Selenium is a strong antioxidant, especially when combined with vitamin E.

- Protects the immune system.

- Assists in regulating the effects of the thyroid hormone on fat metabolism.

- Necessary for the conversion of the T_4 thyroid hormone to the active form T_3 hormone.

- Prevents against the formation of certain types of tumors.

- Necessary for pancreatic function and tissue elasticity.

- Assists vitamin E and zinc in providing relief from enlarged prostate.

- Protects the liver of alcoholics with cirrhosis.

- Enhances the survival of people with AIDS by increasing both red and white blood cell counts.

- Necessary for healthy pancreatic function.

- Most beneficial when taken with vitamin E.

- Deficiency has been linked to cancer, heart disease, high cholesterol levels, exhaustion, infections, liver impairment, pancreatic insufficiency, and sterility.

Sodium

- **Sodium is depleted by:**

    o **ACE inhibitors and other blood pressure lowering drugs**
    o **Acetazolamide™ (a carbonic anhydrase inhibitor)**
    o **Antidepressants (especially SSRI antidepressants)**
    o **Antifungal medication**
    o **Antigout medication**
    o **Aspirin**
    o **Beta-blockers**
    o **Diuretics**
    o **Laxatives**
    o **Muscle relaxants**
    o **Narcotics**

- **Sodium is also depleted by extreme sweating (fever, heat or exercise), severe diarrhea, starvation, and vomiting.**

- Sodium is a water-soluble trace mineral, which means only minute amounts are required. Minerals depend on each other for balance, thus if one is out of balance all mineral levels are affected. If not corrected, this can start a chain reaction of imbalances that leads to illness.

- NOTE: Trace minerals should be taken with an acidic food or drink, preferably in the evening, for optimal utilization and absorption.

- Necessary for maintaining proper water balance and blood pH.

- Necessary for stomach, nerve, and muscle function.

- Assists in the regulation of blood pressure.

- Assists in making the cell walls permeable.

- Deficiency is most common in people who take diuretics.

- Deficiency can produce: abdominal cramps, anorexia, confusion, dehydration, depression, dizziness, fatigue, gas, headache, heart palpitations, low blood pressure, nausea and vomiting, poor coordination, recurrent infections, weight loss, muscle weakness, poor concentration, memory loss.

Zinc

- **Zinc is depleted by:**

    o **ACE inhibitors or Beta-blockers and other blood pressure lowering drugs**
    o **Alcohol**
    o **Antacids and ulcer medication**
    o **Antibiotics**
    o **Aspirin**
    o **All cholesterol-lowering drugs, including statins and bile acid sequestrants (i.e. Questran™, Colestid™)**
    o **Antiseizure medication (i.e. barbiturates, phenytoin)**
    o **Caffeine**
    o **Diuretics**
    o **Estrogen (and oral contraceptives)**
    o **Histamine H$_2$ blockers (i.e. Tagamet™, Pepcid™, Zantac™)**
    o **HIV medication**
    o **SSRI antidepressants**
    o **Steroids and corticosteroids**

- **Zinc is also depleted by diarrhea, perspiration, kidney disease, cirrhosis of the liver, diabetes, food processing, a diet high in fiber, physical and mental stress, and the consumption of hard water.**

- Zinc is a water-soluble trace mineral, which means only minute amounts are required. Minerals depend on each other for balance, thus if one is out of balance all mineral levels are affected. If not corrected, this can start a chain reaction of imbalances that leads to illness.

- Important in prostate gland function and the growth of the reproductive organs.

- Assists vitamin B$_6$ in testosterone production.

- Reduces cholesterol deposits.

- Promotes mental awareness.

- Prevents acne and regulates the activity of oil glands.

- Necessary for the metabolism of protein, fats, and carbohydrates.

- Zinc is a constituent of insulin.

- Necessary for collagen formation.

- Necessary for the conversion of the T$_4$ thyroid hormone to the active form T$_3$ hormone.

- Necessary for proper concentration of vitamin E in the blood.

- Necessary for bone formation.

- Zinc is an antioxidant. It protects the liver from chemical damage.

- A proper ratio (1-10) between copper and zinc levels should be maintained for optimum health.

- Assists in acuity of taste and smell.

- Zinc increases the absorption of vitamin A.

- Vitamin D increases the absorption of zinc.

- Most beneficial when taken with phosphorus, vitamin A, vitamin C, and vitamin D.

- Food (especially milk, dairy products, protein, and fiber) interferes with the absorption of zinc, therefore it is best to take zinc supplements 2 hours after a meal.

- Take zinc and iron supplements at different times, as they interfere with each other's activity.

- Deficiency can produce: loss of taste and smell, loss of appetite, acne, delayed sexual maturation, fatigue, growth impairment, hair loss, high cholesterol levels, night blindness, impotence and prostate problems, infertility, decreased immune system (susceptibility to infection, recurrent colds and flu, slow wound healing), impaired memory, propensity to diabetes.

Carnitine

- **Carnitine is depleted by:**

  o **Antiseizure medication (i.e. barbiturates, phenytoin)**
  o **HIV medication**
  o **Valproic Acid and derivatives (seizure medication)**

- Carnitine is a non-essential amino acid. Although not an amino acid in the strictest sense, it is actually a substance related to the B vitamins (vitamin Bt), with a chemical structure similar to that of amino acids.

- Carnitine is a major source of energy for the muscles.

- Increases the use of fat as an energy source.

- Prevents fatty buildup, especially in the heart, liver and skeletal muscles.

- Useful in treating chronic fatigue.

- Reduces the health risks associated with diabetes.

- Inhibits alcohol-induced fatty liver.

- Increases cerebral blood flow (blood flow to the brain).

- Reduces the risk of heart disorders.

- Reduces damage to the heart from cardiac surgery.

- Lowers cholesterol and blood triglyceride levels.

- Assists in weight loss efforts.

- Improves sperm mobility.

- Improves muscle strength in people with neuromuscular disorders.

- Enhances effectiveness of vitamin E and vitamin C.

- The synthesis of carnitine depends on the presence of adequate levels of vitamin C.

- Assists antioxidants in slowing the aging process.

- Deficiency can produce: confusion, heart pain, muscle weakness and reduced energy, obesity, elevated blood lipids, abnormal liver function, and impaired glucose control.

Glutathione

- **Glutathione is depleted by:**

  o **Acetaminophen (Tylenol™)**
  o **Narcotics (i.e. codeine)**
  o **SSRI and tricyclics antidepressants**

- Glutathione is not an amino acid in the strictest sense, but is a compound produced from the amino acids cysteine, glutamic acid, and glycine.

- Glutathione is a powerful antioxidant, produced in the liver.

- Reduces some of the damage caused by tobacco smoke, ethanol, and overdoses or frequent use of aspirin or acetaminophen.

- Protects the liver from alcohol-induced damage.

- Assists the immune system.

- Assists in maintaining the integrity of red blood cells, while protecting the white blood cells.

- Necessary for carbohydrate metabolism.

- Assists in the prevention and breakdown of oxidized fats that contribute to atherosclerosis.

- Glutathione levels naturally decline with age.

- Deficiency can produce: decreased immune system, hair loss and baldness, lack of coordination, mental disorders, tremors, and increased free radical damage.

- Deficiency contributes to oxidative stress, which plays a key role in the worsening of many diseases including Alzheimer's disease, Parkinson's disease, liver disease, cystic fibrosis, sickle cell anemia, HIV, AIDS, cancer, heart attack, and diabetes.

- Brain glutathione levels have been found to be lower in patients with Parkinson's disease (http://www.raysehalian.com/glutathione.html).

- Note: The lack of glutathione accelerates the aging process.

Tyrosine

- **Tyrosine is depleted by estrogen (and oral contraceptives).**

- Tyrosine is a nonessential amino acid, as it is produced from the amino acid phenylalanine, an essential amino acid.

- Tyrosine is part of the structure of almost all proteins in the entire body.

- Necessary for brain nutrition and the synthesis of the neurotransmitters dopamine, norepinephrine, and epinephrine, which regulate mood, stress response, mental function, and sex drive.

- Suppresses the appetite. Important to overall metabolism. Reduces body fat.

- Assists in the production of melanin, which is responsible for skin and hair color.

- Assists in the functions of the adrenal, thyroid and pituitary glands.

- Necessary for the production of the thyroid hormones.

- Beneficial in treatment of chronic fatigue, anxiety and depression.

- Beneficial in treatment of narcolepsy.

- Beneficial in treating allergies.

- Deficiency can produce: depression and emotional disturbances, low blood pressure, low body temperature (i.e. cold hands and feet), underactive thyroid, disrupted metabolism, and restless leg syndrome

- Low plasma levels of tyrosine have been linked with hypothyroidism.

SAMe (S-adenosylmethionine)

- **SAMe is depleted by Levodopa (treatment for the symptoms of Parkinson's disease).**

- SAMe is a derivative of the essential amino acid methionine, which is formed in the body when methionine combines with adenosine triphosphate (ATP).

- SAMe supplementation promotes the synthesis of glutathione, which is responsible for detoxification in the liver.

- Protects the liver from harmful effects of alcohol, drugs, and cytokines.

- Protects against cholestasis (bile impairment or blockage).

- Protects against the death of neurons caused by lack of oxygen.

- SAMe is an effective antidepressant.

- Beneficial in treatment of disorders of the joints and connective tissue, including arthritis and fibromyalgia.

- Lowers homocysteine levels, which are associated with cardiovascular disease.

- Assists in slowing the aging process.

- Is a cofactor in multiple biochemical pathways.

- Always take SAMe on an empty stomach.

- SAMe is taken as a natural food supplement, with no recommended daily allowance (RDA) set, and no specific deficiency syndrome defined.

Essential Fatty Acids (EFAs)

- **EFAs are depleted by:**

  o **Aspirin**
  o **Antiseizure medication (i.e. barbiturates, phenytoin)**
  o **Bronchodilators (i.e. Alupent™)**
  o **Estrogen (and oral contraceptives)**
  o **NSAIDs (ibuprofen)**

- **EFAs are also depleted by a diet high in saturated fatty foods, heat, food processing or cooking.**

- EFAs consist of the 2 fatty acids Omega 6, Linoleic acid (LA), and Omega 3, Alpha Linolenic Acid (ALA), which must be obtained from the diet, as they cannot be manufactured by the body.

- Reduces blood pressure.

- Assists in the prevention of arthritis, as they "lubricate" the joints.

- Lowers cholesterol and triglycerides levels.

- Reduces the risk of blood clot formation.

- Beneficial for treatment of candida.

- Beneficial for treatment of cardiovascular disease.

- Beneficial for treatment of eczema and psoriasis.

- Assists in the transmission of nerve impulses and necessary for the normal functioning and development of the brain.

- Necessary for rebuilding and producing new cells.

- Improves hair and skin.

- Deficiency can produce: thirst, eczema, asthma, allergies, dry chapped skin, depression, impaired ability to learn and recall information.

- Low levels of EFAs have been linked with behavioral and learning disorders and Attention Deficit Disorder (ADD).

- The balance of these two EFAs in our diet and cells, is essential for the maintenance of optimum cell wall (membrane) structures.

Bifidobacterium Bifidum

- ***Bifidobacterium Bifidum* is depleted by:**

  o **ALL antibiotics (especially steroids and corticosteroids)**
  o **Estrogen (and oral contraceptives)**
  o **Sulfa drugs**

- *Bifidobacterium Bifidum* is the predominant healthy strain of bacteria (intestinal flora) in the large intestine.

- Assists in the syntheses of the B vitamins and vitamin K by creating healthy intestinal flora.

- Beneficial for treatment of cirrhosis of the liver and chronic hepatitis.

- Improves digestion and bowel function, which prevents digestive disorders and food allergies.

- Substantial amounts of these essential bacteria are not found in foods. Best obtained by purchasing commercial probiotic products that contain bifidobacteria.

- Most beneficial when taken with *Lactobacillus Acidophilus.*

- Deficiency can produce: candida yeast infection, digestive disorders, gas and bloating, diarrhea or constipation, decrease in appetite, nausea and vomiting, bad breath, chronic vaginal yeast infections, acidic blood pH.

Lactobacillus Acidophilus

- **Lactobacillus Acidophilus is depleted by:**

  o **ALL antibiotics (especially steroids and corticosteroids)**
  o **Estrogen (and oral contraceptives)**
  o **Sulfa drugs**

- *Lactobacillus Acidophilus* is the predominant healthy strain of bacteria (intestinal flora) in the small intestine.

- The flora in the healthy colon should consist of at least 85 percent lactobacilli and 15 percent coliform bacteria. However, the typical colon bacteria count today is the reverse.

- Reduces blood cholesterol levels.

- *Lactobacillus Acidophilus* produces a natural antibiotic against more than 20 types of harmful bacteria in the gastrointestinal tract. Enhances several aspects of the immune system.

- Produces enzymes that assist in digesting fats, proteins, and dairy products.

- Assists in detoxifying harmful substances.

- Promotes healthy digestion, and enhances the absorption of nutrients.

- Metabolizes cholesterol.

- *Lactobacillus Acidophilus* has antifungal properties.

- Most beneficial when taken with *Bifidobacterium Bifidum*.

- Deficiency can produce: gas, bloating, intestinal and systemic toxicity, decreased immune system, bad breath, constipation, malabsorption of nutrients, and chronic vaginal yeast infections.

- NOTE: It is best to take acidophilus on an empty stomach, one hour before each meal.

CHAPTER THIRTY-THREE
RESOURCES FOR HEALTH PRODUCTS, ALTERNATIVE PROFESSIONALS AND PROCEDURES MENTIONED IN THIS BOOK

None of the manufacturers or distributors mentioned has had any connection with the production of this book. Address and telephone numbers are subject to change.

Health Products

♣ **Armour™ Thyroid**
Sold through *Women's International Pharmacy*
(800) 699-8143
http://www.womensinternational.com/

Women's International Pharmacy
12012 N 111th Avenue
Youngtown, AZ 85363
In Arizona (623) 214-7700

Women's International Pharmacy
2 Marsh Court
Madison, WI 53718
In Wisconsin (608) 21-7800

Or to locate a doctor nearest you who prescribes Armour™ thyroid:
http://www.armourthyroid.com

♣ **Cardio-plus™**
Standard Process™, Inc.
Products only sold through doctors (most often N.D.s)
For a doctor nearest you call:
(425) 882-0700

♣ **Cataplex-B™**
Standard Process™, Inc.
Products only sold through doctors (most often N.D.s)
For a doctor nearest you call:
(425) 882-0700

♣ **Cataplex-E™**
Standard Process™, Inc.
Products only sold through doctors (most often N.D.s)
For a doctor nearest you call:
(425) 882-0700

♣ **Celtic sea salt**
Sold through *The Grain & Salt Society™, Inc.*
273 Fairway Drive
Ashville, NC 28805
(800) TOP-SALT (800-867-7258)
http://www.celtic-seasalt.com/

♣ **EssProL'eve™ Natural Progesterone cream**
Sold through *International Health*
(800) 481-9987
http://www.ihsite.com

♣ **Ezekiel 4:9™ bread**
For a store nearest you contact:
Food For Life Baking Company
PO Box 1434
Corona, CA 92878
(800) 797-5090
In California (951) 279-5090
http://foodforlife.com/info-center-customer-service/store-finder.cfm

♣ **GlucoVita™**
Sold through *Gero Vita™ International*
578 Washington Blvd., #420
Marina del Rey, CA 90292
(800) 678-7860
http://www.gvi.com

♣ **Goji 100™**
Genesis Today™
14101 W Hwy 290
Building 1900
Austin, TX 78737
(512) 858-1977
(800) 916-6642
http://www.genesistoday.com/

♣ **Holistrol™**
Made and sold through *PharmEast, Inc.*
PO Box 1270
Pahoa, HA 98778
(888) 275-3570
http://www.holistrol.com/

♣ **Iodoral™**
Sold through *Women's International Pharmacy*
(800) 699-8143
http://www.womensinternational.com/

Women's International Pharmacy
12012 N 111th Avenue
Youngtown, AZ 85363
In Arizona (623) 214-7700

Women's International Pharmacy
2 Marsh Court
Madison, WI 53718
In Wisconsin (608) 21-7800

♣ **Magnesium (liquid form)**
Sold through *WaterOz*
Route 1, Box 104-B
Grangeville, ID 83530
(800) 547-2294
http://wateroz.com

♣ **Mangosteen 100™**
Genesis Today™
14101 W Hwy 290
Building 1900
Austin, TX 78737
(512) 858-1977
(800) 916-6642
http://www.genesistoday.com/

♣ **Noni juices**
Genesis Today™
14101 W Hwy 290
Building 1900
Austin, TX 78737
(512) 858-1977
(800) 916-6642
http://www.genesistoday.com/

♣ **NOX-3™**
Made and sold by *Universal Nutrition*
(800) USA-0101
or
Sold through *Nutrition Express*
(800) 338-7979

♣ **Poly-MVA**
(877) POLYMVA (877-765-9682)
http://www.polymva.org/

♣ **Serenity** ™
Sold through *Urban Nutrition*
PO Box 1258
New York, NY 10018
(800) 515-1070
http://www.feelserenity.com/

♣ **Super MiraForte with Chrysin**
Sold through *Life Extension Foundation*
PO Box 229120
Hollywood, FL 33022
(800) 544-4440
http://www.lef.org/

♣ **Standard Process™, Inc.**
Products only sold through doctors (most often N.D.s)
For a doctor nearest you call:
(425) 882-0700

♣ **TG100™**
Sold through *Women's International Pharmacy*
(800) 699-8143
http://www.womensinternational.com/

Women's International Pharmacy
12012 N 111th Avenue
Youngtown, AZ 85363
In Arizona (623) 214-7700

Women's International Pharmacy
2 Marsh Court
Madison, WI 53718
In Wisconsin (608) 21-7800

♣ **Thyromin™**
Sold through *Young Living™ Essential Oils*
For a distributor nearest you contact:
Young Living™ Essential Oils
Thanksgiving Point Business Park
3125 West Executive Parkway
Lehi, UT 84043
(800) 371-2928
http://www.youngliving.com

♣ **Uni-Liver™**
Made and sold by *Universal Nutrition*
(800) USA-0101
or
Sold through *Nutrition Express*
(800) 338-7979

♣ **VitaGreen™**
Sold through *Young Living™ Essential Oils*
For a distributor nearest you contact:
Young Living™ Essential Oils
Thanksgiving Point Business Park
3125 West Executive Parkway
Lehi, UT 84043
(800) 371-2928
http://www.youngliving.com

♣ **Vitalzyme™**
Sold through *World Nutrition, Inc.*
Scottsdale Seville
7001 N. Scottsdale Rd., Suite 2000
Scottsdale, AZ 85253
(800-548-2710)
In Arizona (480) 921-1188
http://www.worldnutrition.info

Alternative Professionals and Procedures

♣ **American Association of Naturopathic Physicians (AANP)**
To locate a naturopathic physician nearest you:
(866) 538-2267
http://www.naturopathic.org/findannd.php

♣ **American Board of Clinical Metal Toxicology**
4889 Smith Road
West Chester, OH 45069
To locate a physician nearest you that performs EDTA chelation therapy:
(800) 356-2228
(513) 863-6277
http://www.abcmt.org/

♣ **American Board of Holistic Medicine**
To locate an American Board of Holistic Medicine certified physician nearest you:
http://www.holisticboard.org/D/locate_physician.html

♣ **American College for Advancement in Medicine (ACAM)**
24411 Ridge Route, Suite 115
Laguna Hills, CA 92653
(949) 309-3520
For a list of natural practitioners in your area:
(888) 439-6891
http://www.acam.org

♣ **American Holistic Health Association**
PO Box 17400
Anaheim, CA 92817-7400
To locate a natural practitioner nearest you:
(714) 779-6152
http://ahha.org/ahhasearch.asp

♣ **Cancer Coalition**
9396 Richmond Ave, Suite 307
Houston, TX
(713) 335-5677
http://www.burzynskipatientgroup.org/contribu.htm

♣ **The Cancer Cure Foundation**
PO Box 3782
Westlake Village, CA 91359
(800) 282-2873
(805) 498-0185
http://www.cancure.org/financial_assistance.htm

♣ **Directory of Practitioners Internet Resources (National/International)**
Holistic Medicine Resource Center
To locate a natural practitioner nearest you:
http://www.holisticmed.com/www/directory.html

♣ **Insulin Potentiation Therapy (ITP)**
To locate a physician who practices ITP nearest you:
http://iptforcancer.com/

♣ **International College of Integrative Medicine**
Box 271
Bluffton, OH 45817
To locate a natural practitioner nearest you:
(866) 464-5226
(419) 358-0273
http://icimed.com/member_search.php

♣ **Natural Solutions**
For a directory of natural practitioners nearest you:
http://www.naturalsolutionsmag.com/

♣ **Tahoma Clinic / Jonathan Wright**
801 SW 16th
Renton, WA 98055
(425) 264-0059
http://www.tahoma-clinic.com/

♣ **Whitaker Wellness Center**
4321 Birch Street
Newport Beach, CA 92660
(800) 488-1500
http://www.whitakerwellness.com/

REFERENCES FOR INFORMATION REGARDING DRUG-INDUCED SIDE EFFECTS / NUTRIENT DEPLETION

Any information found in this book regarding drug warnings, interactions, side effects, and nutrients depleted, unless otherwise noted elsewhere, was obtained from the following sources:

- *Anti-Fat Nutrients*, (Dr. Dallas Clouatre, 1993)
- http://ezinearticles.com/?Prescription-Drugs-Can-Lead-to-Vitamin-and-Mineral-Deficiencies&id=69854
- http://forum.bodybuilding.com/archive/index.php/t-716910.html
- http://my.webmd.com/hw/index/index-drug_data-a?orgpath=/hw/index/index-drug
- http://utopia.knoware.nl/~wwitsel/main/artikelen/treatment.cardiomyopathy.heart.failure.5.html
- http://www.accessmednet.com/prescription-drug-information/index.html
- http://www.bigvitamindictionary.com/samples.html
- http://www.bipolarweb.net/lithium.htm
- http://www.bipolarworld.net/Meds_Trt/Medications/druglist.htm
- http://www.diet-and-health.net/Nutrients/minerals.html
- http://www.diet-and-health.net/Nutrients/vitamins.html
- http://www.drugdigest.org/DD/DVH/Uses/0,3915,551194%7CSyntest+H%252ES%252E,00.htm
- http://www.druginfonet.com/index.php?pageID=faq/new/DRUG_FAQ/Aricept.htm
- http://www.estherslegacy.homestead.com/HOWWEDEPLETEOURNUTRIENTS~ns4.htm
- http://www.go2thesite.com/health/Combat_DrugInduced_Nutrient_Depletion.html
- http://www.greatestherbsonearth.com/nsparticles/interaction.htm
- http://www.healingwithnutrition.com/sdisease/sportsinjuries/injurydrugs.html#A1
- http://www.health-net.info/alphabetical-medications.html
- http://www.healthsquare.com/drugmain.htm
- http://www.hypoglycemia.asn.au/articles/rich_sources_nutrients.html
- http://www.jbc.org/cgi/content/full/277/7/5588#SEC2
- http://www.leaflady.com/drugsdeplete.htm
- http://www.medicinenet.com
- http://www.netnutritionist.com/fa12.htm
- http://www.nlm.nih.gov/medlineplus/druginfo/uspdi/202018.html#CATEGORY_SECmy.webmd.com
- http://www.nutrifarmacy.com/alive2.html
- http://www.postgazette.com
- http://www.prescriptions-for-less.com/index.php?product_id=43&language_id=1
- http://www.quantum-life.com/library/gcr/NELSONS_DRUG_CONVERSION_AND_HOMEOPATHIC_ALTERNATIVES.doc
- http://www.rxlist.com
- http://www.sona.ie/information9.asp
- http://www.thedoctorslounge.net/pharmalounge/drugs/
- http://www.umm.edu/patiented/articles/what_medications_used_anxiety_disorders_000028_7.htm
- http://www.vitaminevi.com/Index/Drug_Index-F.htm
- http://www.vitamin-one.com/Know_your_vitamins.htm
- *Naturally Well Today*™ newsletter (2004, Dr. Marcus Laux)
- *Prescription for Nutritional Healing, 3rd Edition* (2000, Balch & Balch)
- *The Drug-Induced Nutrient Depletion Handbook, 2nd Edition* (2001, Hawkins, Krinsky, LaValle, & Pelton)

INDEX

5-HTP · 107, 116

A

ACE inhibitor · 10, 16, 34, 77, 79, 80, 84, 95, 140, 158, 159, 194, 195, 196, 210, 220, 225, 226, 227, 228, 229, 230, 254, 255, 263, 264, 311, 314, 315, 317, 318

Acetaldehyde · 23, 69, 188, 199, 260

Acetaminophen · 196, 208, 321

Acetylcholine · 99, 107, 121, 124, 126

Acid reflux disease · 96, 113, 132, 203, 252, 255, 256, 259, 261, 262, 272

Acidic food · 155, 307, 308, 309, 313, 314, 316, 317

Acidophilus (also see Lactobacillus acidophilus) · 255, 325, 326

Acidosis · 65, 154, 156, 185, 189, 197, 212, 213

ADA (also see American Diabetic Association) · 106, 152, 153

Adaptogen · 43, 50, 86

ADD (also see Attention Deficit Disorder) · 324

Addiction · 18, 68, 69, 83, 84, 86, 100, 102, 110, 118, 128, 166, 167

ADHD (also see Attention Deficit Hyperactivity Disorder) · 12

Adrenal fatigue · 12, 93, 115, 116, 132, 133, 160

Adrenalin · 122, 137, 228

Adrenals · 12, 32, 93, 99, 102, 106, 112, 115, 116, 121, 132, 133, 136, 140, 143, 144, 148, 149, 150, 160, 165, 167, 228, 273, 285, 295, 322

Aerobic · 64, 188, 189, 212

Alanine (L-alanine) · 181, 182

Albuterol (also see Proventil™) · 82, 85

Albuterol (Proventil™) · 59, 82, 85

Alcohol · 18, 23, 29, 33, 41, 42, 61, 63, 68, 69, 71, 79, 83, 84, 86, 89, 90, 93, 94, 95, 96, 97, 99, 100, 101, 102, 114, 117, 118, 119, 137, 139, 140, 141, 144, 148, 154, 155, 156, 157, 158, 159, 160, 161, 164, 166, 167, 168, 173, 177, 182, 188, 190, 192, 193, 194, 195, 196, 198, 199, 208, 209, 210, 213, 215, 227, 252, 253, 254, 255, 256, 260, 262, 264, 281, 282, 283, 284, 285, 286, 288, 290, 291, 292, 293, 294, 295, 297, 299, 301, 305, 309, 311, 313, 315, 316, 318, 320, 321, 323

Alcoholic · 68, 69, 100, 101, 110, 161, 167, 199, 316

Alcoholism · 68, 108, 114

Alfalfa · 50, 155, 231, 250, 269

Algae · 50, 173, 269

Alkaline · 48, 56, 119, 154, 155, 219, 230, 231, 248, 250, 268, 269, 270, 296, 315

Alkalinizing food · 155

Alpha lipoic acid (ALA) · 90, 184, 324

Alupent™ (also see Metaproterenol) · 81, 85, 324

American Diabetic Association (also see ADA) · 106, 152, 153

Amino acids (also see individual names of amino acid) · 10, 15, 34, 41, 101, 105, 106, 107, 109, 112, 113, 114, 115, 116, 119, 130, 131, 140, 144, 147, 148, 159, 166, 167, 175, 179, 180, 181, 182, 196, 203, 204, 212, 221, 223, 225, 229, 232, 240, 249, 252, 254, 256, 258, 267, 280, 283, 309, 320, 321, 322, 323

Ampli chip 450 · 21, 23

Amylase · 155, 262

Anaerobic · 65, 212

Analgesics (also see Painkillers) · 140, 157, 158, 190, 194, 209, 217, 253, 267, 292, 295, 297

Anemia · 74, 78, 79, 165, 203, 215, 217, 220, 226, 231, 242, 246, 247, 249, 250, 256, 257, 259, 285, 287, 288, 289, 290, 292, 299, 300, 308, 310, 321

Aneurysm · 30, 63, 64, 195, 201, 203, 205, 308

Angina · 58, 60, 143, 190, 191, 194, 201, 211, 216, 218, 220, 224, 226, 232, 240, 241, 263, 276, 304

Antacids · 33, 59, 94, 95, 113, 136, 139, 140, 142, 143, 149, 158, 159, 193, 194, 195, 208, 209, 210, 252, 253, 254, 255, 264, 281, 282, 283, 292, 297, 305, 308, 309, 311, 314, 318

Antibiotics · 19, 33, 40, 51, 89, 94, 95, 136, 139, 140, 148, 149, 157, 158, 159, 174, 193, 194, 195, 196, 208, 209, 210, 252, 253, 254, 255, 264, 281, 282, 283, 284, 286, 288, 290, 292, 293, 295, 297, 299, 301, 305, 309, 311, 315, 318, 325, 326

Antidepressant · 3, 8, 12, 13, 14, 15, 16, 19, 20, 21, 22, 23, 33, 34, 41, 46, 68, 69, 70, 73, 74, 77, 79, 81, 83, 84, 89, 93, 94, 95, 96, 97, 98, 100, 103, 104, 105, 107, 108, 109, 111, 112, 113, 115, 116, 117, 120, 129, 130, 131, 132,

90, 95, 96, 106, 115, 122, 126, 134, 140, 142, 143, 158, 159, 164, 165, 166, 171, 185, 188, 189, 194, 195, 196, 197, 199, 200, 205, 206, 207, 208, 209, 210, 211, 212, 213, 214, 215, 216, 217, 218, 219, 220, 221, 222, 223, 224, 225, 226, 227, 228, 229, 230, 231, 232, 233, 235, 236, 239, 247, 250, 253, 254, 255, 257, 258, 259, 263, 264, 283, 284, 287, 288, 291, 295, 299, 303, 304, 305, 306, 311, 312, 313, 314, 315, 317, 318, 322, 324

Blood sugar · 3, 32, 41, 48, 50, 59, 70, 78, 83, 86, 89, 97, 100, 106, 114, 115, 118, 119, 121, 122, 126, 128, 132, 134, 135, 141, 150, 151, 152, 153, 154, 155, 156, 157, 158, 159, 160, 161, 163, 164, 165, 166, 167, 168, 169, 170, 171, 172, 173, 174, 175, 177, 178, 179, 180, 181, 182, 183, 184, 185, 186, 189, 190, 197, 205, 219, 220, 232, 236, 258, 259, 261, 266, 284, 290, 307, 309, 313

Blood type · 51, 100, 154, 171, 175, 182, 189

Blood type diet · 51, 154

Blood vessel · 34, 47, 63, 64, 83, 106, 156, 157, 189, 190, 194, 201, 206, 207, 208, 209, 214, 217, 223, 230, 231, 232, 233, 241, 259, 295

Blood-brain barrier · 115, 119, 125, 126, 199, 246

Bloodstream · 76, 82, 90, 91, 125, 126, 137, 151, 154, 164, 169, 171, 173, 174, 177, 181, 184, 188, 199, 203, 211, 212, 213, 219, 225, 228, 230, 260, 272, 315

Boomer Coalition · 26

Brain · 10, 12, 16, 18, 26, 29, 30, 31, 38, 39, 41, 47, 49, 56, 58, 63, 71, 76, 77, 83, 86, 88, 90, 92, 93, 95, 96, 97, 98, 99, 100, 101, 102, 103, 106, 107, 108, 109, 112, 113, 114, 115, 116, 117, 118, 119, 120, 121, 122, 123, 124, 125, 126, 128, 129, 130, 135, 145, 154, 160, 165, 166, 167, 172, 179, 181, 182, 184, 185, 190, 191, 193, 196, 199, 200, 202, 203, 205, 206, 207, 212, 214, 217, 220, 221, 222, 223, 224, 225, 226, 227, 228, 229, 231, 232, 233, 246, 247, 248, 271, 274, 275, 276, 279, 286, 291, 292, 320, 321, 322, 324

Brain chemistry · 97, 274, 275

Breast · 22, 30, 32, 50, 70, 79, 116, 147, 250, 257, 259, 263, 297, 313

Bromelain · 267

Bromine · 116, 135

Bronchodilator · 51, 81, 82, 83, 95, 114, 196, 210, 324

Bronchospasms · 82

Fiber · 90, 140, 151, 152, 159, 160, 161, 169, 170, 171, 172, 173, 174, 175, 177, 184, 205, 255, 261, 318, 319
    insoluble · 172
    soluble · 169, 172
Fibromyalgia · 19, 45, 266, 267
Fish oil · 89, 113, 119, 173, 184, 230
Flax oil (also see Flax seed oil) · 90, 113, 174
Flax seed · 86, 90, 113, 131, 169, 172, 173, 174, 184, 230, 267, 271
Flax seed oil · 86, 90, 113, 131, 173, 174, 184, 230, 267, 271
Flax seeds · 169, 172, 174, 184
Fluid retention (also see edema) · 9, 21, 22, 38, 62, 73, 79, 82, 85, 122, 132, 154, 163, 166, 207, 214, 215, 220, 223, 226, 230, 231, 259
Fluorescent lighting · 111, 138
Fluoride · 86, 95, 97, 116, 119, 135, 138, 141, 155, 158, 188, 194, 195, 209, 210, 227, 248, 254, 264, 305, 311
Fluoxetine (also see Prozac™ or Sarafem™) · 70, 71
Folic acid · 33, 59, 61, 70, 75, 78, 80, 87, 94, 113, 177, 179, 180, 190, 193, 217, 247, 249, 253, 256, 257, 267, 285, 288, 289, 291, 292, 294, 296, 304
Food combining · 203, 255, 260, 272
Free radicals · 48, 49, 65, 91, 102, 156
Fructose · 119, 161, 162, 165, 169, 176, 191, 251, 308
Fruit drinks · 119, 162

G

GABA (Gama-aminobutric acid) · 114, 115, 121, 130
Garlic · 50, 90, 149, 155, 185, 231
Gastro-esophageal reflux disease (GERD) · 45, 251, 255, 259, 261, 272
GLA (gamma linolenic acid) · 173
Glandulars · 144, 149
GLO (Gulonolactone oxidase) · 178
Glomeruli · 207, 225, 230
Glucomannan · 172
Glucosamine · 268
Glucose · 41, 49, 65, 89, 90, 97, 128, 134, 135, 141, 150, 151, 152, 153, 154, 155, 156, 158, 159, 161, 162, 164, 165, 167, 168, 169, 170, 171, 173, 176, 178, 179, 180, 181, 182, 183, 184, 185, 186, 189, 219, 223, 248, 257, 272, 274, 299, 301, 307, 313, 315, 320

Glutamic acid (L-glutamic acid) · 181, 182, 321
Glutathione · 70, 87, 179, 180, 182, 184, 196, 321, 323
Glycemic index · 153, 162, 164, 168, 169, 170, 171, 174, 176, 177
Glycine (L-glycine) · 130, 182
Goji Berry · 45, 48, 49, 50, 51, 52, 53, 54, 55, 86, 92, 112, 113, 115, 130, 167, 180, 182, 184, 212, 232, 239, 248, 261, 266, 267, 328
Good fats · 151, 161, 169, 173, 174, 178
Grapefruit · 22, 23, 97, 144
Guar gum · 172
Guggul · 89
Gulonolactone oxidase (also see GLO) · 178
Gymnema sylvestre · 167, 183, 184, 186

H

Halide · 135, 138
Hawthorn · 240
HCL (also see hydrochloric acid) · 155, 184, 251, 254, 258, 259, 262, 309
HDL (high-density lipoprotein) · 29, 89, 90, 91, 211
Health insurance (also see Insurance) · 278
Healthcare · 3, 10, 12, 14, 15, 34, 38, 42, 67, 109, 149, 197, 203, 242, 243, 244, 279
Heart attack · 9, 26, 27, 33, 38, 49, 58, 59, 71, 74, 79, 80, 89, 91, 92, 106, 136, 142, 143, 151, 165, 183, 187, 189, 190, 191, 192, 194, 195, 196, 197, 198, 200, 201, 202, 203, 204, 209, 210, 211, 212, 214, 218, 220, 221, 224, 226, 230, 231, 235, 257, 258, 276, 299, 312, 321
Heartburn · 60, 61, 62, 75, 79, 82, 251, 260
Heavy metals · 116, 188, 194, 198, 212, 213, 295
Herbs · 10, 12, 14, 20, 43, 44, 50, 51, 89, 90, 116, 129, 147, 149, 155, 167, 168, 184, 203, 204, 214, 229, 231, 232, 233, 240, 250, 265, 267
High blood pressure (also see Hypertension) · 8, 26, 33, 35, 38, 47, 48, 49, 58, 64, 70, 73, 74, 75, 79, 81, 83, 84, 85, 89, 140, 143, 164, 165, 171, 188, 189, 195, 196, 197, 205, 207, 208, 209, 210, 211, 213, 217, 218, 219, 229, 231, 232, 233, 247, 250, 253, 259, 283, 287, 288, 291, 304, 306, 312, 313, 315
High fructose corn syrup · 119, 162, 191
High-density lipoprotein (also see HDL) · 29, 211
Histadelia · 123, 124

341

N

O

P

Pneumonia · 79, 226

Policosanol · 90

Potassium · 33, 56, 58, 77, 78, 80, 81, 82, 87, 95, 116, 119, 122, 123, 127, 128, 140, 147, 148, 155, 159, 165, 181, 183, 185, 188, 196, 209, 210, 211, 217, 219, 222, 223, 227, 228, 229, 230, 253, 286, 288, 315

PPA (also see Phenylpropanolamine) · 197

Prednisone · 46

Pregnenolone · 89, 118, 130

Prevention · 10, 30, 40, 43, 46, 52, 97, 123, 149, 150, 153, 165, 181, 183, 192, 194, 195, 204, 209, 210, 212, 217, 218, 237, 242, 244, 257, 258, 261, 266, 267, 269, 277, 286, 295, 297, 299, 305, 312, 315, 321, 324

Procrit™ (also see Epoetin Alfa) · 246, 247, 249

Progesterone · 32, 89, 192, 267

Proline (L-proline) · 182, 212

Prostate · 50, 83, 116, 147, 258, 299, 316, 318, 319

Protease · 61, 75, 76, 89, 262

Protein · 23, 34, 48, 69, 89, 93, 95, 96, 99, 105, 106, 113, 118, 126, 130, 136, 140, 141, 144, 146, 148, 152, 155, 159, 161, 162, 164, 169, 171, 172, 173, 175, 178, 182, 184, 187, 189, 194, 205, 209, 211, 213, 217, 222, 227, 230, 245, 251, 252, 253, 254, 255, 256, 257, 258, 259, 260, 262, 264, 267, 268, 281, 283, 284, 285, 286, 288, 290, 292, 293, 294, 301, 305, 308, 311, 313, 318, 319, 322, 326

Protein-binding · 23, 69, 93, 141

Protein-digesting · 89, 213, 230, 245, 267

Protolytic (also see protein-digesting) · 89, 213, 230, 245, 267

Prozac™ (also see Sarafem™ or Fluoxetine) · 8, 12, 15, 16, 19, 20, 21, 23, 41, 68, 69, 70, 71, 73, 83, 84, 85, 86, 93, 95, 97, 98, 99, 100, 101, 102, 103, 104, 105, 111, 113, 115, 116, 118, 119, 120, 121, 122, 127, 129, 131, 132, 133, 135, 137, 138, 141, 142, 149, 156, 188, 194, 209, 254, 264, 279, 305, 311

Pyridoxine (also see Vitamin B_6) · 94, 139, 148, 165, 193, 209, 252, 264, 286, 287

Pyroles · 101

Pyroluria · 126

Q

Quantum medicine · 189

R

Radiation therapy · 95, 242, 244, 245, 246, 247, 248, 250, 294

Ranitidine (also see Zantac™) · 259

Receptors · 16, 29, 32, 86, 100, 102, 107, 113, 116, 120, 121, 129, 137, 142, 150, 153, 154, 173, 181, 184, 185, 199, 226, 228, 261

Red blood cells · 45, 48, 49, 51, 64, 65, 114, 164, 165, 217, 247, 249, 250, 256, 257, 258, 283, 286, 288, 294, 300, 308, 309, 321

Reductase inhibitor · 39, 60

Relora™ · 118, 149

REM sleep · 102, 111, 217, 288

Renal sodium wasting · 123

Rhodiola · 117, 186

Riboflavin (also see Vitamin B_2) · 139, 148, 164, 208, 211, 217, 252, 283

Ritalin™ (also see Methylphenidate) · 12, 279

S

SAD (also see Seasonal Affective Disorder) · 111, 118, 119

SAMe (S-adenosylmethionine) · 113, 115, 116, 180, 267, 323

Sarafem™ (also see Prozac™ or Fluoxetine) · 70

Seasonal Affective Disorder (also see SAD) · 111, 119

Selective Serotonin Reuptake Inhibitors (also see SSRIs) · 41, 70, 72, 93

Selenium · 70, 87, 135, 140, 144, 148, 172, 196, 198, 300, 316

Sequestrants · 33, 34, 59, 94, 95, 139, 140, 158, 159, 193, 194, 195, 209, 210, 253, 254, 255, 264, 281, 288, 292, 297, 299, 301, 303, 305, 308, 309, 311, 314, 318

Serenity™ · 130

Serine (L-serine) · 182

Serotonergic · 99, 100, 102, 103, 105

Serotonin · 16, 31, 41, 47, 70, 72, 73, 77, 86, 93, 98, 99, 100, 101, 102, 103, 104, 105, 107, 109, 111, 112, 113, 115, 116, 117, 118, 119, 120, 121, 126, 127, 130, 141, 142, 154, 166, 167, 207

Sertraline (also see Zoloft™) · 12, 19, 23, 41, 63, 93, 113, 115, 132, 141, 156

Shortness of breath (also see Dyspnea) · 18, 58, 59, 60, 62, 66, 74, 76, 82, 85, 142, 166, 201, 228

B₅ (also see pantothenic acid) · 94, 157, 159, 165, 177, 252, 253, 281, 285, 287, 289, 294, 296

B₆ (also see pyridoxine) · 33, 70, 73, 78, 81, 82, 87, 94, 101, 113, 119, 137, 139, 148, 165, 177, 180, 182, 193, 209, 217, 231, 249, 252, 264, 284, 286, 287, 289, 290, 296, 312, 318

C · 30, 59, 70, 73, 78, 80, 81, 82, 87, 89, 90, 96, 149, 155, 156, 157, 159, 166, 167, 177, 178, 182, 183, 184, 193, 194, 209, 211, 217, 231, 248, 249, 253, 257, 268, 281, 282, 287, 295, 296, 298, 300, 302, 304, 306, 308, 309, 312, 313, 319, 320

D · 31, 59, 61, 70, 73, 75, 78, 81, 82, 87, 118, 135, 140, 148, 153, 156, 158, 177, 183, 194, 218, 232, 257, 273, 281, 297, 298, 306, 319

E · 59, 61, 75, 87, 96, 135, 148, 154, 156, 158, 159, 167, 177, 183, 194, 209, 230, 241, 250, 257, 281, 299, 300, 303, 313, 316, 318, 320

K · 40, 41, 59, 60, 61, 62, 63, 64, 75, 87, 125, 136, 153, 156, 158, 183, 210, 213, 214, 219, 225, 255, 257, 301, 313, 325

W

Warfarin (also see Coumadin™) · 22, 61, 62, 71, 74, 76

Weight gain · 58, 61, 62, 70, 73, 75, 76, 78, 113, 154, 156, 162, 220, 224, 226, 228, 229, 259, 260, 289, 291

X

Xylitol · 168

Y

Yeast Infection (also see Candida yeast infection) · 23, 47, 95, 140, 253, 254, 255, 256, 259, 260, 292, 294, 303, 309, 324, 325

Z

Zantac™ (also see Ranitidine) · 33, 94, 95, 139, 140, 158, 159, 171, 193, 194, 195, 209, 253, 254, 255, 256, 259, 261, 262, 264, 288, 292, 297, 305, 308, 309, 318

Zocor™ (also see Simvastatin) · 22, 28, 41, 57, 58, 59, 60, 61, 62, 64, 65, 67, 75, 84, 85, 92, 196, 213, 235

Zoloft™ (also see Sertraline) · 12, 19, 23, 41, 63, 93, 113, 115, 132, 141, 156